Praise for *The Mindfulness Solution*

"Down-to-earth and helpful, Dr. Siegel offers genuinely practical training in the transformative art of mindfulness."
—Jack Kornfield, PhD, author of *The Wise Heart*

"Mindfulness is an innate capacity that, when cultivated, can awaken us to true health and happiness. Dr. Siegel's book is a clear and comprehensive guide for anyone who wants to apply the power of mindful awareness to challenging emotions, physical pain, or relational difficulties. Filled with wisdom that is both practical and deep, this book is an invitation to live the real moments of our life with presence and heart."
—Tara Brach, PhD, author of *Radical Acceptance*

"In your hands is a readily accessible book that can walk you step by step to a better life. Being present in the moment with acceptance is more than just a practice—it is a key research-proven strategy that promotes health in the body, in the mind, and in our relationships with one another. Now is the time—and here is the invitation—to step into a new way of being that can reduce anxiety, stress, and fear, and enhance joy, gratitude and well-being in your life."
—Daniel J. Siegel, MD, author of *Mindsight*

"This clear and practical guide can help you discover your own potential to develop mindfulness. It offers guidance for building a formal meditation practice as well as tools for coping in everyday life."
—Sharon Salzberg, author of *Lovingkindness*

"Dr. Siegel offers us an abundance of exercises, transformative practices, and the skillful means to live a mindful life of conscious awareness and meaningful connection. I applaud and recommend his unique perspective, gleaned from a life of meditation and psychotherapeutic practice and research. This wonderful book is a real contribution to the field of happiness studies and spiritual development."
—Lama Surya Das, author of *Awakening the Buddha Within*

"Talk of 'mindfulness' brings up images of monks spending years on end doing something mysterious. But Dr. Siegel shows how to bring the simple wisdom of acceptance and mindfulness into the everyday actions of ordinary living. Gentle, genuine, and wise, this book coaxes, cajoles, and guides the reader into looking with clear eyes at how we humans get in our own way, and provides simple, powerful, step-by-step methods for learning how to live the kind of lives we want."
—Steven C. Hayes, PhD, author of *Get Out of Your Mind and Into Your Life*

"Both accessible and persuasive in showing how mindful awareness can help us take care of ourselves and stay centered as we navigate life's inevitable challenges."
—Zindel V. Segal, PhD, coauthor of *The Mindful Way through Depression*

the mindfulness solution

everyday practices
for everyday problems

RONALD D. SIEGEL

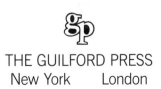

THE GUILFORD PRESS
New York   London

To Gina, my support, inspiration, and love

And to my parents, Claire and Sol,
my most important teachers

© 2010 Ronald D. Siegel
Published by The Guilford Press
A Division of Guilford Publications, Inc.
72 Spring Street, New York, NY 10012
www.guilford.com

Printed in the United States of America

This book is printed on acid-free paper.

Last digit is print number: 9   8   7   6   5   4   3   2   1

Library of Congress Cataloging-in-Publication Data

Siegel, Ronald D.
  The mindfulness solution : everyday practices for everyday problems / Ronald D. Siegel.
    p.   cm.
  Includes bibliographical references and index.
  ISBN 978-1-60623-294-1 (pbk. : alk. paper)
  ISBN 978-1-60623-456-3 (hardcover : alk. paper)
  1. Meditation. 2. Meditation—Buddhism. 3. Mental healing. 4. Self-help techniques.   I. Title.
  BF637.M4S54 2010
  158.1′2—dc22

                                                        2009031139

The names, characteristics, and details of individuals described and quoted in this book have been changed to protect their privacy.

Contents

Preface

*W*hen I first took up mindfulness practice in college, I was impressed. Learning to attend to and accept the present moment—to really stop and smell the roses—had immediate benefits. Worries about getting good grades, finding a girlfriend, and being cool began falling away. Boredom practically disappeared. I imagined that after a few years of practice I'd be free of hurt, pain, and worry—blissfully enjoying the rest of my life.

I'm sorry to report that things didn't quite turn out that way. I soon learned that mindfulness practice isn't a very good narcotic—it doesn't really make pain disappear. But don't put this book down yet. Mindfulness practice actually offers something even more valuable: instead of anesthetizing us, it helps us see more clearly the habits of our minds that create unnecessary suffering—and offers a way to change them. In my own practice, it didn't take long to see how my mind was constantly drawn to fantasize about the next party and dread the next research paper, rarely appreciating the moment. I also noticed how thoughts about being smart or dumb, attractive or ugly, good or bad, a success or failure, were my constant companion, coloring my moods and keeping me stressed. I realized too that despite my continued efforts, the highs that came from getting a good grade, making out with a new flame, or winning a tennis match never lasted very long—I soon found myself chasing the next victory or comfort.

Luckily, along with showing me how these mental habits were making me unhappy, mindfulness practice offered an alternative—a way to live my life with more ease—less concerned with chasing after highs and trying to avoid lows. I could use the practice to notice the trees as I walked to class, taste my food in the dining hall, and connect more intimately with my friends. I could watch thoughts and feelings come and go without getting so caught up in them. Paying attention to the present moment in this way began to transform my relationship to life's ups and downs. Even difficult moments—like when my girlfriend moved away to be with the other guy—felt more manageable as I learned how to attend to rather than escape from my anger, sadness, and vulnerability.

As my own college-age children are fond of pointing out, nearly 40 years into this, on the surface I still don't look like a poster child for mindfulness practice. In the car running late for an appointment, I often get tense and start to use what my kids affectionately call *that voice.* And when they say, "Dad—don't you teach people how to live in the moment? Doesn't mindfulness practice help you accept the things you can't change?," I don't always appreciate their wisdom.

Now that my daughters are old enough to understand the scientific method, I'm able to point out that we don't have a good control group. We don't know with certainty how distressed I'd be by everyday problems without mindfulness practice. And I'm convinced from both my own experience and from research findings that the answer is *a lot more distressed.* In my early days of practice I hoped that it would give me a whole new personality. I've discovered that instead mindfulness practice has actually helped me enjoy the one I have while giving me effective tools to work with life's inevitable challenges—tools without which I'm afraid I'd really be in bad shape.

Mindfulness practice has not only been enormously useful for me personally, but is proving to be helpful for a remarkable number of people dealing with an equally remarkable range of everyday problems. Research is showing that it can help us work effectively not only with worry about being late for appointments and other anxieties, but also with sadness and depression; stress-related medical conditions such as insomnia, digestive difficulties, sexual problems, and chronic pain; and addictions to everything from alcohol and drugs to food, gambling, and shopping. It can help us get along better with our children, parents, friends, coworkers, and romantic partners. It can even help us age more gracefully and find happiness that doesn't depend on fickle fortunes.

How can one practice possibly help with so many different problems? The answer is that they're all made worse by the same natural tendency: in our effort to feel good, we try to avoid or escape discomfort, only to discover that this in fact multiplies our misery. As you'll see in the coming pages, an astonishing variety of problems actually stem from our attempts to get rid of problems. By helping us be with our moment-to-moment experience in a new way, mindfulness offers us a surprising solution.

Many of us are so busy that the thought of adding one more thing—no matter how potentially beneficial—is just too much. The good news is that mindfulness practice can be taken up in different ways to suit different lifestyles. While making time for formal meditation is important, mindfulness can also be practiced as part of our ordinary routine, while brushing our teeth, driving to work, walking the dog, or waiting in the check-out line. Most people actually feel as though they have *more* time in their lives once they begin practicing mindfulness—they become increasingly focused and efficient while feeling more rested and less stressed. There are even specific mindfulness practices we can use during crises when we're about to "lose it"—when we're so aggravated, upset, or overwhelmed that we're at risk of saying or doing something we will regret. These practices make life easier by helping us create fewer messes that we need to clean up later.

My own journey with mindfulness practice has continued unbroken from my college years through my training and career as a clinical psychologist. It provided the backdrop for my study of psychology. Early in my training, few mental health professionals were interested in mindfulness practice. I was fortunate in the early 1980s to join a group of like-minded clinicians who were all practicing personally. For many years we met regularly and discussed what mindfulness traditions had to offer conventional psychology and what conventional psychology had to offer mindfulness traditions. We didn't speak much about this in the wider professional community since meditation and related practices weren't highly valued in those days. Nobody wanted to be accused of having *unresolved infantile longings to return to a state of oceanic oneness*— what Freud saw as the unconscious motivation behind meditation.

In the late 1990s, things began to change. My colleagues and I began presenting in workshops some of what we had been discussing privately. Gradually, larger and larger numbers of mental health providers took interest. The pace soon accelerated, and practically overnight mindfulness practice became one of the most researched and discussed treatment approaches in the mental health field. Suddenly my colleagues and I were being invited to write and teach everywhere about how these practices could be used both inside and outside of psychotherapy to resolve all sorts of emotional and behavioral difficulties. All over the world, mindfulness-based treatments were being developed and tested for every imaginable problem—and they were proving to be remarkably effective.

While relatively new to us in the West, Asian cultures have been refining mindfulness practices for thousands of years. These ancient teachings have informed my colleagues' and my work throughout our careers. This book therefore includes the fruits of many people's efforts. It includes wisdom passed down from the traditions that originally developed mindfulness practices, insights developed by my colleagues who have been exploring mindfulness and psychotherapy together for several decades, and recent innovations by researchers and clinicians who have been developing mindfulness-based approaches to working with a wide range of psychological conditions. It also includes lessons I've learned both personally and from my patients who have used mindfulness practices to work with common and not-so-common difficulties.

Since very little of this book is actually my own invention, there are many people I'd like to thank for making it possible. My long-time friends and colleagues at the Institute for Meditation and Psychotherapy contributed immeasurably to my understanding of this topic and have been wonderfully supportive of my teaching and writing: Phillip Aranow, whose energy and leadership brought the Institute to life before his untimely death, and board members Paul Fulton, Trudy Goodman, Sara Lazar, Bill Morgan, Stephanie Morgan, Susan Morgan, Andrew Olendzki, Tom Pedulla, Susan M. Pollak, Charles Styron, and Janet Surrey, each of whom contributed their unique perspectives and expertise, and particularly Christopher Germer, who encouraged The Guilford Press to ask me to write this book and encouraged me to accept the invitation.

For teaching me about mindfulness practice and helping me understand its transformative potential, I'd like to thank all of the teachers from whom I've had the privilege of learning, in particular His Holiness the Dalai Lama, Jack Kornfield, Joseph Goldstein, Sharon Salzberg, Chogyam Trungpa, Thich Nhat Hahn, Shunryu Suzuki, Ram Das, Pema Chodrin, Tara Brach, Surya Das, and Larry Rosenberg. I'd also like to thank some of the pioneers who have advanced our understanding of mindfulness practices and how they can help with both everyday problems and more serious disorders, including Jon Kabat-Zinn, Marsha Linehan, Zindel Segal, Steven Hayes, Alan Marlatt, Liz Roemer, Susan Orsillo, Jack Engler, Daniel Goleman, Daniel Siegel, Richard Davidson, Mark Epstein, Barry Magid, and Jeffrey Rubin.

Closer to home, I'd like to thank all of my teachers, friends, students, and colleagues at the Graduate School of Applied and Professional Psychology at Rutgers University, Harvard Medical School/Cambridge Health Alliance, the Cambridge Youth Guidance Center, and the South

Shore Counseling Center for helping me learn about clinical psychology, along with all of the patients who have trusted me with their troubles over many years and have taught me so much about human suffering and happiness. I'd also like to thank my colleagues who have provided me with opportunities to develop many of the ideas in this book through teaching others, including Ruth Buczynski, Richard Fields, Rob Guerette, Gerry Piaget, Judy Reiner Platt, and Rich Simon.

For their enthusiastic and unwavering support in shaping this book and seeing it through to completion, I'd like to thank everyone at The Guilford Press, and in particular my editors Chris Benton and Kitty Moore. It has been a privilege and a treat to work with professionals with their level of experience, intelligence, and psychological sophistication who are also genuinely kind people with great senses of humor.

Finally, I am indebted to my friends and family, who have supported me throughout my life generally and this project specifically. While there isn't room here to acknowledge them all, I'd like to particularly thank my parents, Sol and Claire Siegel, for providing the foundation of a loving, supportive childhood home and unwavering care to this day; my brother, Dan Siegel, for his continuing companionship and friendship; and my daughters, Alexandra and Julia Siegel, for their love, understanding, and encouragement.

I owe my greatest debt to my wife, Gina Arons, who encouraged me to take on this project despite knowing full well what she would be giving up. She has been present throughout with loving support, practical and editorial assistance, food, tolerance of my emotional ups and downs, patience while waiting for me to reemerge from countless hours in front of the computer, and innumerable other sacrifices putting up with yet another book-writing project.

PART I

Why
Mindfulness
Matters

CHAPTER 1

Life is difficult,
for everyone

*D*o you ever wonder, "Why is my life so difficult?" I wonder about this a lot. Compared to the vast majority of the six billion people on the planet, I've had it pretty easy. Good parents, no really serious diseases so far, plenty of food and shelter, a loving wife and children, caring friends, even an interesting career. Still, not a day goes by without my mind generating some sort of subtle or not-so-subtle emotional suffering:

> "Am I starting to get a cold? I really don't want to be sick over the weekend."
> "I hope my daughter does well on today's test—she was so upset after the last one."
> "I wish this traffic would clear up; I can't be late again."
> "If only I had ... "
> "Getting old really sucks. Who knew?"

Why does my mind fill with thoughts like these all day long? Do I just have bad genes? Perhaps—but if so, I seem to have plenty of company.

Emotional suffering comes in all shapes and sizes. We might worry about the future, be angry or sad, feel guilty or ashamed, get upset about physical pain, or just feel bored or stressed. Sometimes it's pretty subtle—we "don't feel great" or are "out of sorts." Other times we can get so taken over by anxiety, depression, addictions, pain, or stress-related symptoms that it's hard to even function. A remarkable amount of the time, being human isn't easy.

3

Happiness is possible—but optional

The problem may be that we did not evolve to be happy. Natural selection, the process that guides evolution, favors adaptations that help us reproduce successfully. This means surviving long enough to mate, snag a partner, and then support our children's survival. Evolutionary forces don't particularly "care" whether we enjoy our life—unless this increases our survival or mating potential. And they really don't "care" about what happens to us after our childbearing and protecting years are over.

But we care. While most of us think the survival of humanity is a good idea, we would also like to be able to enjoy *our* lives while we're here. It doesn't seem like a lot to ask.

Yet we struggle. As a clinical psychologist, I've had a window into the lives of many other people, and they all find life to be difficult. Of course, my patients might be an unusual lot. After all, aren't people with problems the ones that seek psychotherapy? While there is some truth to this, I suspect that most of them are actually in no more distress than people who are not in therapy—they're just more motivated and able to do something about it. On top of this, every friend, colleague, and family member that I've ever known well—whether or not they've been in therapy—seems to find life emotionally challenging too.

What's wrong with us? Life is so remarkable. The natural world and human culture are astonishingly complex and interesting, and by historical standards almost everyone in developed countries lives privileged lives full of riches. Most of us never experience the tragedies that we see on the news, like losing a family in a natural disaster, being attacked by a hostile army, or barely surviving a horrible accident—and yet we all experience a surprising amount of stress and emotional pain.

Have we actually evolved to be *un*happy? In a sense, yes. What counts in natural selection is the survival of the *species*. Certain instincts and intellectual abilities that have helped our species prosper over the past few million years have created some pretty negative consequences for us as individuals. Let's look at an example from the past:

Fred and Wilma were early *Homo sapiens* living on the plains of East Africa about 40,000 years ago. They had evolved quite a bit from their *Homo erectus* ancestors, developing enormous brains. In fact they each needed to eat 400 calories a day—a fifth of their normal diet—just to keep these going. The couple used their brains to do all sorts of marvelous things that helped them survive: to think abstractly, plan for their future, find novel solutions to problems, and trade with their neighbors.

They were even able to make cave paintings and stone jewelry in their spare time.

But all was not well on the savannah. Fred's and Wilma's brains also gave them trouble. They worried about rhinoceroses and lions, were envious of their neighbors who had a bigger cave, and got into arguments over who should haul the water on hot days. When it was cold and rainy, they both got irritable, remembering how much better they liked the sun. They noticed changes around them, fretting when there wasn't as much fruit on the trees, roots to eat, or insect larvae (a favorite treat) to snack on. When neighbors got sick or died, they were distressed to realize that this could happen to them too. Sometimes Wilma got upset when Fred looked at other women. Then she wouldn't have sex with him—which upset *him*. Sometimes they both thought about their dog that was eaten by the hyenas. And they felt terrible whenever their son was hurt by the bully from over the hill.

Even when everything was going well, they had thoughts about what had gone wrong in the past or what might befall them in the future. Fred and Wilma were surviving pretty well, and their son had a good chance of making it too, but they still had a lot on their minds.

In some regards, things haven't changed much over the last 40,000 years. Our brains—marvelous as they are—continue to give us trouble. Fortunately, though, some of the same abilities that helped our ancestors survive have also enabled us to develop effective practices to deal with our troublesome brains and enhance our happiness. Luckily these techniques have come a long way since Fred and Wilma's time.

Mindfulness: an antidote

Mindfulness is one of these practices. It developed through thousands of years of cultural evolution as an antidote to the natural habits of our hearts and minds that make life much more difficult than it needs to be. Mindfulness is a particular attitude toward experience, or way of relating to life, that holds the promise of both alleviating our suffering and making our lives rich and meaningful. It does this by attuning us to our moment-to-moment experience and giving us direct insight into how our minds create unnecessary anguish.

When our minds topple forward into worries about being attacked or running out of food, mindfulness practice helps bring us back to the relative safety of the present moment. When our minds make envious or competitive comparisons with our neighbor's husband, wife, or home, mindfulness practice helps us see that these are just symbols and no lasting victory is possible. When our minds protest against the heat or cold, mindfulness helps us notice that it is actually the protesting—not the temperature itself—that causes our suffering. Even when illness or death visits us or our loved ones, mindfulness helps us understand and accept the natural order. By helping us observe exactly how we create our own distress, mindfulness practices teach us how to let go of painful mental habits and replace them with more useful ones.

Various cultures have developed their own ways to cultivate mindfulness, each shaped by particular philosophic or religious views. Despite differences in approach, all of these practices evolved to deal with psychological difficulties similar to those we face today. In the East, mindfulness developed in Hindu, Buddhist, Taoist, and other traditions as a component of yoga and meditation practices, designed to free the mind of unwholesome habits. In the West, mindfulness is an element in many Jewish, Christian, Muslim, and Native American practices designed for spiritual growth. Secular artists, athletes, writers, and others have also developed techniques involving mindfulness to "clear the mind" and facilitate their work. While some of these practices take exotic forms, others are very simple and practical.

Over the past decade or so, researchers and mental health professionals have been discovering that both ancient and modern mindfulness practices hold great promise for ameliorating virtually every kind of psychological suffering—from everyday worry, dissatisfaction, and neurotic habits to more serious problems with anxiety, depression, substance abuse, and related conditions. They're even proving useful for enhancing romantic, parenting, and other interpersonal relationships and for fostering overall happiness. Research and clinical practice are beginning to demonstrate what ancient cultures have long proclaimed—that mindfulness provides insight into what causes our distress and offers effective ways to alleviate it. Lucky for us, it is a skill that can be learned by almost everyone.

Fortunately, too, there are ways to cultivate mindfulness without huge new time commitments. You can actually learn to develop mindfulness while engaged in normal, everyday activities such as walking, driving, showering, and doing dishes. But if you can also set aside regular times for formal mindfulness practice, you may end up actually feeling less pressured and better able to deal with obligations as your mind becomes clearer and your body becomes less stressed.

This book will show you how to cultivate mindfulness in the midst of your daily routines, as well as how to develop it through a step-by-step program of formal practices. Either way, learning mindfulness will help you enrich good times and work more effectively with bad ones.

To understand how mindfulness can be so worthwhile, you need to understand a bit more about why life as we normally live it can be so hard. Let's start with the obvious.

Our prognosis is terrible

In the workshops on mindfulness and psychotherapy that I conduct for mental health professionals, I sometimes ask the audience, "Who here is going to die?" No more than half the hands ever go up. Everything changes, and everything that is born dies. We know this, yet we don't like to think about it. A great Zen master renowned for his wisdom was once asked, "What's the most remarkable thing you've learned in all of your years of meditation and study?" He answered, "The most remarkable thing is that we're all going to die but we live each day as though it weren't so."

He was on to something important. In fact, we can understand much of our emotional suffering by looking at how we react when things change:

"I don't want to give up my pacifier."
"I don't want to use the potty—I like my diapers."
"I don't want to go to school."

Our resistance to change starts very early in life and continues with every subsequent transition—moving, losing friends and loved ones, changing life roles. Who really wants to grow up and drive a minivan? I cried when my twin daughters went off to college. After all that effort, and so many intimate moments together, why did they have to leave home? (My wife wisely pointed out that the alternative—not being emotionally or intellectually able to go off to college—might be even more upsetting.) Looking forward, something tells me I won't be too thrilled when it's time to enter an assisted living facility, or say good-bye to this world entirely.

Resisting these inevitable changes causes us considerable unhappiness. Judith Viorst wrote a groundbreaking book that many psychotherapists read in the 1980s called *Necessary Losses*, which points out that *most* of what makes us unhappy involves difficulty dealing with the inevitability of change. This certainly fits my experience—both personally and professionally. Could it be true for you too?

A RESISTANCE TO CHANGE INVENTORY

Take a moment to make two short lists on the lines below. First, list a few of the more emotionally difficult changes that have happened over the course of your life—the ones that you really didn't welcome. Second, list the most recent few changes, no matter how small, that you found yourself resisting. Now next to each item, jot down what emotions the change brought up at the time.

Most Difficult Changes	*My Emotional Reaction to Each Change*
_____	_____
_____	_____
_____	_____
_____	_____

Most Recent Unwelcome Changes	*My Emotional Reaction to Each Change*
_____	_____
_____	_____
_____	_____
_____	_____

You may have noticed that your life has been full of unwelcome changes, both big and small. Perhaps you've run out of lines. Do the changes that came to mind have anything in common? Did similar emotions arise in response to each of them? Since we all find some changes easier than others, the answer to these questions may hold clues as to which you find most challenging, and which feelings arise most often.

These clues will help you later choose the mindfulness practices that are most suited to your needs.

Hooked on pleasure

Have you ever wondered why doughnuts are so irresistible? Nutritionists speculate that we are attracted to doughnuts—despite their deadly biological effects—because sweet and fatty tastes were associated with getting nutrients when food was both natural and scarce. It's no surprise that we're hardwired to enjoy those things that historically have helped us survive and reproduce. For the same reason that our cars just seem to steer themselves to the doughnut shop, we're fond of love, sex, and comfortable temperatures. And we typically do what we can to avoid pain and discomfort. These sensations, after all, are generally associated with harm to the body: putting a hand too close to a fire, being bitten by a saber-toothed tiger, and freezing in the snow are all both unpleasant and dangerous.

The problem is that our wonderfully adaptive tendency to seek pleasure and avoid pain, while great for our collective survival, locks us into shopping for pleasure and running from pain all day long. The species thrives, but as individuals we live each day perpetually stressed. So on top of the inevitability of change and loss, we have here another built-in source of emotional pain.

Both ancient philosophers and modern psychologists have pondered our tendency to seek pleasure. Freud described it as the "pleasure principle" and pointed out that it explains a lot of our behavior. Later, behavioral psychologists observed that we continue to repeat those actions that are followed by rewards (which are generally experienced as pleasurable). These forces play a role in everything we do. Our whole economy revolves around producing and selling goods and services designed to bring us pleasure.

Unfortunately, the pleasure principle also makes it difficult for us to just *be*. In virtually every moment we're attempting to adjust our experience, trying to hold on to pleasant moments and avoid unpleasant ones. This makes it very difficult to relax fully and feel at ease or satisfied. We become like Goldilocks—reacting to almost everything as too hot, too cold, too large, too small, too hard, or too soft. Take a minute right now to review the past 24 hours. During how many moments were you truly content, appreciating the moment-to-moment unfolding of your life? For most of us these moments are the exceptions—they stand out in our memory. The rest of the time we're restlessly pursuing some goal or another, trying with limited success to maximize pleasure and minimize pain or discomfort. This difficulty really being content is then amplified considerably by another accident of our evolutionary heritage.

Too smart for our own good

As humans, we have other faculties besides the instinct to pursue pleasure and avoid pain that have helped us survive. It's a good thing, too. Magnificent as they are, our bodies are pathetic for life in the wild—no sharp claws, big teeth, or swift feet. Just imagine trying to frighten off a lion or tiger by baring your teeth and claws or to escape from one by running away. Our hide also offers virtually no protection, and our fur is truly comical—a few tufts on top, under arms, and around sexual organs. Our eyesight and hearing aren't great compared to other creatures either, and our sense of smell is absolutely pitiful (just ask a dog).

What we do have, of course, is an extraordinary capacity to reason and plan. This ability enabled us to survive in the wild by *thinking*. Fred, Wilma, and our other ancestors figured out how to hunt animals and avoid being eaten themselves. They learned how to gather and cultivate plants. They developed the culture and technology that have enriched our lives and brought us to the point of dominating (and, if we're not careful, destroying) the planet.

But here we find another adaptive mechanism—so well suited to our survival—that often makes us unhappy. Thinking and planning, wonderful and useful as they are, are at the heart of our daily emotional distress because, unlike other tools, we can't seem to put these down when we don't need them. They keep us worrying about the future, regretting the past, comparing ourselves to one another in thousands of ways, and forever scheming about how to make things better. This makes it very difficult to be truly satisfied for more than a brief time. Our constant thinking can make it impossible to wholeheartedly enjoy a meal or listen to a concert, to fully listen to our child, or to fall back asleep in the middle of the night. It can send our emotions on a nonstop roller coaster as our mood soars and sinks based on thoughts. One day we're smart, attractive, popular, or successful—the next we're dumb, ugly, unwanted, or a failure. Even a casual observation of our minds reveals that we are compulsive thinkers.

THOUGHT STOPPING

I'd like you to try a little experiment right now. *Close your eyes for about a minute and stop your thoughts. See if you can keep words from forming inside your head.* (Please don't cheat—try this before you continue reading.)

What happened? Most people find that they can't stop thinking for more than a few seconds.

Now jot down a few of the thoughts that came to mind.

_____

_____

_____

_____

_____

_____

If you examine the content of your thoughts, you may notice that many of them are about the past or the future and involve wishes to increase pleasure and decrease pain.

For example, I'm writing this right now on an airplane, which left very early in the morning. Before getting on the plane, I was deciding whether to get a granola and yogurt parfait. Hmm, 400 calories—that's a lot. But what if I get hungry on the plane? Remember, they usually don't serve food anymore.

Once on the plane, I wondered, "Should I nap or should I write? I'm pretty tired; will I be exhausted later if I don't sleep? But maybe I'll feel better if I make some progress on the book." (So far this idea is winning.) These are all perfectly reasonable thoughts. The problem is, when I close my eyes to rest for a few minutes, they don't stop. My mind keeps planning how to maximize pleasure and minimize pain, unless I'm lucky enough to fall asleep.

We live most of our lives this way—lost in thought, more often thinking about life than experiencing it. But missing out on the moment-to-moment richness of life isn't our biggest problem. Unfortunately, our thoughts frequently make us unhappy. We're all susceptible to a kind of *thinking disease.* In our attempt to ensure that we'll feel good, we think of all the possible developments that might make us feel bad. While sometimes this is helpful, just as often it generates needless suffering, since every negative anticipatory thought is associated with a bit of tension or painful feeling.

The number of at least mildly negative thoughts that arise in a day is extraordinary—even on good days.

NEGATIVE THOUGHTS INVENTORY

Take a moment right now to review the thoughts that have passed through your mind so far today. Try jotting down all of the unpleasant, worried, or concerning ones that have arisen so far (it may take you a moment to recall them—we sometimes try to forget these).

_____

_____

_____

_____

_____

What did you find? Has your mind been actively working to ward off disaster, by anticipating all the bad things that could befall you or your loved ones?

Just so you don't feel alone in this, here are my results for this little exercise. At the moment I'm on a different airplane, revising this chapter after visiting my daughter at college for parents' weekend. Starting from the most recent, remembering backward, here are the greatest hits from my negative thoughts of just the past hour:

- What if the guy in front of me tilts his seat back—will it damage my laptop?
- My head hurts a little—hope I don't develop a headache.
- Did the pilot extend the wing flaps? I just read that pilots have forgotten to do this 55 times over the past eight years—most recently causing a fatal crash in Spain.

- I wonder if I'll get to visit my daughter at college again—she's a sophomore now and may feel too old after this to have me come for another parents' weekend.
- Damn—a patient just canceled *again* only 24 hours before his appointment. I bet I won't be able to reschedule someone else in time, and the economy is not looking good.
- I hope my daughter is making good choices about her major—is she really interested in the subject or just picking these classes because she thinks she should?

And this is a good day!

Filtering out our lives

By constantly thinking, trying to maximize pleasure and minimize pain, we filter out much of life's potential richness. We gravitate toward things we like, try to avoid things we don't like, and ignore the things we don't feel strongly about either way. This incessant pursuit of goals makes it difficult to appreciate the fullness of the world—and easy to miss important information.

If I'm walking down the street, I might come out of my thoughts enough to notice people I find attractive (such as cute little children or beautiful women). I might also notice people that I find threatening—either because they remind me of my vulnerability (such as very old or disabled people) or because I fear they might hurt me (such as teenage gang members). I'll basically ignore everyone else. In a sense, we're always shopping—either literally, for goods or services that we imagine will make us happy, or figuratively, for attractive sights, sounds, tastes, and other sensations. This narrows our focus and makes us miss out on a lot.

You can observe the tendency of the mind to evaluate everything we encounter as pleasant, unpleasant, or neutral, and gravitate toward the pleasant while recoiling from the unpleasant, with the simple exercise on the following page. Please take a look at it now.

If you are attentive, it won't take long to complete a column. Our minds are constantly evaluating our environment, noting what might bring us pleasure or pain, ignoring everything else.

This takes a toll. We can see the problem clearly when traveling. Have you ever visited a new region or country with a list of "must see" sights—things you really want to do—but not have enough time to fit

ATTRACTION/AVERSION TALLY

This is easiest to do when going for a walk or when literally shopping for food or other items. Take a small pad or notebook with you. Make two columns, labeled "Attraction" and "Aversion." Every time you see something you like or find attractive, put a tally mark in the "Attraction" column. Every time you see something you don't like or find unattractive, put a mark in the "Aversion" column. Notice the feeling of each impulse to hold on to the pleasant or push away the unpleasant. See how long it takes for a column to fill up.

them all in? As we rush from place to place, our minds are focused on maximizing our pleasure and avoiding the disappointment of missing something. But in the process, we fail to take in the little things—the boy in the park, the grocer selling fruit, the man holding lottery tickets. Experienced travelers learn that this goal-oriented, pleasure-seeking approach is actually less interesting and fulfilling than taking time to just *be* in a new environment, attending to the random sights, smells, and sounds. The same turns out to be true for daily life, but most of us have difficulty relaxing our pleasure seeking and goal orientation long enough to appreciate this.

And it's not just the richness of the world we miss. We might trip over a curb and sprain an ankle while eyeing someone attractive or absentmindedly miss a highway exit while fantasizing about the weekend. Ever find yourself feeling nervous, sad, or irritated and not know why? It might be because of leftover emotions from something that happened earlier—when you were too busy pursuing a goal to notice your feelings. Maybe you have lingering remorse because you were worried about your to-do list and didn't really listen to your son when he was telling you something important. Or perhaps you've got some resentment left from when—focused on some important objective—you glossed over the fact your boss was rude to you.

While mindlessly pursuing the myriad goals woven into the fabric of our everyday lives, we can miss simple, important things happening here and now—like the curb, the exit ramp, and other people. And, as we'll soon see, by distracting us from important emotions, mindlessness even sets us up for problems such as anxiety, depression, and addictive behaviors.

All things must pass

Since everything changes, and we incessantly think about how to maximize pleasure and minimize pain, it's no wonder we find life difficult. No matter what we do, pleasure will pass and pain will recur (of course, pain also passes and pleasure recurs—we'll discuss this later). Being intelligent creatures, we soon learn that everything is transient. This knowledge creates a pervasive sense of dissatisfaction. Even in the midst of pleasant moments, we're aware that they will end. Soon the ice cream cone will be finished, summer camp will be over, our girlfriend or boyfriend will leave. We may not get an A on the next test, our job may be eliminated. Children eventually realize that their parents will die. Most of us fear running out of money, getting sick, or dying ourselves. Once we notice that all things really must pass, the pleasure principle combined with incessant thinking becomes a real problem. One of my patients found this out on a much-needed vacation.

Alex worked hard running a successful import/export company. While it was stressful, he liked his job and rarely took time off, fearing that things might fall apart when he wasn't around. But after months of cajoling from his wife, he finally took the plunge and made plans for a weeklong vacation in the Caribbean. He did lots of research, wanting to choose the right island so that his wife would be happy.

When the day of departure arrived, Alex was stressed. He was nervous about leaving unfinished business, and concerned about having chosen the right vacation spot. He started to feel better when they got to the hotel, though. The beach and ocean were beautiful, and his wife really liked the place.

The first days were exciting. They discovered all sorts of new delights and were looking forward to more. "It'll be fun to eat at that restaurant." "We should go on the snorkeling trip." Soon, though, Alex realized that a week isn't very long. By the third day, he was thinking, "Damn—almost halfway through—we'll never have time to really take full advantage of this place." The last few days were still nice, but tinged with uneasiness. When it rained, Alex got upset because they had so little time left. Thoughts of work intruded more and more.

The trip made Alex realize that he needed a change in attitude. Even though the Caribbean was great, he couldn't fully enjoy it knowing he would soon have to leave.

Most of us experience Alex's problem in small ways all the time. Who hasn't looked forward to the weekend, only to get irritated when Sunday rolls around? And thinking about the big endings is so painful that we usually try to block them out of our awareness entirely.

An Ancient Problem

Mindfulness practices were developed to address this predicament. In fact, the central legend of the Buddhist tradition, in which many mindfulness practices were refined, is about the problem of the pleasure principle meeting the reality of impermanence.

The story goes more or less like this: It's said that the historical Buddha was born a prince in a small kingdom in what is now Nepal. Following the custom of the day, his father had Brahmins come to evaluate the new baby. Instead of the Apgar scores of modern pediatricians, the priests looked for 32 signs of greatness—and found them. This meant that the prince was destined to become either a great worldly leader or a great spiritual teacher. Wanting, like many fathers, that his son should follow in his footsteps, the king sought to prevent his son from becoming interested in spiritual matters. To this end, he kept his son cloistered on the palace grounds, surrounded by pleasant things. The idea was that if his son didn't experience pain, he wouldn't be motivated to become a spiritual teacher.

On the rare occasions when the prince would leave the palace, the king made sure that upsetting things were kept out of sight—like they do nowadays when the Olympics come to town. As the prince grew older, however, he became restive and curious, and one day convinced his chariot driver to take him on an unsanctioned visit outside the palace gates. It's said that on this first trip, the young man saw an old person. He asked his driver, "What's that?"

"Old age," replied his driver.

"And who does that happen to?" asked the prince.

"The lucky ones," said his driver.

Disturbed by this discovery, he returned to the palace. On a second unauthorized tour, they saw a sick man. "What's that?" asked the prince.

The driver replied, "Illness."

"And who does that happen to?" asked the prince.

"Most everyone eventually."

On a third visit they saw a corpse. "What's that?"

"Death."

"And who does that happen to?"

"Everyone, I'm afraid."

Now the prince was really shaken, and even more energized to learn about the world. So he convinced his driver to take him on one more trip outside the palace. They came across a wandering spiritual seeker (these were common in the kingdom at the time). "What's that?" asked the prince.

"Someone trying to figure out how to deal with what we've seen on our earlier visits," his driver might have said.

That did it. Illusions shattered, the prince was no longer satisfied with his life. He (like us) had to figure out how to live with reality.

So our central problem is that old age (if we're lucky), illness, and death are inevitable. Add to this the millions of small disappointments when we don't get what we want and it's clear that pain is unavoidable. Since we spend most of our moments thinking about how to maximize pleasure and avoid discomfort, no wonder we wind up dissatisfied.

The failure of success

It gets worse. We also seem to be hardwired to try to enhance our self-esteem. Robert Sapolsky is a neuroscientist at Stanford University who studies the physiology of stress. I heard him interviewed on NPR several years ago by Terry Gross. As I recall, he was explaining that he had spent the last couple of decades hiding with his colleagues behind blinds of vegetation in the African savannah, watching baboon troops. The scientists would wait for a particularly dramatic soap-opera interaction among the baboons and then shoot anesthetic darts into all of them to put them to sleep. Then they drew blood and studied the baboons' physiological response to stress.

Terry Gross asked him, "What did you learn?"

"It's actually very complex, and hard to make generalizations," he replied.

"Were there any findings that really impressed you?"

"Well, we did discover one thing repeatedly: *It is particularly bad for your health to be a low-ranking male in a baboon troop.*"

Yes, we're not baboons. But as the "smart monkeys," our concerns are remarkably like those of other primates. It is no accident that kids in middle school and junior high (who are perhaps closest to our simian ancestry) refer to their insults as "ranking" on one another or "ranking out" other kids. As adults, we're a bit more subtle.

Do you ever compare yourself to others? Have feelings of either envy or superiority? Ever notice who is better liked, earns more money, has the nicer car or home, is more attractive, has the more desirable partner or family, is healthier, smarter, or gets more respect? The list goes on and on and occupies a remarkable number of our waking moments. To see how pervasive this tendency is, try the following exercise.

RANKING CRITERIA

Jot down the criteria you use to establish your rank. This can be a little embarrassing, but it is also instructive. List in rough order of importance the qualities that grab you the most when comparing yourself to others (such as wealth, strength, intelligence, attractiveness, generosity, etc.).

1. _____

2. _____

3. _____

4. _____

5. _____

6. _____

7. _____

8. _____

Looking at your list, you may find that these are also the issues that cause you the most unhappiness.

As humans, we can never really achieve a stable rank in our social order. This is because our minds have the remarkable ability to rethink our situation and to change whom we include in our troop. When a smart girl is in high school, she's proud to do better than most of her peers. But when she gets to a selective college, suddenly she's disappointed to find herself in the middle of the new pack.

We also constantly adjust the level of pleasure or comfort that we consider to be "enough." As young adults, being able to afford our own small apartment feels like an accomplishment; a few years later, we "definitely need" a bigger house. The scale by which we measure our success or satisfaction is continuously being recalibrated.

ATTAINED GOALS

Take a moment to think of an event in your life that you once imagined would provide a lasting feeling of well-being. Sometimes our goals are small: all I want is for this toothache to go away; all I need is for my child to sleep through the night. Other times, they're big watersheds, such as earning a degree, meeting the right person, getting a good job, reaching a new level of wealth, or having a child. Jot down a few goals that you focused on for some time and then managed to achieve.

- _____
- _____
- _____
- _____

Did reaching your goals provide lasting satisfaction? Or, in each case, did you become accustomed to your new accomplishment or level of comfort and start looking for something more? Does your mind continue to imagine happiness lying somewhere in the future—"I can't wait until I finish school, get married, buy a house, or retire"?

A patient I saw many years ago taught me a great lesson about how this works. He had just sold his oil trading business for $30 million cash. He kept using that phrase, "*30 million dollars cash*," and I kept imagining the wheelbarrow full of bills. But he was depressed. He had devoted his life to international energy sales, and now that he was no longer making deals, he felt at loose ends, without meaning or purpose. Being philosophically inclined, I was excited to work with him. I imagined that he was at a vital turning point in his life and I could help him awaken to important human values and find new meaning to his existence.

As often happens when a psychotherapist gets attached to his or her own agenda, the first few sessions didn't go well. I just wasn't connecting with him. At about the fourth meeting, however, he came in looking much happier. I asked what had happened, and he said, "The other day I came up with a business plan by which I think I could parlay my thirty million dollars into a fifty-million-dollar business. I think that if I could establish a fifty-million-dollar business, I'd feel as though I had finally succeeded."

He was completely serious, and that was the last I saw of him.

As a young psychologist, I had plenty of concerns about my own professional, social, and romantic success. My patient had given me a real gift. I realized that day that no matter what I accomplished, the tendency to compare myself to others would probably continue—I'd just pick new peers with whom to compete. We don't tend to compare ourselves passionately to others of very different rank—the attorney doesn't compete professionally with the janitor; the young fashion model doesn't compete with the old woman—but rather we compare ourselves to people who have a bit more or a bit less. Our comparison group keeps shifting, but our restless concern about our rank in the troop continues.

This concern with "success" causes repeated difficulty because we win some and lose some. (I was once talking about this at a workshop and asked, "Who here always wins?" One hand went up. I thought, "Better avoid him at lunch.") Not only do we win and lose the small daily competitions in which we compare ourselves to others, but we become sick, old (again, if we're lucky), and die.

DEFEATS BIG AND SMALL

I'd like you to make two lists again. In the first column, make note of the more significant moments in your life when you felt unhappy or inadequate about losing a competition or feeling "less" than someone else. In the second column, jot down when this has happened, even in very small ways, over the past few hours or days.

Biggest Defeats   *Most Recent Defeats*

_____   _____

_____   _____

_____   _____

_____   _____

If we're honest with ourselves, most of us can find quite a few items for both lists. Do you see any patterns or themes? It can be interesting and freeing to see if the incidents share common features and if they are related to the items you listed in the *Ranking Criteria* exercise. While we all seem concerned with our rank in the primate troop, we tend to measure that rank by different yardsticks. Our experiences of winning and losing depend on how we create our identity. We'll explore this further in Chapter 6, where we examine how mindfulness practice can help us gain perspective on these mental habits (which get particularly out of hand when we feel defeated or depressed).

Love hurts

So here we are: smart monkeys who are instinctually programmed to seek pleasure and avoid pain, trying to enhance our rank in the troop, living in a world in which illness, aging, and death, along with myriad smaller disappointments, are unavoidable. On top of this we have the capacity to imagine things going wrong all the time. It's a wonder we don't find life *more* difficult than we do.

As though this weren't enough, there is yet another hardwired evolutionarily adaptive mechanism that has helped us survive but adds to our troubles: our predisposition to love. While adult humans are physically pitiful animals in the wild (with no big teeth or claws), our children are even less well endowed. A human infant wouldn't last more than a few minutes in the jungle or on the savannah without a parent. Luckily, we have evolved powerful emotional responses that prompt parents to take care of their kids and prompt kids to seek care from their parents. Related feelings connect sexual or romantic partners to one another. These emotions bind us together in couples, extended families, tribes, and larger cultural groups. They enable us to nurture and protect one another, dramatically increasing our chances of survival.

But these emotions also set us up for a host of painful experiences. On top of thinking constantly about seeking pleasure and avoiding pain for ourselves, we have the opportunity to worry about the well-being of our loved ones. I have a patient who recently became a father—an event he'd been dreading for some time. At the heart of his concern is feeling too "emotionally sensitive." He is deeply affected by every pleasurable or painful event and lives in fear of disappointment. The thought of now also being vulnerable to his son's ups and downs is almost too much to bear.

His fear is justified. For those of us with children, safety is even more elusive now than it was before they were born. We now not only worry about disappointing or tragic events in our own lives but also are deeply affected by our kids' experiences of pleasure and pain. And it doesn't stop there. To varying degrees we're affected by the ups and downs of other family members, friends, and people in our wider community. In general, the more we're able to love, the more everyone's pleasure and pain become our own. While this capacity for attachment and empathy is a wonderful part of being human, it makes the project of trying to hold on to pleasure and avoid pain even more impossible.

THE TROUBLE WITH LOVE INVENTORY

Once again I'd like you to make two short lists. In the first, jot down a few significant incidents from the past in which your concern for a loved one or other person made you feel worried, angry, or sad. In the second list, note a few times that this has happened, even subtly, during the past few days.

Big Pain for a Loved One   *Recent Pain for a Loved One*

_____   _____

_____   _____

_____   _____

_____   _____

Here too, most of us find that these thoughts occupy our minds quite regularly. Even when everyone we know is doing pretty well, we know it's just a matter of time before something unfortunate happens to someone dear.

Pain over pleasure

As though all this weren't enough, we seem to have evolved to notice and remember negative experiences more vividly than positive ones. Nancy

Etcoff, an evolutionary psychologist at Harvard Medical School, points out this makes good sense for survival. We can think of our emotional system as a smoke detector—we won't die from a false alarm, but if the alarm doesn't go off during a real fire, we're toast (literally). Research shows, for example, that our taste buds respond more strongly to bitter tastes than to sweet ones. This may have evolved to protect us from poison—which is much more important than being able to fully enjoy a piece of fruit. Since we evolved in a world full of immediate dangers—snakes, tigers, cliffs, and poisonous plants—it's no wonder that we would be better at remembering and learning from negative experiences than positive ones. Missing one opportunity for a tasty morsel or sexual encounter probably won't end our line of DNA, but missing one tiger or cliff will.

This doesn't bode well for our moods. Since we tend to remember painful experiences, we also tend to anticipate them in the future. Each unpleasant memory, worried thought, and pessimistic conclusion is associated with a bit of emotional hurt—even when nothing is actually going wrong. So as long as we're living in our heads, lost in narratives about the past and the future, we're going to experience a lot of pain.

And it's all my fault

Ironically, many of us put icing on the cake of our suffering with a uniquely human addition—concluding that our dissatisfaction is our own fault. Living in a more or less free-market economy exacerbates this. (I'm not advocating the other systems—they all have their problems.) The way I can motivate you to buy my goods or services is by suggesting that they will bring you more pleasure and less pain. Entrepreneurs and marketers are smart—they know that this is what makes us tick. When we see the happy couple in their new convertible, or the sexy surfer with his beautiful babe holding a beer, we draw the conclusion that we would feel great if only we had that car or brew.

Besides creating a remarkable amount of wasteful, environmentally destructive consumer spending, such marketing contributes to our personal suffering. Growing up with our minds marinated in these messages, most of us come to believe that if we're not happy, either we must have made bad decisions or there is something fundamentally wrong with us. "If only I had chosen the right career, spouse, diet, plastic surgery, shampoo, or jeans—then I'd be happy. Why do I keep getting it wrong?"

MY MISTAKES INVENTORY

One way to see how this works is to take an inventory of your supposed "mistakes." Take a moment to jot down some choices you regret—instances where you've imagined at one time or another that you'd be happier if only you had chosen differently.

_____

_____

_____

_____

_____

Complete the inventory above and then look at your list. Would the other choice really have worked to bring lasting satisfaction?

Of course, sometimes we don't think we made bad decisions. The alternative belief, that I made good choices but am still unhappy, is even worse: it means there must be something so wrong with me that even the right choices don't work.

Either way, we're left blaming ourselves rather than noticing that most human suffering derives from our evolutionary history, biological makeup, and existential predicament. By not noticing that suffering stems from universal habits of mind rather than our personal failings, we compound our difficulty.

The belief that our suffering is our fault also keeps us from telling other people about it. We fear that admitting to others that our life is difficult will lower their view of us, and no one wants to be thought of as a "loser." So we tend to minimize our suffering when speaking to others, making ourselves feel inadequate or defective because _our_ life is challenging, while everyone else seems to be doing fine. This sometimes shows up as a sinking sensation when we ask someone, "How are you?" and he or she answers annoyingly, "_Awesome!_"

Since we're hardwired to continually compare ourselves to others, these feelings of inadequacy can really color our lives. They're behind a lot of our competitive urges and even underlie the experience of what the Germans call schadenfreude—our secret delight in others' misfortunes.

Mindfulness practice to the rescue

Fred and Wilma's painful concerns about wild beasts and food shortages, tensions over coveting their neighbor's cave and spouse, irritation with the heat and cold, worries about illness and death, and distress about their son's welfare were all the natural consequence of their enormous brains working to perpetuate their DNA. Like the rest of us, they suffered because everything changes, yet they evolved to seek pleasure and avoid pain, analyze the past to prepare for the future, keep up their social rank, and care for their children and one another.

Luckily, we humans evolved not only mental habits that lead us into emotional difficulty but also faculties through which we can free ourselves from them. The same skills we have used for millennia to understand and thrive in our environment can help us understand how our minds create unnecessary suffering and how to free ourselves from it.

The rest of this book is about cultivating mindfulness. This deceptively simple way of relating to experience that has been practiced for thousands of years can alleviate precisely the kind of psychological suffering we've been discussing. Mindfulness can help us embrace, rather than resist, the inevitable ups and downs of life and equip us to handle our human predicament. It can help us come to grips with being mortal beings with a propensity to seek pleasure and avoid pain, while living in a world full of both. It can also help us see the folly of our concern with how we compare to others and our inability to stop thinking about the past or future for more than a few seconds. And it can deepen our capacity to love others, even as this makes us vulnerable not only to our personal successes and failures, but to their joys and sorrows as well.

CHAPTER 2

Mindfulness

A solution

*I*f only Fred and Wilma had learned to practice mindfulness. While they still wouldn't have had indoor plumbing or air conditioning, they would have found it easier to deal with daily irritation and discomfort, worried less about illness, aging, and death, cared less about how they compared to their neighbors, fretted less about success and failure, and taken everything less personally. This might have saved Fred from developing stomach problems, Wilma from needing more and more fermented berry juice to sleep at night, and their son from spending so much time in the cave, hiding from the animals that he was sure were going to devour him. It would have allowed them all to really notice and savor the present moment, feel connected to their neighbors, natural environment, and one another, and work more creatively with everyday threats and disappointments. They might have even become *Homo sapiens sapiens*—truly wise human beings.

We have the opportunity that they lacked—to benefit from mindfulness practices developed over thousands of years. To take full advantage of it, we need to look further into how our minds normally operate.

Sounds So Simple

What do we mean when we say "mindfulness"? It doesn't refer to a particular state of mind (such as being peaceful or joyous) or to particular contents of the mind (such as positive thoughts or feelings), but rather to a particular *attitude* toward our experience—whatever that experience may be. This is difficult to convey fully in words, because mindfulness is essentially a nonverbal attitude. Nonetheless, words can help point us toward mindfulness, and they can also teach us how to cultivate it.

The working definition of mindfulness that my colleagues and I find most helpful is *awareness of present experience with acceptance*. This sounds pretty simple, so you may be thinking, "Hey, I'm already aware and accepting of my present experience." We often think this until we take a careful look at our normal mental states, most of which turn out to be anything *but* mindful. In fact, researchers find that they can most reliably measure our level of mindfulness by asking us to examine our moments of everyday mind*less*ness.

Everyday mind*less*ness

Would you like to guess the leading cause of emergency room visits to hospitals in Manhattan on Sunday mornings? Take a moment to imagine what it might be. (Don't peek.) It's *bagel-cutting accidents*. While schmoozing with family members on Sunday mornings, scores of people are so distracted by their loved ones that their bodies cut bagels on automatic—and their bodies aren't very skilled at this without guidance from the conscious mind.

The frequency of bagel-cutting accidents shouldn't be a surprise. Even casual introspection reveals that our typical mental state—particularly if we live a busy life in modern society—is pretty mindless. We spend most of our time lost in memories of the past and fantasies of the future. More often than not, we operate on "autopilot," in which our mind occupies one space and our body another. It's as though the mind has a mind of its own.

Let me give you an embarrassing example. This happened to me recently when driving to present a workshop on—of all things—*mindfulness and psychotherapy*:

I was in a rush and running late. Suddenly, a few minutes into my drive, I realized I was heading in the wrong direction on the Massachusetts Turnpike. Now the "Mass Pike" is a toll road in which the exits, when you miss one, seem to be spaced about 100 miles apart. Heading the wrong way, and behind schedule, I had plenty of time to ponder, "Who was driving the car?" I certainly had no recollection of deciding to go west instead of east. I could recall the sights as my car entered the right lane instead of the left, but had no memory of deciding to go west.

My mind had been preparing my presentation, while my body was driving the car—entirely on autopilot.

Other examples of everyday mindlessness abound. Ever notice how often, when you're at a restaurant, the conversation turns to where you have eaten in the past or where you might eat in the future? We sit with our friends or family, engrossed in memories of past meals or fantasies of future ones, only occasionally tasting the food actually on our plates. Or have you ever found yourself daydreaming about vacation while at work, only to think about the work piling up on your desk when you're on vacation?

You may even be able to observe some everyday mindlessness right now. As you read this book, where has your mind gone? Have you had thoughts like "I wonder if this book is actually going to be useful," "I wonder if I'll be any good at this mindfulness stuff," or "I hope this chapter isn't going to be as depressing as the first one"? Perhaps you've left the book entirely and begun thinking about what you'll do later or what happened earlier today. Any of these thoughts would have taken you away from the experience of reading these words here and now. In fact, the very act of reading this has probably taken you away from awareness of the position of your body, the temperature of the air around you, whether it's night or day, or whether you happen to be hungry or thirsty.

Becoming mindful involves observing where our attention goes minute by minute. This includes noticing the many ways in which our minds become distracted or preoccupied. Most of us are so in the habit of being mindless that we are like a fish in water—we don't notice that our minds are leaving the present moment because they do it all the time. You can see for yourself when you are most mindless by completing the *Mindlessness Inventory* on the facing page.

If you're like most people, you probably notice that much of the time your mind is anything but fully *aware of present experience with acceptance.*

What matters most

The pervasiveness of everyday mindlessness is particularly striking when we think about what matters most to us. Try the *What Really Matters* exercise on the facing page to do this.

Now recall where your mind was during this important moment. Was it focused on recalling the past or imagining the future? Or was it focused on the moment-to-moment experience at hand? (The correct answer is: *it was focused on the moment-to-moment experience at hand.*)

A MINDLESSNESS INVENTORY

1–Rarely   2–Sometimes   3–Often   4–Very often   5–Most of the time

Using this scale of 1 to 5, rate how often each of the following happens:

- I break or spill things (_____)
- I run on automatic without much awareness of what I'm doing (_____)
- I rush through things without being really attentive to them (_____)
- I get so focused on goals that I lose touch with what I'm doing right now (_____)
- I listen to someone with one ear, doing something else at the same time (_____)
- I become preoccupied with the future or the past (_____)
- I snack without being aware that I'm eating (_____)
- I get lost in my thoughts and feelings (_____)
- My mind wanders off and I'm easily distracted (_____)
- I drive on "automatic pilot" without paying attention to what I'm doing (_____)
- I daydream or think of other things when doing chores such as cleaning or laundry (_____)
- I do several things at once rather than focusing on one thing at a time (_____)

WHAT REALLY MATTERS

Take a few seconds to recall a moment you have really valued. Perhaps it was a special time with a loved one or a special experience in nature. Maybe it was a time that you held a child, hiked up a mountain, or supported a friend in need. Jot down what was happening at the time.

_____

_____

_____

Despite the fact that our most meaningful experiences involve being present, our minds habitually try to escape the moment—usually wanting to get to the "good stuff." This is a particularly pervasive form of mindlessness:

- Do you ever find yourself rushing through the dishes to get to your cup of tea, book, or television program?
- Do you ever find yourself checking the clock at work, wanting it to go faster?
- Does your mind ever sound like a kid on a car ride, asking, "When are we going to get there?"

When we reflect honestly, we notice that very often we're rushing, actually trying to get rid of *this* life experience to arrive at a better moment. This is the result of the pleasure principle guiding our lives. Our incessant drive to seek out pleasure and avoid discomfort leaves us toppling forward toward what we imagine will be a better next moment. Bizarrely, this leaves us hurrying toward death, missing out on the moments that we're actually alive.

Another form of mindlessness—also driven by the pleasure principle—causes us to miss out on life because we're trying so hard to get it to go according to our plans:

Susie always looked forward to Christmas. It was the one time of year that everyone would be together, and she wanted it to be perfect. She started preparing right after Thanksgiving—buying presents, decorating the house, and planning menus.

But this year when Christmas came she felt unsettled. The house wasn't totally ready, and she still didn't have a great present for her daughter. When everyone arrived, she felt distracted. She wanted to enjoy her family's company but couldn't quite relax—she kept thinking of what she still needed to do and what wasn't quite right.

When it was all over and everyone had left, Susie felt like a failure. She had been so concerned about things turning out well that she hadn't really enjoyed being with her family.

We've all had similar experiences. It can happen throwing a party, preparing a meal, giving a talk, or taking a child to the zoo. To paraphrase the philosopher Voltaire, "The best becomes the enemy of the good."

Early in my training, a senior supervisor told me that people near the end of their lives rarely think, "Darn—I should have spent more time at the office." Very few regret not having achieved more, become richer or more powerful, or reached other external goals. Rather, people more often regret not having tended more to important relationships—and not having been more present in the ordinary everyday moments of their lives. We can notice this even when we don't think we're imminently facing death. When our children are leaving home or someone we love is dying, who hasn't looked back and lamented missing out on the small moments?

The alternative to mindlessness is to actually experience what is happening in the moment: to be attentive to what we're doing rather than operating on automatic, to appreciate the present moment rather than wishing it away. This means noticing our body and the sensations of holding a bagel when we cut it. It means being aware of our minds and bodies when we drive and noticing whether we're heading east or west. It means tasting our food when we eat and paying attention to our friends and loved ones when we're with them. *Right now* it means noticing the position of your hands as you hold this book, being aware of the physical experience of your body in space, and noticing how your mind reacts to these words. As my colleague Metta McGarvey puts it, "Mindfulness is *single*tasking." It means being wholeheartedly present in our lives.

The origins of mindfulness

"Mindfulness," as we currently use the word in Western psychological circles, stems mostly from 2,500-year-old Buddhist teachings. While many different cultures have developed methods to cultivate mindfulness, hundreds of these techniques have been continuously described and refined over 25 centuries in the Buddhist tradition. (This doesn't mean that you have to become a Buddhist to benefit from these practices. Rather, you can take advantage of the tradition's detailed instructions for mindfulness practice, and descriptions of insights that develop from it, and apply these to your own life regardless of your personal beliefs.)

To pick up where we left off in the legend of the Buddha in the last chapter, you may recall that the young prince became distressed when he realized the inevitability of old age, sickness, and death. His life of ease and indulgence now felt unsatisfactory given his awareness of our collective prognosis. So he decided to leave the palace and seek a different path to contentment.

As the story goes, for five or six years he practiced strict asceticism, nearly starving to death. Despite mastering all manner of spiritual practices, he found this approach also to be unsatisfactory—he continued to feel discontented as conflicts and desires persisted. One day he was so weak that he nearly drowned, and he realized that he was on the wrong track. He decided to start eating more normally again to nourish his mind and body. The prince then committed himself to sitting under a tree and meditating until he found a way to deal with his (and our) existential predicament. It's said that after 49 days and nights, he "woke up." He had found a way to alleviate psychological suffering.

This awakening came through carefully observing the workings of his own mind and enduring a host of pleasant and unpleasant mental states. He engaged in some of the same sort of mindfulness practices that we will be discussing here and that are turning out to be remarkably useful in dealing with a wide range of contemporary psychological difficulties.

What exactly did the prince do under that tree? *Mindfulness* is often said to be an English translation of a Pali term, *sati,* which connotes awareness, attention, and remembering (Pali is the language in which the stories and teachings of the Buddha were originally recorded). The words *awareness* and *attention* are used in this definition pretty much the way we normally use them in English—to know that something is happening and to attend to it. The "remembering" part is different, however— it's not so much about recalling past events, but rather about continually *remembering* to be aware and pay attention.

I had the privilege of attending a lecture by John Donne, a scholar at Emory University who studies Pali texts. He pointed out that the way we currently use the term *mindfulness* in the West actually goes considerably beyond awareness, attention, and remembering. He used the example of a sniper poised on the top of a building aiming a high-powered rifle at an innocent victim. The sniper would be very aware and attentive, and each time his mind wandered, he'd remember to return his attention to watching his victim through the telescopic gun sight. This kind of focus, while useful for tasks such as shooting people at a distance, is not really the attitude of mind that will help most of us deal with life's challenges.

What is missing for the sniper is acceptance, or nonjudgment. This adds warmth, friendliness, and compassion to the attitude. For many of us, cultivating an accepting attitude toward our experience is both the most important and the most challenging aspect of mindfulness practice. Acceptance allows us to be open to both pleasure and pain, to embrace both winning and losing, and to be compassionate with ourselves and others when mistakes are made. Acceptance allows us to say "yes" to the parts of our personality we want to eliminate or hide. It is at the heart of how mindfulness allows us to work effectively with fear, worry, sadness, depression, physical pain, addictions, and relationship difficulties—all of which, as we will soon see, are perpetuated by our refusal to accept some thought, feeling, or other experience. Ultimately, it's acceptance that allows us to embrace both our ever-changing life and the ever-present reality of death.

Mindfulness *practice*

While it can be disturbing to notice how frequently we are mindless, how many moments of our lives we wish away, and how much grief we cause ourselves and others by not accepting things as they are, there is good news: *mindfulness can be cultivated.* The benefits of cultivating mindfulness are far reaching. By providing an effective way to deal with our human predicament, discussed in the last chapter, it can greatly improve our everyday experience.

Mindfulness can help us see and accept things as they are. This means we can come to peace with the inevitability of change and the impossibility of always winning. The concerns about things going wrong that fill our minds each day begin to lose their grip. The traffic jam, rained-out picnic, misplaced keys, and lost sales are all easier to accept. We become more comfortable with the reality that sometimes we'll get the date or the promotion and other times we won't. By letting go of our struggle to control everything, we become less easily thrown by life's daily ups and downs—and less likely to get caught in emotional problems like depression and anxiety or stress-related physical problems like chronic pain and insomnia.

Mindfulness also helps us loosen our painful preoccupation with "self." Most of what makes reality so painful is its implications for *me*. Mindfulness can help us all be less concerned with what happens to this *me*. Worries about my health, wealth, beauty, and self-esteem fall into perspective. Having a cold, the car breaking down, a bad hair day, and being afraid I just sounded like an idiot all become easier to bear. Becoming less preoccupied with *me* is a great relief—especially given what we know will inevitably happen to each of us.

In addition to reducing suffering in these ways, mindfulness allows us to experience the richness of the moments of our lives. We actually smell the roses, taste our food, notice the sunset, and feel our connections to others each day. Boredom disappears as we awaken to the rich complexity of each moment. Everything becomes alive as our attention moves out of our thoughts about living and toward noticing how it actually feels to walk, stand, sit, or drive. As we see that no two moments are alike, they all become valuable and interesting.

Finally, mindfulness frees us to act more wisely and skillfully in our everyday decisions as we become less concerned with the implications of our actions for our particular welfare and more focused on the bigger picture. This allows us to live each day with a sense of dignity and appreciation. We actually find that our minds operate more clearly when they're not so burdened by anxiety about what others will think about us or whether we'll get what we want. It becomes fun to watch our minds work freely while our creativity unfolds.

Support from the laboratory

If you haven't had much experience with mindfulness practice, all this could sound too good to be true. Can simply cultivating a different attitude toward our daily experience so profoundly change our lives?

A wealth of scientific evidence says it can. Research documents changes in both inner experience and outward behavior resulting from mindfulness practice. Recently, studies demonstrating the effects of mindfulness practice on brain function and structure have also created quite a stir among scientists. These studies involve a form of practice that we'll be discussing shortly: formal mindfulness meditation.

Effects on Brain Function

One of my favorite lines of research comes from the Laboratory for Affective Neuroscience at the University of Wisconsin. Let's start with some background: Dr. Richard Davidson and his colleagues have demonstrated that people who are typically distressed have more activity in the right prefrontal cortex of the brain (an area behind the forehead) than in the left prefrontal cortex. This right-side activation is seen most in people who are anxious, depressed, or hypervigilant (scanning their environment for danger). On the other hand, people who are generally content and have fewer negative moods tend to have more activity in the left prefrontal cortex.

Dr. Davidson and his colleagues have gathered data about brain activity on hundreds of people. Strikingly, the person who showed the most dramatic left prefrontal cortical activation of all the subjects tested was a Tibetan monk with many years of experience in mindfulness (and other) meditation practices. The effect wasn't limited to one case. Dramatic shifts toward left prefrontal activation were found in the brains of a number of Tibetan monks who had 10,000 to 50,000 hours of meditation practice.

As a researcher, Dr. Davidson had to consider the possibility that perhaps people who naturally have more left-sided activation choose to become meditators or monks—so the greater left-sided activity seen in these subjects might not be caused by the meditation practice, but might instead have caused them to take up meditation in the first place. To test this, Dr. Davidson and Dr. Jon Kabat-Zinn recruited a group of pressured workers in a biotechnology firm and taught half of them mindfulness meditation for three hours per week over an eight-week period. They compared this group to a similar group of coworkers who were not taught meditation. On average, all of the workers tipped to the right in their prefrontal cortical activity before taking up meditation. However, after taking the eight-week course, the meditating group now had more left-sided activation than the nonmeditators. The meditators also reported that their moods improved and they felt more engaged in their activities.

While these results were impressive, the researchers also discovered something very interesting when they measured the subjects' responses to influenza vaccines. It turned out that the meditating group had a greater immune response (their bodies created more desired antibodies) than the nonmeditating group. The degree of this difference corresponded to the degree of their shift toward left prefrontal cortical activation. This means that not only did meditation make one group of workers feel better, but the changes brought on by meditation were measurable in their brains and the meditation practice also seems to have strengthened their immune response.

Effects on Brain Structure

Another exciting area of mindfulness meditation research involves changes to the actual physical structure of the brain. Many of us worry about our hair thinning or graying as we age. This isn't such a big deal when we realize that our cerebral cortex also thins and our brains actually lose gray matter over time. Luckily, mindfulness meditation may help.

A friend and colleague of mine, Dr. Sara Lazar, is a biological researcher at Massachusetts General Hospital in Boston. She has been studying magnetic resonance images (MRIs) of long-term Western meditators and nonmeditator control subjects. One of her studies took the scientific community by storm. She looked at a group of people with an average of nine years of meditation experience, averaging six hours of practice per week. She then compared them to age-matched controls. It turned out that the meditators had thicker cerebral cortexes in three areas: the anterior insula, sensory cortex, and prefrontal cortex. All three of these areas are involved in paying attention to the breath and other sensory stimuli, as one typically does during meditation practice. The prefrontal cortex is also involved in what is called working memory—holding thoughts in our head long enough to reflect on them, make decisions, and solve problems. The differences in thickness were more pronounced in older subjects, and the degree of thickening was proportional to the amount of time a person had spent meditating over a lifetime. While the implications of these results for preserving our cognitive abilities are still being studied, they are promising. (I had the privilege of being one of the meditating subjects in Dr. Lazar's study, and while I often think that I'm losing my mind as I age, I trust that things might be worse had I not been meditating.) Other research has shown less loss of gray matter with age among meditators, which corresponded to less loss in their ability to sustain attention—an important component of many mental tasks—compared with nonmeditating controls.

In yet another encouraging study, Dr. Lazar also found measurable changes in a part of the brain stem involved in the production of serotonin, a mood-regulating neurotransmitter. This area became denser after just 8 weeks of mindfulness practice. The increase in density was greatest for subjects who did the most practice. These same subjects were the ones that reported the greatest increases in sense of well-being after taking up mindfulness meditation.

Effects on Thoughts and Feelings

These changes in brain function and structure offer exciting support for what mindfulness practitioners have been reporting anecdotally for thousands of years—these practices dramatically change our minds. As Western psychotherapists and psychological researchers enthusiastically design treatments that incorporate mindfulness meditation, similar discoveries are being made about the effect of mindfulness practice on feelings and behavior. These are far reaching and explain both why mindfulness practice is attracting so much professional attention and why it can help us deal with so many different problems.

As you'll see in Part II of this book, mindfulness meditation has been shown to be useful in working with depression, anxiety, substance abuse problems, eating disorders, anger and other relationship difficulties, back and other chronic muscular skeletal pain, and a wide variety of other stress-related medical problems. It even leads people to act more compassionately.

One problem or many?

Despite accumulating evidence that mindfulness can change brain function and structure, it can be hard to imagine how it could help with such a wide variety of everyday issues. Might it be that they all have something in common?

When I first trained as a psychologist in the 1970s, our diagnostic system was relatively simple. Most patients seemed to have one of a few different diagnoses, such as anxiety, depression, substance abuse, or, less commonly, major mental illnesses such as schizophrenia or manic-depressive (bipolar) disorder. There was relatively little experimental evidence to support different treatments, so our professors and supervisors taught us techniques based on their own training and subsequent clinical successes and failures.

As years passed, research in mental health exploded. The field developed more and more detailed diagnostic systems, designed to help us determine which therapies will be useful to different patients. As the number of possible diagnoses multiplied, the probability that a given individual would be suffering from more than one disorder also increased.

Researchers currently revising the diagnostic system are wrestling with an issue that has turned into a political battle between two factions: The *Splitters* contend that our diagnostic system isn't refined enough—we're still combining apples and oranges—and we need to subdivide categories further to better test new medications and psychotherapies. The *Lumpers* feel instead that we've lost our way and become so enchanted by our labels that we no longer understand the common factors underlying human emotional distress. Most practicing clinicians tend to agree with the Lumpers, while many researchers are in the Splitters camp.

The Lumpers say the idea that different forms of psychological distress do have something in common is in fact borne out by a review of the research. And the common ingredient is both simple and surprising.

Experiential Avoidance

The Lumpers contend that most of our psychological suffering stems from our attempts to avoid psychological suffering. It is actually the things we do to get away from pain—either consciously or unconsciously—that are at the heart of our difficulties. They call this *experiential avoidance*. It includes everything we do to try to block out, avoid, deny, deaden, or otherwise rid ourselves of discomfort.

Of course it's not surprising that, given the choice, most of us will choose to do things that we think will make us feel better rather than those that we imagine will make us feel worse. This is after all the essence of the *pleasure principle* described in Chapter 1. The problem is that many things that make us feel better in the short run actually make us feel much worse in the long run.

The *Diver Dan* approach

Long before the term *experiential avoidance* came into use, a friend of mine called this the *Diver Dan* approach to life. Like the old-fashioned divers who put on bulky suits with big steel helmets to insulate themselves from the cold seawater, we try to insulate ourselves from everything that might bother us. We do this in many different ways.

Mother's Little Helper

Many of us medicate discomfort one way or another. Alcohol is very popular of course. Even normal social drinking involves using alcohol to "relax" or "have fun." We don't drink only because alcohol "tastes good" (though humans have done a remarkable job of flavoring this particular drug). Rather, we like the psychopharmacological effects—mostly the way alcohol lessens anxiety or tension and can alleviate sadness, frustration, and anger. Milder drugs, such as caffeine, are so much a part of daily life that most of us don't think of them as drugs at all—until they're not available. And then there is the host of legally prescribed and illegally acquired mind-altering drugs that the pharmaceutical industry promotes and drug dealers distribute. All of these are designed to shift our experience away from something unpleasant and toward something more pleasant; they all involve blocking out uncomfortable thoughts or feelings.

Most of us know the perils of self-medication when taken to excess. Drugs can interfere with our functioning, messing up our lives in ways that bring on new painful feelings—which we then medicate with more drugs. Sometimes drugs harm us physically; other times they can just keep us from maturing. By turning to substances whenever difficult feelings arise, we never learn to handle those feelings very well. (We'll see how to use mindfulness practices to work with intoxicants and related issues in Chapter 9.)

The Joys of Distraction

Many of the "drugs" we use to feel better aren't chemical. Almost all of us become hooked on one activity or another because it helps distract us from unpleasant thoughts or feelings. The U.S. Bureau of Labor Statistics collects data not only on what we do at work but also on what we do in our leisure time. Would you like to guess what the most popular leisure activity in America is? Most of us can get this right just by thinking about our own lives: it's watching television. Now try to guess the second most popular nonwork activity. These days a lot of people imagine it's surfing the Internet. Actually, that's a subset of the number two activity: *shopping*. We're fortunate to live in a culture that seamlessly blends our favorite endeavors. While watching TV, every few minutes we're generously offered suggestions for things we might buy while shopping.

And then there's that little problem with obesity in our culture. This arises partly because we spend so much time comforting ourselves with television and partly because we spend so much time comforting ourselves with food. Almost everyone eats, at least sometimes, to soothe themselves. Sometimes we even combine our vices, eating while watching TV or shopping.

As with many drugs, we tend to develop tolerance over time for our distractions, so that we need higher and higher doses for them to work. When I was young, there was a TV show about a lawyer named Perry Mason who investigated his cases to uncover the secret truth. If you're too young to recall it, the show was a bit like *Law & Order*. The difference was that on *Perry Mason*, a really, really intense moment would involve seeing an arm holding a gun, which would then fire—pop. We wouldn't see the victim or any blood, and the action all took place on a small black-and-white screen. Nonetheless, at the time it was very intense and engrossing.

Because we tend to become accustomed to a given level of stimulation and need more and more to distract ourselves from the contents of our minds, *Perry Mason* no longer holds our attention. Now if we're watching *Law & Order: Hideous Events*, even though there's a doe-eyed child being dismembered while his siblings watch, we think, "Ho-hum, just another sadistic child abuse episode—I wonder if there's anything more interesting on." Similarly, the tendency to multitask entertainment—to listen to an iPod while walking, or work on a laptop while watching TV, speaks to our constant efforts to turn up the volume on stimulation to avoid being with our thoughts and feelings.

I'm not suggesting that there's anything inherently depraved about watching TV, listening to an iPod, shopping, or eating. But if you approach these activities with mindfulness, you'll probably notice that at least at times you use them to distract yourself from something uncomfortable.

Sometimes we describe the unwanted feeling as "boredom." This is a popular word in our culture for an unpleasant emotion that we can't quite identify. Consider, however, the experience of blissfully sitting on a beach watching a sunset. How is this different from moments of inactivity in which you feel "bored"? You may discover that the "boredom" involves some restlessness, irritation, anxiety, sadness, or other unwanted emotion. The things we do to feel better are usually designed to distract us from these sorts of underlying feelings.

Self-Imprisonment

Experiential avoidance causes trouble beyond prompting us to use too many intoxicants, watch too much TV, buy too many things, or eat too much food. It also plays a big role in maintaining anxiety, depression, chronic pain, and other forms of distress. In the case of worry or anxiety, experiential avoidance limits our life as we try to avoid the activities that we fear will make us more anxious. The shy young man who stays home alone because he's afraid he'll feel awkward at the party only grows more fearful and reclusive. The nervous flier who spends all day taking the train to a meeting is that much more reluctant the next time he has to fly.

One aspect of depression involves feeling dead and cut off from the world as we try to avoid sadness, anger, or other emotions that threaten to envelop us. The "nice guy" who never wants to argue winds up bored at work and irritable at home after his coworker treats him badly. The "tough guy" who won't let himself cry wonders why he's lost interest in his life after a terrifying car accident. Chronic headaches, backaches, and digestive troubles also get worse as we try to block out unpleasant emotions and limit activities in an attempt to feel better. And a lot of fights start when one party raises an issue that the other would rather avoid.

Experiential avoidance has paradoxical effects: Like the Chinese handcuffs we played with as children, the harder we try to escape from our troubles, the more ensnared we become. Who knew that so many of our efforts to alleviate pain—which on the surface seem so sensible— would lead to something worse? In Part II you'll learn how avoidance can trap us in every manner of psychological and physical difficulty—and how mindfulness practices can help you deal effectively with them.

> The reason that mindfulness practice is useful for working with so many different problems is because experiential avoidance plays a role in them all—and mindfulness is its antidote.

Learning to be with our experience

When we practice mindfulness meditation, we practice being with whatever is occurring at the moment without doing anything to try to change or escape it. We pay attention to how things actually are rather than how we want them to be. This is very different from our usual approach to discomfort. Instead of trying to make it go away, we work on increasing our capacity to bear it.

Our ability to handle things, or to bear our experience, is very variable. Imagine that you have a bad cold and you haven't slept well for a few nights. You wake up groggy and stuffy and start getting ready for work or school. It's raining and you have a long day ahead. You're moving slowly, so you're behind schedule. On the way out the door you have an argument with your spouse. As you are driving down the road, you feel a thumping and realize you have a flat tire. Know the feeling? "I just can't take one more thing."

Now imagine a different day. You've been healthy—eating, exercising, and sleeping well. You wake up refreshed, and the sun is shining. You have a relatively light day of work coming up, and you're right on schedule. On the way out the door you have a nice, connected moment with your spouse. Driving down the road, someone runs a red light and crashes into your car. Luckily, no one is injured. You feel startled but relieved that the only damage is to metal and plastic, and you exchange papers with the other driver. Your car is drivable; you decide you'll call your insurance company in the afternoon.

What happened in these two examples? On the first day, the intensity of the difficulty—a flat tire—was relatively low, but your capacity to bear it was very limited, so you felt overwhelmed. On the second day, the intensity of the difficulty—a car crash—was much higher, but your capacity to bear it was stronger still, so you weren't overwhelmed. These examples illustrate that what matters for our sense of well-being is our capacity to bear experience relative to the intensity of that experience.

> We usually try to feel better by decreasing the intensity of painful experiences; in mindfulness practice, we work instead to increase our capacity to bear them.

In mindfulness practice, we change our *relationship* to difficult experiences—instead of trying to escape or avoid them, we move toward them. Over time, difficult experiences become much easier to bear and we're less readily overwhelmed. This principle will guide our use of mindfulness practice to deal with whatever life brings.

Sounds pretty good, huh? Ready to sign up? There are a number of ways to begin.

The varieties of mindfulness practice

There's an old joke: A tourist is lost in Manhattan. He is becoming increasingly frantic because he's late for a concert. Finally he spots a police officer on the corner and hurries toward him. Breathless, he pleads, "Officer, officer, how do I get to Carnegie Hall?" The policeman pauses thoughtfully and studies the tourist very carefully. Several seconds go by during which the man can hardly contain his agitation. Finally the officer looks him in the eye and says, "*Practice, practice.*"

There are many ways to cultivate awareness of present experience with acceptance. Just as with other skills, all of them involve repeated practice. Think of mindfulness the way you think of physical fitness. Just as you can become more fit through regular physical exercise, you can become more mindful by engaging in deliberate mindfulness practices. For example, if you wanted to improve your cardiovascular health, you might begin by informally integrating exercise into your everyday routines—taking the stairs instead of the elevator or riding a bicycle instead of driving to work. If you wanted to become even more fit, you might set aside time to exercise formally, perhaps at a gym or health club. To really accelerate the process, you might even go on a hiking or bicycling trip or go away to a fitness spa.

Analogous options are available for cultivating mindfulness: informal mindfulness practice, formal practice, and retreat practice.

Informal Mindfulness Practice

Informal mindfulness practice involves reminding ourselves throughout the day to pay attention to whatever is happening in the moment. It's like taking the stairs instead of the elevator; bicycling instead of driving. Practicing mindfulness in this way means noticing the sensations of walking when we walk, noticing the taste of our food when we eat, and noticing the clouds and the trees as we pass them.

The Vietnamese Zen teacher Thich Nhat Hanh suggests a number of informal techniques to develop mindfulness. They are all designed to counteract our tendency to multitask or to do things on automatic while lost in our thoughts. For example, when your telephone rings (or chirps, or plays the national anthem), try just listening to the first few rings, attending to the detail of the sound as you might listen to a musical instrument. Or when the red taillights of another vehicle force you to slow down as you drive, try appreciating their color and texture as you might a beautiful sunset. When you wash the dishes, try noticing the feeling of the soapy water on your hands, the color and texture of the food scraps, the shine on the dishes when they are clean. Opportunities for informal mindfulness practice are infinite. At every moment when it's not necessary to be planning or thinking, we can simply bring our attention to what is happening in our sensory awareness.

Formal Meditation Practice

Formal meditation practice involves setting aside time to go to the mental "gym." We dedicate a certain period of time, ideally each day, to sit quietly in meditation. This is the kind of practice that has been studied scientifically.

Unlike informal practice, in which we're accomplishing another task such as walking, driving to our destination, or cleaning dishes while practicing mindfulness, during formal practice we dedicate a period of time entirely to cultivating it. Many types of meditation can be used. Most initially involve choosing an object of attention such as the breath or another sensation and returning our attention to that object each time the mind wanders. This develops a degree of concentration, which enables us to better focus the mind on a chosen object. Once some concentration is established, mindfulness meditation per se entails directing the mind to whatever begins to predominate in awareness—usually focusing on how the event is experienced in the body. These objects of attention can be physical sensations such as an itch, an ache, or a sound; or emotional experiences as they manifest physically, such as the tightness in the chest that comes with anger or the lump in the throat that comes with sadness. Regardless of the object of attention, we practice being *aware of our present experience with acceptance.* Classically, this kind of formal mindfulness meditation is practiced in four postures: sitting, standing, walking, and lying down. As we'll see, each tends to have somewhat different effects. Other related forms of meditation are designed to cultivate mental qualities that support mindfulness practice, such as empathy or compassion.

Retreat Practice

Retreat practice is a "vacation" dedicated entirely to cultivating mindfulness. You can think of it as taking your mind to the spa. There are many styles of meditation retreats. Most involve extended periods of formal meditation practice, often alternating sitting meditation with walking meditation, eating meditation, and other activities. They are usually conducted in silence with very little interpersonal interaction, except for occasional interviews with teachers. All the activities of the day—getting up, showering, brushing teeth, eating, and doing chores—are done in silence and used as opportunities to practice mindfulness. As one observer put it, the first few days of retreat practice are "a lot like being trapped in a phone booth with a lunatic." We discover how difficult it is to simply be present. Initially, the mind is often alarmingly active and restless, spinning stories about how well we're doing, how we compare to others on the retreat (with whom we never speak), and other concerns. Memories of unresolved emotional events enter the mind, along with elaborate fantasies about life in the future. During a retreat, we get to vividly see how our minds create suffering, despite being in an environment in which all of our needs are tended to. Most people find that even a single intensive mindfulness meditation retreat of a week or more is transforming—the insights one gains about the workings of the mind last a lifetime.

How should I start?

As you read about these different forms of practice, what reactions did you have? Did you think "I could try informal practice, but this other stuff isn't for me"? Or "I've wanted to develop a regular meditation practice for years—I really want to start now"? Maybe you even thought "My life is so chaotic and stressful—I'd love to go on a retreat." Everyone is different. Some of our lives are so busy that the thought of adding one more thing immediately makes us feel sick. Others of us are so tired of being caught up in distressing mental habits that we're eager to set aside time so that we can jump in immediately with both feet.

Your approach will depend in part on why you are drawn to mindfulness practice. If you're feeling stressed or have developed stress-related medical symptoms such as headaches, stomachaches, or chronic muscle pain, you may be very motivated to establish a regular formal practice to help you begin to slow down today. Similarly, if you're suffering with excessive worry, tension, and anxiety, feeling overwhelmed by sadness or depression, or struggling with self-defeating habits, you may be tempted to devote more time to a regular formal mindfulness practice. If you are feeling pretty good, don't have much free time, but still want to be more present in your life, you may be tempted to enter into this more lightly, focusing more on informal practice. On the other hand, if this is a time when you are searching to really grow psychologically or spiritually, you may be ready to try an intensive retreat.

A beauty of mindfulness practice is that we can take it up at whatever level of intensity suits our particular life. That said, most people find that at least some formal practice is usually needed to get a feel for what mindfulness is. While anyone will benefit from trying to be more present each day through informal practice, formal practice allows us to see more clearly how distracted the mind is ordinarily and how it feels to be really present. The particular balance of practices that you choose will be up to you and will likely change over time.

You'll see once you begin that each form of practice supports the others. If you take the time to regularly practice formal meditation, you will find it considerably easier to do informal practice at other times because your attention will be more concentrated. (If we're working out at the gym several times a week, we usually find it much easier to climb the stairs.) Similarly, if you do informal mindfulness practice throughout the day, you'll find it much easier to sit down and meditate formally when you have the time, because your mind will be in the habit of noticing what is happening in the present moment.

Most people who take up mindfulness practice will choose to do a mix of informal and formal practice. How often and how long you meditate will be up to you. Both scientific studies and informal reports suggest that the effects of these practices tend to be "dose" related, meaning the more time you dedicate to them, the more profound their effects will likely be. Regularity also helps. As with the gym, doing formal practice at least several times a week will help you see its cumulative effects. For one person this may involve setting aside 20 minutes at a time; for another 30 or 45. But again, if you don't have the time or inclination for such a commitment right now, simply entering each day with the intention to do informal practice will also be useful.

Just as formal and informal practice support one another, retreat practice can support both. Of course most people won't sign up for a retreat unless they have first found the other practices beneficial. But once you've tasted for yourself the benefits of mindfulness in your daily life, a retreat can be very useful for deepening and reinforcing your practice.

In the next two chapters you'll learn several formal and informal mindfulness practices to get you started. Then, in Part II, you'll learn how to put these together with other practices designed for specific challenges such as worry and anxiety, sadness and depression, stress-related physical problems, relationship challenges, destructive habits, difficulties dealing with illness and aging, and more. A general mindfulness practice can help all of us deal better with the inevitable challenges of life. But if you feel plagued by a particular problem—getting stuck in bouts with the blues, caught up in attacks of nerves, visited by headaches, digestive troubles, or back pain, confused by relationships going poorly despite all of your efforts, or mysteriously driven to visit the refrigerator—there are ways to customize your mindfulness practice to address these directly.

We'll explore practices that can break the grip of entrenched problems and also ones that are useful in the moment when you need a "life preserver" to deal with a torrent of anxiety that broadsides you, a wave of depression that knocks you down unexpectedly, irresistible urges to scream at your child, cravings for a drink or doughnut, and other ambushes. We'll discuss practices that work best when we are tired, practices that can help when we feel overwhelmed, practices to use when our minds are full of critical thoughts, those that help with pain and illness, and others that support making healthy choices. As you come to understand mindfulness better, you'll be able to decide when to use these different practices and how to modify them to suit your particular needs.

Avoiding confusion:
what mindfulness practice is *not*

I've had the privilege of introducing mindfulness practices to patients, colleagues, and lots of other people over many years. Perhaps because these practices originated in non-Western cultures and are associated with all sorts of exotic images, misconceptions about them abound. These misconceptions can create confusion, make people wonder if they're practicing incorrectly, or make mindfulness practices difficult to embrace. To help get you off on the right foot, let's clear some of these up in advance.

Not Having a Blank Mind

Jon Kabat-Zinn, who made great strides introducing mindfulness practices to Western audiences, tells the following story: A participant in one of his workshops brought to him a Bazooka Joe comic (the kind that comes in bubble gum). In the comic, Joe is sitting in full lotus meditation posture, talking to his friend Mort. Joe says, "Since I've discovered meditation, my mind has become a complete blank." Mort replies, "That's funny, I thought you were born that way." While there are indeed many concentrative meditation practices designed to empty the mind of thought, this is not the aim of mindfulness practice. Nor is it designed to make us stupid or make us lose our analytical abilities. Instead, mindfulness practice involves noticing what the mind is doing at all times, including being aware that we're thinking when we're thinking. Rather than eliminating thoughts, it brings a certain perspective, an ability to notice that our thoughts are just thoughts, instead of believing they necessarily reflect external "reality." Mindfulness practice also helps us stop pursuing thoughts that we have come to see are irrational or unhelpful, while at the same time teaching us that deliberately trying to avoid or block out thoughts only makes them return with a vengeance. We come to see that struggling to stop thoughts is like agitating a glass of muddy water to get it to clear.

> Mindfulness practice helps us see our thoughts clearly.

Not Becoming Emotionless

Many people imagine that mindfulness practice will relieve them of their painful emotions. Especially when we're upset, the fantasy of becoming emotionless is quite appealing. In reality, mindfulness practice usually has the opposite effect. Because we practice being aware of whatever is occurring in the mind each moment, we actually notice our emotions quite vividly. In fact, we generally become *more* sensitive.

We all engage regularly in psychological defenses. These can take many forms—trying to build ourselves up to compensate for feelings of inadequacy, rationalizing unethical behavior, distracting ourselves by turning on the television, or eating to self-soothe. Mindfulness practices make us aware that we're trying to feel better when we do these things. As a result, we tend to notice the feeling that's behind the defense.

> Mindfulness practice enables us to more fully and poignantly bear a full range of emotional experience.

Not Withdrawing from Life

Because monks, nuns, and hermits originally developed and refined meditation practices, people often assume that they involve withdrawing from living a full, interpersonally rich life. While there are certainly benefits to be derived from going on a meditation retreat or joining a monastery, even when meditating in these settings one isn't exactly withdrawing. Instead, the ups and downs of life are experienced more vividly, because we're taking time and putting in effort to pay attention to them.

For example, most people find while participating in meditation retreats that their minds are full of thoughts about other people. During a day of silence with no eye contact, it's not unusual to find oneself thinking, "Wow—she looks so beautiful when she serves herself oatmeal" or "Doesn't he see there are other people here? I can't believe

> Mindfulness practice attunes us to others, helping us feel more connected.

he's taking five prunes!" Even when we're far from our normal activities, mindfulness practice reveals our minds to be thoroughly tuned in to the interpersonal world.

Not Seeking Bliss

How disappointing! The image of the spiritual master blissfully smiling instead of struggling with everyday reality is very appealing. When we first start to practice mindfulness, most of us are very upset to discover that our minds continue to wander. We then become agitated about feeling agitated. Students regularly complain to their teachers, "Everyone else seems to be at peace in their meditation—why am I having so much trouble?" While from time to time pleasant, even blissful states do arise, in mindfulness practice one works on

> Mindfulness practice helps us accept all of our experiences instead of just clinging to pleasant ones.

allowing these to come and go—neither clinging to blissful states nor rejecting unpleasant ones. It is important not to view moments of irritation, frustration, or restlessness as failures. Of course, like most aspects of mindfulness practice, this is easier said than done.

Not Escaping Pain

This sounds even worse—perhaps it's time to return this book and get one that promises something better. Rather than escaping pain, mindfulness practices help us increase our capacity to experience it. They all involve deliberately abstaining from things we usually do to relieve pain. For example, if we are meditating and an itch arises, a typical instruction is to observe the itch and notice any impulse that arises (such as the urge to scratch)—but not act on that impulse. So we actually come to experience pain and discomfort *more* vividly. As we will see later, this attitude extends beyond itches and physical pain to include the vivid experience of emotional pain as well. As we practice *being with* these unpleasant experiences, our capacity to bear them steadily increases. We also come

> Mindfulness practice helps us embrace pain, which actually lessens suffering.

to see that painful sensations are distinct from the *suffering* that commonly accompanies them. We notice that the suffering arises from our reactions to the pain (we will return to this theme later). When we practice responding to pain with acceptance rather than resistance, pro-test, or avoidance, our suffering diminishes.

Not Converting to a New Religion

A concern that comes up repeatedly when people consider taking up mindfulness meditation is whether this might somehow run counter to their religious beliefs. After all, many mindfulness practices derive from Buddhist and other religious traditions. Let's return again to the Buddha legend to address this issue:

When the prince "woke up" after 49 days and nights of meditation practice, he began to teach what he had learned. The people he encoun-tered noticed that he was unusual—he was happier and less preoccupied with himself than other people. They asked him questions appropriate to their time: "Are you a god?" "Are you a ghost?" The prince would reply, "No, I'm just a man, but I've woken up" (the word *Buddha* means "one who is awake"). They would also ask him cosmological questions about the origins of the world. He is said to have replied, "I don't teach about such matters. I am a physician of the mind. I teach about the origins of psychological suffering and how to alleviate it." Elsewhere in this tradi-tion we see a strong emphasis on what is called in Pali *ehipasiko*—which roughly translates "come and see for yourself." The idea is not to take any teachings on faith but rather to try the practices and see if the teachings turn out to be true in your own experience.

As secular scientific researchers and mental health professionals are adopting mindfulness techniques, they are doing it in this spirit. Rather than suggesting that people abandon their religious beliefs and take up new ones, they're inviting their clients or patients to experiment with mindfulness meditation and observe its effects for themselves.

Interest in mindfulness meditation extends beyond the scientific community into the religious community as well. When I first became involved in these practices in the 1970s, I went on a 10-day meditation retreat at the then newly established Insight Meditation Society in Barre, Massachusetts. I was surprised to see Trappist monks meditating next to me. These monks found that mindfulness meditation was a great help to their Christian spiritual practice, and some of them went on to teach what is now called centering or contemplative prayer in the Catholic tra-dition. Similar adaptations are springing up all the time in the Jewish, Muslim, and other faiths.

The bottom line is that mindfulness meditation practice is being adopted successfully by nonreligious people interested in enhancing their personal psychological development, as well as by adherents of a wide variety of religious traditions who are

Mindfulness practice can support our efforts in almost any spiritual or psychological tradition.

finding it supports their spiritual as well as psychological growth. Its overarching principle—that by seeing things as they are, and learning to accept them, we can experience well-being—knows no bounds.

In the next chapters you'll find detailed instructions for a variety of mindfulness practices along with suggestions for weaving them together into a program that fits your particular life and needs. As soon as you're ready, turn the page and "come and see for yourself" what they can offer.

CHAPTER 3

Learning to practice mindfulness

*H*as anyone ever taught you how to concentrate? Given how useful concentration is for so many things—whether studying for a test, driving a car, or remembering a telephone number—it's striking that most of us are never taught how to do it. We're told to "pay attention" in school and not disrupt the class, but we're not taught *how*. In fact many children whose minds tend to wander are medicated for attention deficit disorder, but relatively few are taught nonpharmacological methods of cultivating attention.

Developing concentration is an important part of all three forms of mindfulness practice: informal practice, formal meditation practice, and intensive retreat practice. All three train the mind to be *aware of present experience with acceptance*. Until we have learned how to focus the mind somewhat, however, it's very difficult to be really aware of our experience. When we're operating on automatic—daydreaming about one thing while our body is involved in another, or restlessly craving the next little treat—we don't really notice what we're doing.

And if we're not aware of our experience from moment to moment, it's very difficult to gain insight into and interrupt the mental habits that create suffering—which is ultimately the point of practicing mindfulness. Without seeing how it happens, we miss out on smelling the roses, get trapped in all sorts of unhealthy habits, spend needless energy proving that we're lovable, capable, or righteous, and alienate important people by not noticing their needs in the moment. Concentration, as a foundation for mindfulness, is a key step on the path to greater sanity.

are somewhat coarser or more vivid for most people than the sensations of the breath. Therefore, when our mind is very busy or distractible, it might be easier to notice walking sensations than breathing sensations. On the other hand, when our mind is relatively calm, we may be able to cultivate more refined levels of concentration by attending to the subtler sensations of the breath.

The key to engaging in concentration practices is finding the right kind of effort. If we try too hard and are overly strict with ourselves, we quickly get tied up in knots and can't concentrate. Most of us are rather alarmed when first meditating to discover just how frisky the mind can be. If we try to strong-arm it into obedience, the mind usually rebels. On the other hand, if we're too loose or relaxed, and don't put sufficient effort into concentrating, the mind just fritters about and never develops very much sustained attention. An optimal balance is found through trial and error.

In the early classical descriptions, finding this balance is compared to tuning a lute. If a string is too tight, it breaks and you can't make any music. If it's too loose, it's out of tune. A musician discovers the right tension by listening carefully and making regular adjustments.

The first few times Jerry tried formal meditation practice he got very frustrated. Even though he was told that the goal wasn't to make his thoughts stop, or even to relax, he kept feeling like he was failing. He would more or less follow his breath for a few seconds and then think, "I don't think I'm very good at this—nothing much is happening." So he'd try to concentrate harder, only to get irritated each time he lost contact with his breath. When he became so tense and unhappy that he was ready to quit, it dawned on him that maybe he was trying too hard to get it right. He needed to focus more on accepting whatever arose in his awareness and less on rigidly following every breath.

George had the opposite problem. When he sat down to meditate, his mind filled with all sorts of entertaining daydreams and plans. He would follow these and spin out great stories about clubs he'd like to visit, women he'd like to date, and movies he'd like see. Sometimes he would think about problems with his car or computer and how he might fix them. While this was pleasant enough, and even provided him with some good ideas, he eventually realized that he wasn't trying at all to bring his mind back to the present. He needed to put more effort into attending to the sensations of the moment instead of following all of his thoughts and fantasies.

In seeking a balance, it's most important to be nice to ourselves. You

Focusing the lens

You might think of mindfulness practice as taking a photograph. To get a clear picture, you first have to focus the camera lens (at least this used to be necessary, before the invention of automatic lenses). Learning to concentrate is like focusing the mind's lens—it allows us to see clearly whatever we turn our attention to. We can then use this skill to see how our minds work and to free ourselves from the patterns that cause suffering.

Because concentration is a necessary foundation for mindfulness, the best way to begin mindfulness practice is by learning how to concentrate. While both informal and formal practices can support our efforts, most people find it necessary to start by learning formal concentration exercises.

Like most skills, concentration can be developed through practice. Most concentration practices follow the same formula. First we choose an object of attention. Then, every time we notice that the mind has wandered from that object, we gently bring it back. The object we choose can be nearly anything that can be perceived:

- A visual object—perhaps a candle, statue, or picture
- A sound—such as a bell ringing or the gurgle of running water
- A sensation in the body when we are sedentary—often the breath
- Sensations in the body when we are moving—such as the feet touching the ground as we walk
- An image in our mind—such as a mandala
- A sound in our mind—perhaps a silently repeated phrase or mantra
- A spoken word—as in chanting

When we are doing informal mindfulness practice, the object of our attention is usually central to the task at hand: the changing image of the road and cars while we drive; the feeling of water droplets striking our body when we shower; the feeling of the broom or vacuum in our hands as we clean the floor. Different objects of attention tend to have different effects on the mind. Depending on our temperament and mood, we may find one or another more appropriate for a given practice period.

We can think of these various objects of attention as differing in degree of subtlety or coarseness. For example, the sensations of walking may find that concentration practices are harder than you imagine they should be—so you'll have to practice patience and self-acceptance as you attempt them. As a respected meditation teacher famously told his students, "If you have a mind, it's going to wander."

Don't just do something; sit there

The next sections of this chapter will introduce you to a number of meditation practices, each requiring between 20 and 30 minutes. Try a few of them in sequence if you have the time or explore them one by one when you can.

If you have about 30 minutes now during which you won't be interrupted, I invite you to try a basic formal concentration exercise (it will help to have a clock, watch, or timer nearby). The meditation can be done either sitting up or lying down—though if you're at all sleepy, you'll be better off sitting. (Some people find it easier to learn new practices by listening to guided meditation instructions. You can access these for this and many of the other practices in this book at *www. mindfulness-solution.com.*)

——————— *Breath Awareness Meditation* ———————

If you choose to sit up, you can use a chair, a meditation cushion, or a meditation bench. If using a chair, find one that allows you to sit comfortably with a more or less straight spine. This posture helps us pay attention—having a straight spine increases alertness. You can use the back of the chair for support if you like, or sit a bit forward, finding a balanced position in which your spine supports itself.

If using a meditation cushion, place the cushion on a folded blanket or carpet to create a soft surface and sit cross-legged on it. The cushion needs to be tall enough so that your knees can touch the floor, forming a stable triangle between your two knees on the ground and your buttocks on the cushion. You can place one foot on top of the opposite ankle or calf or simply allow both feet to lie on the floor, one just in front of the other, without actually crossing them. The idea is to find a posture that feels comfortable and stable with a relaxed, yet erect spine.

If using a meditation bench, place it on a folded blanket or carpet. Begin by kneeling, with your knees, shins, and feet against the ground. Then place the bench under you so that it supports your buttocks and most of your weight. You may also want to put a cushion or folded blanket on top of the bench to give yourself more height and padding. Here, too, the idea is to find a posture that feels comfortable and stable with a more or less straight spine.

Regardless of how you choose to sit, you may find it helpful to imagine that a string is attached to the top of your head, pulling you gently toward the ceiling or sky, lengthening your spine. Next gently rock your head forward and back and from side to side to find a position where it balances naturally. The idea is to arrive at a relaxed yet dignified and alert posture. You can rest your hands comfortably on your thighs or knees to add to a sense of stability. Don't use your arms to support your torso or to keep from falling backward, as this creates a lot of tension.

While this is not a physical exercise, it will be useful to try to remain as still as possible while meditating. If an urge arises to scratch an itch or adjust your position, experiment with just observing the urge without acting on it. While you don't have to be heroic or stoic about this, exercising some restraint with the urge to move will enhance your concentration. It will also illustrate an important principle about how the mind habitually reacts to discomfort—a principle at the heart of mindfulness practice (more about this later).

Once you're sitting in an alert, comfortable position, close your eyes (obviously you'll need to read the rest of these instructions first). If all is going well, you'll be able to notice that you're already breathing. Your assignment for the first 20 minutes of this meditation will be to bring your attention to the sensations of your breath. While there are several places in the body where you might observe the breath, for this first exercise, try bringing your attention to the rising and falling sensations in your belly that accompany each inhalation and exhalation. See if you can observe the breath through its entire cycle—from the beginning of an in-breath, to the point where the lungs are relatively full, back down to the point where they are relatively empty, and on to the beginning of the next cycle. You won't be trying to control the breath in any way—this is a concentration practice, not a breathing exercise. The breath may be short and shallow or long and deep. It may be one way one minute, and different the next. There is no need to regulate or change it. You're simply using the sensations of the breath in the belly to practice paying attention to what is happening right now.

Unless you've got a very strong natural talent for this, pretty soon you'll notice that your attention wanders, either to other sensations in the body or to thoughts. You may discover that your mind leaves the breath entirely for long stretches during which you are thinking about other things entirely. This is perfectly normal (remember, "If you have a mind, it's going to wander"). When you notice that this has happened, just gently return your attention to the breath. You might even congratulate yourself on becoming aware. This is sometimes described as being like puppy training—the puppy wanders off, you bring it back; the puppy wanders off again, you bring it back again. We don't get upset with the puppy—we expect it to be frisky.

So, before you read any further, I invite you to try this concentration exercise for 20 minutes. You can use a timer or just open your eyes and check your clock or watch periodically. Please try this now and then continue to the next paragraph when the time is up.

Now that you've followed your breath for 20 minutes, take a few moments to experience your environment. Start with the ocean of sound that surrounds you. Listen to all of the sounds striking your ears right now as you might listen to a symphony, or as you might listen to the birds, crickets, or wind on a summer evening. Try to listen as a musician might—not labeling the sounds but hearing them as music. Close your eyes again and do this for a few minutes before reading on.

Next notice the sensations of contact between your body and the chair, cushion, bench, ground, or other surface. Observe the hundreds of sensations coming from each point of contact—your feet, your buttocks, anywhere else that your body touches something firm. Notice how these sensations are actually not solid but are made up of hundreds of small sensations strung together. Explore these sensations with your eyes closed for a little while.

Now turn your attention to the sensations of contact with the ocean of air that surrounds you. Observe the sensations wherever your skin is exposed—your face, hands, or other body parts. Notice whether the air feels warm or cold, still or breezy. Notice the sensations of your breath at the tip of your nose, how it is cool when you breathe in and warmer when you breathe out. Again closing your eyes, just feel the air for a few minutes.

Finally, in a moment, you'll bring your attention to your visual field, noticing the colors, shapes, and textures of your environment. Try to take them in as an artist might—putting aside for a moment the usual habit of labeling objects. Please look up from the book for a few minutes now to do this before reading on.

WHAT DID YOU DISCOVER?

Each of us has a different experience when we try concentration meditation. In fact, the same person will usually have very different experiences each time he or she does it. Take a couple of minutes now to jot down what you noticed during each phase of the exercises, as though you were telling a friend about the experience.

_____

_____

_____

_____

_____

_____

Now let's see how your observations compare with some common experiences.

It was harder than I had expected.

Most of us are so busy and so constantly entertained by TV, radio, iPods, magazines, books, and other people that we find it quite difficult to sit silently and concentrate on one set of sensations for very long. We are visited by *restlessness*, in which staying still is difficult, and *doubt*, in which we wonder why we are doing this. Sometimes intense feelings or images arise—perhaps sadness or anger of which we weren't fully aware or memories of painful past events. Sometimes these experiences are so intense that we want to quit the exercise early.

If you felt overwhelmed by feelings or memories during this exercise, you may wish next time to try an externally focused concentration practice—one that uses the sensations of walking, the taste of food, or an object in your environment. I'll present instructions for these shortly.

Sometimes, too, the exercise can be physically painful, producing soreness or stiffness in the body. Perhaps you are unaccustomed to the posture. In addition, tensions that you may not have been aware of can surface, creating pain in the back, neck, knees, or shoulders. When this happens, try exploring the pain sensations for a while without adjusting your posture—you may find that they change by themselves. We'll discuss further how to use mindfulness to work with physical pain in Chapter 7.

I became very sleepy.

Many of us are chronically sleep deprived, and as soon as we give up external entertainment or goal-oriented activity, we start to nod off. And, of course, when we're asleep, it's difficult to redirect our attention to the breath. Because of this dilemma, sleepy students have historically been offered a radical solution: try meditating at the edge of a deep well or high cliff! Luckily, less drastic alternatives exist, such as keeping your eyes open, gazing a few feet ahead at around a 45-degree angle, or meditating standing up.

I enjoyed this—it was very relaxing.

One aim of concentration practices is to calm and slow the mind. While this doesn't always happen, sometimes it does, and this can be quite pleasant. It becomes a problem only if we develop the expectation that concentration practice *should* always be calming or feel good. Such expectations tend to jinx the experience and cause agitation the next time we meditate and find the mind more active.

The colors, sounds, and sensations were intense.

A common effect of cultivating concentration is heightening of the senses. This effect is generally dose related, meaning that a little concentration practice produces a subtle enhancement of sensory experience, while sustained concentration practice brings a rather dramatic intensification. I remember vividly my first extended meditation retreat. After a couple of days it was time for a shower. I wasn't expecting what happened and could scarcely believe what I felt. I stepped into an ordinary shower stall and found that the sensations of thousands of water drops hitting my skin, combined with the feeling of the slippery, sensual soap gliding over my body, was almost overwhelming. That shower was more vivid and absorbing than gourmet meals, amusement park rides—even moments of sexual discovery. While sensory enhancement isn't the primary goal of concentration practice, it can feel really nice and is one way in which concentration meditation enriches our lives.

I'm no good at this.

This is often the result of wanting meditation to be peaceful or relaxing. Our judging, evaluating minds get into the action and become relentless in their criticism. Since most of the time our minds wander quite a bit, we get very disappointed if we expect them to hold still. Given our preoccupation with self-esteem related to concerns about our rank in the primate troop, meditation can be a rich territory for self-torture. We end up convinced that everyone else is much saner—they can control their minds, but we can't control ours. One reason that the image of puppy training helps in this practice is that most of us are forgiving toward puppies—who can blame a puppy for being frisky and unruly? They're young, untrained, and don't know any better. Just like us.

Pointing the camera

Some meditation traditions have concentration as their primary aim. The goal is to develop a calm and steady mind by becoming really skilled at focusing. *Transcendental meditation*, which was very popular in the United States and Europe during the 1960s and 1970s, is one such tradition. It gives people a secret mantra to use as an object of attention in order to develop a state of deep rest and relaxation. Similarly, the *Relaxation Response* described by Harvard Medical School cardiologist Dr. Herbert Benson uses concentration practices to gain control over physiological arousal in order to get relief from stress-related medical problems.

If you've been trained in one of these practices, it's important to know that, while they are clearly valuable, they are not by themselves mindfulness exercises. Rather, they are useful techniques that prepare us for mindfulness practice. Concentration practices teach us to focus the mind so as to be able to observe mental phenomena clearly. *Mindfulness* practices then use that concentration to actively examine how the mind works—in particular to observe how the mind creates unnecessary suffering. Through mindfulness we see our habits of living in thoughts of the past or the future, trying to bolster our sense of self through comparisons to others, and making ourselves unhappy by constantly seeking pleasure and trying to avoid pain. We also learn to undo these habits by attending to and learning to accept the moments of life as they unfold.

Formal mindfulness meditation usually begins with concentration practice. Once this is established, however, the meditation instructions change. The idea becomes to turn our attention toward whatever predominates in awareness—whether that is the breath, another body sensation, a sound, a sight, an emotion, an intention, or even a thought.

> Mindfulness is like having the freedom to point our camera at all sorts of interesting objects once we know how to focus it.

Even early in our meditation practice, however, while we're still developing concentration, we can begin cultivating some mindfulness—*awareness of current experience with acceptance.* There are several ways that a mindful attitude can begin to inform our concentration meditation. First, when the mind wanders away from the breath, we can notice where it went before returning our attention to the sensations of breathing. So we might silently note "thinking" or "hearing" or "fantasizing," before coming back to the breath. Second, mindfulness involves an attitude of interest or curiosity toward whatever is occurring. So as we practice concentration, we can try to bring this attitude of interest or curiosity to each breath—to notice the texture, depth, and rhythm of each inhalation and exhalation—treating our object of attention as though it were both fascinating and precious. Finally, we can endeavor to accept everything that we notice while doing concentration practice—the myriad sensations that arise, as well as all of the thoughts and feelings that inevitably come to visit.

Cultivating Mindfulness during Concentration Practice

- Notice (and perhaps label) where your mind goes when it drifts away from the breath.
- Be interested in and curious about the qualities of each breath and whatever else arises.
- Try to welcome everything you notice.

One breath, many ways to follow it

As mentioned above, anything that can be perceived can be used as an object of attention in concentration meditation. Even within the realm of breath meditation, many variations are possible. Each of them has its unique qualities and tends to produce its own effects. Just as the breath offers more subtle sensations than walking, different ways of attending to the breath provide subtler or coarser sensations. You'll probably find that some of the following techniques are more useful when the mind is agitated, while others work better when the mind is already calm:

Focus on the sensations at the tip of the nose instead of the rising and falling of the belly. You can concentrate on the more subtle sensations that occur at the tip of the nose as you inhale and exhale (as you did at the end of the first meditation exercise). Try this right now for a few moments. You may notice that the breath is a little cool as it enters the nostrils and a little warm when it leaves. Sometimes focusing on the breath here is very difficult—the sensations are too subtle and the mind too distractible, so attending to sensations in the belly is preferable. Other times, by challenging the mind to tune in to these more refined sensations, focusing on the tip of the nose allows for deeper levels of concentration.

Use silent self-talk. This is a good way to help focus an agitated mind. It's useful when the mind is so active that the rising and falling sensations of the breath fail to capture your attention. For example, when noticing the sensations of breathing in the belly, you can silently say "rising" each time the belly rises and "falling" each time it falls. The idea here is to have most of your awareness directed to the actual sensations in the body and to use the repetition of words to keep the mind focused on those sensations. Similarly, when using the tip of the nose as a point of attention, you can silently repeat "in" and "out" with each breath.

Count breaths. This is a related approach you might use when the mind is agitated. Try counting only the in-breath or the out-breath. People often report that counting the in-breath tends to be more energizing, while counting the out-breath tends to be more calming. The breath can be counted silently until you reach 10, at which point you begin the counting cycle again. Alternately, breaths can be counted until you reach 100.

Play "catch." If you are readily motivated by goals, you can try this game: count each breath, attempting to reach 100, but begin the count over whenever you notice that your mind has wandered. This is a little like playing catch and seeing how many times you can throw the ball back and forth without dropping it.

A little experimentation will reveal which variation of these methods—noting "rising, falling" or "in, out"; counting the in-breath or out-breath; counting to 10 or 100; or structuring the meditation as a game— seems to enhance your concentration most during different mind states. One way to get a feel for this is to dedicate a session of formal meditation to practicing a number of these variations in sequence. You'll need about 30 minutes for this exercise, so if this isn't a good time, please return to it later.

——————————— *Breath Practice Sampler** ———————————

Begin as you did in the first concentration practice by finding a comfortable, alert posture. Unless you're sleepy, you may find it easiest to stay focused if your eyes are closed (after reading the instructions, of course).

In sequence, try following the breath in the ways listed below, each for about five minutes (using a watch or timer will help). If you feel it might help you reflect on your experience, when you're done come back to the book and jot down what you noticed about each variation and what moods or mind states you imagine each one might best suit:

1. Observe the breath in the belly without words.

————————————————————————————

————————————————————————————

————————————————————————————

2. Observe the breath in the belly, silently labeling "rising," "falling."

————————————————————————————

————————————————————————————

————————————————————————————

3. Observe the breath at the tip of the nose without words.

————————————————————————————

————————————————————————————

————————————————————————————

4. Observe the breath at the tip of the nose, labeling "in," "out."

————————————————————————————

————————————————————————————

————————————————————————————

———————————————

*Available in audio at *www.mindfulness-solution.com*.

5. Observe the breath in either place, counting out-breaths to 10 and repeating.

_____

_____

_____

6. Observe the breath in either place, trying to count out-breaths to 100 but starting over each time you realize your mind wanders.

_____

_____

_____

_____

Were some forms of breath meditation easier for you than others? Might some be better suited to one or another state of mind?

Making practice part of your life

Now that you've tried breath meditation in these different forms, how do you integrate it into your life? Many people develop concentration by just working with the breath, even though there are many other varieties of formal and informal practice available, several of which we'll discuss shortly. What's important is to make a commitment to a practice pattern and try to stick with it over a period of days or weeks.

It's relatively easy to commit to informal practice since this doesn't require taking time away from other things. We can decide to just try to pay more attention to our moment-to-moment experience when we shower, drive, or brush our teeth. Committing to formal meditation practice, however, is a different story. Many of us are strapped for time. You may cringe at the thought of taking on "one more thing" and think it might therefore be best to start light. Surprisingly, many people actually find it easier to practice more than to practice less. This is because more practice, whether in the form of longer practice sessions, more frequent periods, or both, tends to create more noticeable changes to our state of mind. These changes in turn become self-reinforcing and can even make the rest of our lives feel less pressured.

> The effects of regular formal practice can make us feel as though we have more time in our day.

It's like any other skill. If we practice the piano for only a few minutes every few weeks, we're unlikely to feel as though we're learning to play very well and will get frustrated and quit. On the other hand, if we practice often and long enough for the songs to start to flow, we may really come to enjoy and value our time at the piano.

While it can be helpful to do even a few minutes of meditation, most people find they need at least 20 minutes at a time to begin to develop some degree of concentration. People often report that 45 minutes is ideal, as it allows the mind to settle, but is not so long as to produce a great deal of physical discomfort.

Probably the most widely known program teaching formal meditation practice in the United States is the mindfulness-based stress reduction program started by Jon Kabat-Zinn at the University of Massachusetts Medical Center. They teach a variety of concentration and mindfulness practices and typically ask participants to do 45–60 minutes of formal practice each day, six days a week. While this is a significant commitment, participants report that at this level of practice they experience tangible improvements in their sense of well-being. The transcendental meditation program, which has a long history of teaching concentration meditation around the world, typically asks participants to meditate for 20 minutes twice daily.

If you can possibly carve out the time, I'd recommend starting with one of these rhythms—either one 45-minute session or two 20-minute sessions of *Breath Awareness Meditation* daily. You can also start to develop the habit of using certain everyday activities as informal practice opportunities. If you try this, you'll likely notice significant carryover into the rest of your day—feeling more present and more able to accept everyday ups and downs.

Starting a Practice Routine

- Try to do one 45-minute breath meditation practice or two 20-minute sessions a day, as many days each week as you can.
- Consider picking at least one routine activity—showering, shaving, washing dishes, brushing your hair, getting ready for bed, going up or down stairs, driving to work—to use for informal mindfulness practice.

If this degree of commitment isn't practical for you, a smaller "dose" of practice will still have very beneficial effects—they just may not be as dramatic. I would still recommend trying to do the breath meditation for at least 20 minutes at a time, even if less often. Whatever frequency and intensity you decide to try, it will help to choose consistent days of the week and times of day to practice. (Other tips for establishing a practice pattern to fit your particular situation are provided later in the chapter.)

Just as different forms of breath meditation may be more suitable at different moments, each type of formal meditation has its place. All of the following varieties can be used to develop concentration and also be used for mindfulness practice. Some of them also double nicely as informal practices, since you can engage in them while accomplishing other things. With a number of techniques at your disposal, you can adapt your practice to changing circumstances and needs.

Meditation in motion: walking practice

Walking meditation is a very nice complement to breath meditation that can serve as both a formal concentration practice and an informal practice. As a formal practice, this technique is particularly useful when the mind is agitated, when the body is stiff, or when we are sleepy. It's therefore a good one to learn next to support the development of concentration. You can use this at times instead of breath meditation or can split a meditation session between sitting with the breath and walking.

As with breath meditation, to do formal walking meditation it's necessary to set aside time in a relatively quiet environment. Perhaps the most convenient technique involves choosing a path, approximately 15–30 feet in length, that you can traverse back and forth without disturbing or being disturbed by anyone.

As you did with the breath meditation, first read these instructions and then put down the book and give them a try. You might set aside about 20 minutes to do this for the first time. (Again, if now isn't a good time, please return to this later.)

—————————— *Walking Meditation* ——————————

Begin by standing at one end of your path, closing your eyes, and allowing your body to settle into just being here. This can be done wearing shoes, but you may find the experience richer with bare or

stocking feet if conditions allow. Start with a few moments of standing meditation: Notice the sensations of your feet on the ground
and gravity pulling down on your body. Notice the feeling of the air
surrounding you, where it touches your face, hands, and any other
exposed areas. Listen to the sounds that surround you. Notice your
breath, either in your belly or at the tip of your nose.

After you've settled into the experience of standing for a few
minutes, open your eyes and allow your gaze to be cast down comfortably, a few feet in front of you. As you did after the breath meditation, take in the visual field as an artist might—observing the
colors, textures, and shapes.

Once you feel as though you're relatively present to the experience of standing, it's time to begin walking. This can be done either
rapidly or slowly. Under most circumstances, walking more slowly
allows for better concentration. Begin by carefully lifting one foot,
noticing the sensations of lifting in your foot, leg, and rest of your
body. Gradually move the foot forward through space, noticing all
of the sensations of moving. Next attentively place the foot on the
ground in front of you, noticing all of the sensations that arise as
it makes contact with the ground. As you lift, move forward, and
place your foot, try to bring an attitude of interest or curiosity to the
experience—as though you were walking for the first time.

Once your foot is placed firmly on the ground, it's time to move
the other foot. Again, begin with attentively lifting, then pay attention to the feeling of moving the foot forward, and finally notice all
the sensations involved in placing it back on the ground. You'll need
to experiment to find a pace that works well for you. (I usually practice this quite slowly, with the lifting-forward-placing sequence of
each foot taking about five seconds—just fast enough to keep from
falling over.)

Continue these slow, attentive movements until you reach the
other end of your path. At that point, pause for a few moments of
standing meditation—feel the sensations of standing still, attending
again to your feet on the ground, the air, sounds, and visual field.
Once you feel fully present, turn around gradually, noting all of the

sensations associated with this, and then head back in the other direction. Continue slowly walking back and forth along your path, pausing at each end to be fully present, for the next 20 minutes.

WHAT DID YOU DISCOVER?

Just as breath meditation can unfold very differently for different people or even for the same person at different times, each session of walking meditation is unique. Take a few moments to reflect on how walking meditation compared to breath meditation for you and jot down your observations.

_____

_____

_____

_____

_____

To some extent, we can influence our experience of walking meditation by varying the technique. For example, it can be interesting to notice the effects produced by different walking speeds. The very slow and deliberate style of walking meditation just described tends to be calming and to enhance concentration. However, when sleepy, or otherwise having trouble mobilizing energy for meditation, you might choose a brisker pace in order to energize the mind. As with slow walking, the instruction for fast walking is to bring your attention to the sensations of the feet making contact with the ground and the legs moving through space. Walking quickly, we usually cannot attend to sensations with quite the same precision, but this approach can still develop concentration and provide an opportunity for mindfulness practice.

Also, because in the course of daily life we normally walk more quickly, brisk walking meditation provides an excellent opportunity for informal practice. You can get into the habit of using ordinary moments of walking during the day as meditation opportunities.

As with most forms of practice, there is no one "right" way to do walking meditation. Rather, it is useful to experiment and note the effects of the different styles, seeing when it seems more useful to practice one way or the other.

Like the breath meditation, both rapid and slow walking meditation can be done with or without silent narration. Should you find it difficult to remain attentive to the sensations of walking when doing the slow practice, you might try saying silently to yourself, "lifting," "moving," and "placing" as you perform each of these movements. Alternatively, you can count footsteps—to 10, 100, or as a counting game. Here again, the idea is to have most of our attention on the sensory experience, allowing the silent words to be a support.

When the mind is very distracted, another way to develop focus is to coordinate the breath with your footsteps. Depending on the pace at which you are walking, this might be done by breathing in slowly when moving one foot and breathing out slowly when moving the other. If you are walking very slowly, you might try inhaling when lifting your foot and exhaling when placing it. If you are walking more rapidly, you might take several steps with each breath. With a little experimentation, you'll come to see which approach seems to work best for you under different circumstances.

Modifying Walking Practice for Different States of Mind

- Use slow walking to calm and concentrate an agitated mind.
- Use brisk walking when sleepy or low in energy and for informal practice.
- Use silent labeling, counting, and playing "catch" with your footsteps to enhance attention.
- Coordinate your breath with your footsteps when particularly distracted.

As you did with the breath meditation, you might want to experiment with different forms of walking practice. You'll need about 30 minutes for this, so if now isn't a good time, please return to it later:

———— Walking Practice Sampler ————

This exercise divides a 30-minute period of walking practice into different segments, each lasting for about five minutes. Here again, if it might help you reflect on the experience, jot down at the end what you noticed about each style of walking meditation.

1. Walk slowly without words.

_____

_____

_____

2. Walk quickly without words.

_____

_____

_____

3. Walk slowly, silently labeling "lifting," "moving," "placing."

_____

_____

_____

4. Walk quickly, silently labeling "lifting," "moving," "placing."

_____

_____

_____

5. Walk slowly, coordinating the breath with your footsteps.

_____

_____

_____

6. Walk quickly, coordinating the breath with your footsteps.

_____

_____

_____

Were some types of walking meditation easier for you than others? Do you imagine that one or another would be better suited to different states of mind?

Bottom to top meditation: the body scan

Another meditation technique, called the *body scan,* can be practiced while sitting but is also often done lying down (this usually works best on a relatively firm surface, so as to help you remain alert rather than fall asleep). Like walking meditation, this technique can be particularly useful when the mind is having difficulty remaining with a subtle object of attention. It serves primarily as a concentration practice since it dictates where we place our attention. You might want to try it first with this book open, and later, once you have a sense of how it works, try it with your eyes closed. You'll probably need about 30 minutes to do this without feeling hurried. Try it now if you have the time.

---

*Body Scan Meditation**

Start with a few minutes of breath meditation—noticing the rising and falling sensations in the belly with each breath. Next bring your attention to the sensations of contact with the chair and the floor if you are sitting, or with the floor, couch, or bed if you are lying down. Allow the breath to be in the background as you notice the complex sensations of your body being supported while gravity gently pulls it downward.

Once you have a sense of your body in space, bring your attention to the toes of one foot. Notice all the sensations coming from these toes. Observe whether they seem warm or cold, relaxed or tense. See if you can notice how the sensations coming from your toes are not solid, but rather are made up of a series of momentary micro-sensations strung together over time. Try to bring an attitude of interest or curiosity to these sensations, observing how they subtly change from moment to moment. Should you notice at some point that your mind has wandered into thoughts or been drawn to

---

*Available in audio at *www.mindfulness-solution.com.*

other sensations, gently bring it back to the sensations in your toes. Allow your attention to remain with your toes for several breaths, or until you feel as though you've attended to them fully.

Next direct your attention to the top of the same foot. Feel all the sensations occurring there. Notice which are pleasant and which are unpleasant. Again, notice whether the area is warm or cold, relaxed or tense. If at some point you notice that your mind has wandered away, gently bring it back to the sensations at the top of your foot. Try to stay with these for several breaths or until you've attended to them fully.

When you are ready to move on, bring your attention to the sensations arising in the bottom of your foot. Stay with the sensations arising in this area for several breaths, exploring them as you did the others.

The meditation proceeds in this manner. The order in which you scan body regions isn't crucial, though it's easiest to sustain attention if you do this systematically, moving progressively from one end of the body to the other (people usually start at the feet to be as far as possible from where thoughts arise). So after the foot, you might bring your attention to your ankle, calf, shin, knee, thigh, and groin of the same leg. This can be followed by a slow, systematic survey of the other foot and leg, beginning again at the toes. After this you can move on to your belly, chest, and neck, followed by your buttocks, and lower, mid, and upper back. The arms can be explored much like the legs, beginning with the fingers of one hand, moving on to the palms and back of the hand, and then to the wrist, forearm, upper arm, and shoulder. This can then be repeated on the other hand and arm. Finally, bring your attention to the front and back of the neck, the chin, mouth, cheeks, nose, and eyes, and then the forehead, ears, and finally the top and back of the head.

You may find that you can give more detailed attention to areas of the body that are rich in sensory nerves, such as the face. While you may take in the entire middle back or abdomen as one area, the lips, nose, eyes, and cheeks can each be explored separately. Throughout this exercise, try to cultivate an attitude of curiosity, interest, and investigation toward all the sensations coming into your awareness. Also practice accepting whatever you discover, whether it's a pleasant sensation or an unpleasant one. As in other forms of meditation, whenever you notice that the mind has wandered away from the particular area you're exploring, gently bring it back—like training a puppy.

WHAT DID YOU DISCOVER?

After trying the body scan, take a few moments to reflect on the experience. How did it compare with the breath and walking meditations? Jot down your observations.

_____

_____

_____

_____

If you're familiar with Edmund Jacobson's *progressive relaxation*, you may notice parallels with the body scan. Unlike progressive relaxation, however, this meditation practice doesn't involve tensing and relaxing muscles, and it is not designed specifically to promote relaxation. Instead, like the other practices described here, it's a concentration exercise that can be used as a first stage of mindfulness practice. By shifting the object of attention to different body parts, the mind tends to remain more interested, and may therefore be less distracted, than during single-focus techniques such as breath or walking meditation. Also, by exploring the entire body, there is a tendency to become less lost in thought and more aware of physical sensations in the here and now.

Getting more for less: eating meditation

How would you like to enjoy eating more while taking in fewer calories? Sound like a good deal? All it takes is some discipline and a shift in approach.

Eating meditation is a particularly engrossing form of concentration practice that has enormous potential for helping us eat healthfully. It also vividly illustrates the power of concentration for making our life richer and more rewarding. We're often "absent" during meals, lost in thoughts about the past and future (including past and future meals), rather than attentive to the moment-to-moment sensations of eating. This meditation both illustrates how busy the mind is normally when we eat and gives us the opportunity to actually taste and savor our food. Like walking meditation, it also converts very nicely from a formal to an informal meditation practice.

The first few times that you try this meditation, it's best to start with a small, simple bit of food. Meditation teachers often choose a raisin, since they are easy to find and yield interesting surprises that reinforce our motivation to eat with awareness. While this exercise is usually done with eyes closed, since these instructions are written, you can try it first with your eyes open so that you can follow them. You'll need one raisin and about 20 minutes of uninterrupted time.

Raisin Meditation*

Begin practicing with 10 minutes of breath meditation. After this, open your eyes and pick up the raisin. All of the following instructions should be followed very slowly—try to resist the urge to rush.

Hold the raisin in your hand and carefully examine it with your eyes. Notice its texture, color, and patterns. See where it is shiny and where it is dull. Notice too any thoughts or feelings that arise as you hold it.

Next, use your thumb and forefinger to explore the raisin's texture (you might wish to close your eyes for this to better concentrate on the touch sensations). Observe its hills and valleys, whether it is soft or hard, smooth or rough.

Once you've explored it thoroughly in your hand, remaining aware of the sensations of your arm moving through space, lift the raisin to your ear. Hold it just outside of your ear canal and roll it between your thumb and forefinger, exerting a little bit of pressure

---

*Available in audio at *www.mindfulness-solution.com*.

(resist any urge that may arise to insert the raisin). See if you can hear the faint sound a raisin makes as you manipulate it.

After listening to the raisin for a few moments, slowly and consciously bring it beneath your nostrils. Breathe in and see if you can detect any raisin aroma. Also notice your feelings in reaction to whatever you smell—do you find it pleasant, unpleasant, or neutral? Inhale deeply several times to really take in the smell of the raisin.

Now for the really exciting part. Bring the raisin in front of your lips and allow your tongue to reach out and capture it (as only your tongue knows how to do). Just let the raisin lie between your tongue and the roof of your mouth for a while. Notice any reactions that your mouth has. Notice again any feeling responses that arise. Continue to cradle the raisin like this for a minute or two.

Next begin to use your tongue to explore the raisin. See how these sensations are similar to or different from those you experienced when exploring it with your thumb and forefinger. Notice too how the raisin changes as it spends time in your mouth.

Once you feel that you've thoroughly explored the raisin with your tongue (this will require a couple of minutes), gently position it between your upper and lower molars. Just hold it there for a bit and see what that feels like. Notice any urges to bite down, or perhaps even to protect the raisin.

Now, allow your molars to come together once—but only once. Observe what happens. Notice whatever taste sensations, urges, and feelings arise. Just stay with the experience of the raisin crushed between your teeth as your mouth and mind react to it.

Next use your tongue to capture the raisin again and explore your handiwork. See all of the ways in which it has changed and notice how it continues to change as you explore it further. Once the raisin has fallen apart, allow yourself to continue chewing, noticing all the different sensations and urges that arise. Observe the swallow reflex and how the sensations in your mouth continue to change. Wish the raisin well as it continues its journey down your alimentary canal.

WHAT DID YOU DISCOVER?

A first session of eating meditation, particularly if done very slowly, usually brings up all sorts of reactions. Take a moment to jot down what you noticed.

_____

_____

_____

Now see how your responses compare with some of the common ones that people have when they try this for the first time.

Where did you get those raisins?

Many times this exercise marks the first time we really taste a raisin. The flavor can be remarkably intense. Children led through this exercise often ask, "Where did you get those raisins?" Of course, it's not the raisins that are unusual, but our level of attention. We begin to see how much of life we miss by being distracted.

A single raisin is actually satisfying.

We don't usually think of a single raisin as a gourmet experience. But eaten mindfully, it can be. It's not that the raisin fills our belly, but it can still be very _ful_filling. The implication for eating problems is obvious. If we're able to experience the richness of a single raisin, we might be content with an appropriately sized meal and less driven to eat more than is good for us. This also raises the possibility that other small things in our life could be much more rewarding were we to really pay attention to them. We'll explore this further in Chapter 9 when we discuss using mindfulness to work with troublesome habits.

I didn't want to hurt the raisin.

Sometimes people feel that they've developed a relationship of sorts with the raisin by looking at it, listening to it, touching it, and exploring it with their tongue. We can feel almost cruel chewing it. This experience reminds me of the way Native Americans historically honored their food before eating it—thanking an animal for giving up its life. While a raisin probably doesn't have the same emotional reactions as a buffalo, we can develop a similar feeling of respect and appreciation by attending closely to the experience of eating it.

I wanted to chew it already.

Usually when we eat, we're only partially aware of the taste of our food. While chewing one bite, we're already gathering another on our fork or spoon. It can be difficult to slow this process down, because when we do we feel our impatience. Like all mindfulness exercises, eating meditation is designed to illuminate how the mind works. Here we get to see our propensity to topple forward psychologically—how we neglect the experience of the present moment as we rush forward in pursuit of the next one.

I wanted more.

While a single raisin can be gratifying, the enjoyment of eating it can trigger urges to have more. These impulses can be powerful, making it difficult to stay with the experience of eating *this* raisin. Observing them helps us see how the mind endlessly seeks to repeat pleasurable experiences. Mindfulness meditation not only illuminates this but, as we will see, also gives us the freedom to decide whether or not to act on these urges.

Mindfully eating a meal

While it's usually not practical to eat an entire meal with the care and attention we just put into eating a single raisin, it is possible to eat much more mindfully than usual. Most people find mindfully eating a meal quite rewarding.

Choose a meal during which you won't be rushed, when you can either eat alone or with others who wish to practice eating meditation. Pick a time and setting where you'll have at least a half hour without interruption. The procedure is simple. If you're with others, agree to eat in silence and not make eye contact. If you're alone, don't turn on the TV, radio, or iPod; don't talk on the phone or read. The goal will be to attend as fully as possible to your food. When you serve yourself a portion, be aware that you may feel full sooner when eating mindfully than you normally would, so don't take too much.

Eating Meditation

Start by becoming aware of sitting. Close your eyes for a few moments and notice your breath. Feel your body making contact with the chair, your feet with the floor. Settle into being present.

Next look at your food. Notice its texture, color, and position on the plate. Try to take it in as a work of art. Think for a moment about how it got there. Who planted the crops or raised the animals, cared for them, and brought them to you? Take note of the effort that went into producing this food and the remarkable natural processes that enabled it to happen.

Once you've studied it carefully, and considered its origins, take a first bite. It usually helps to put down your fork or spoon before you start to chew. Throughout the meal, try to do one thing at a time: looking at the food, lifting it up, placing it in your mouth, and chewing. When you lift the food to your mouth, let the lifting motion be the object of your attention. When you chew, let this be your focus. As with other meditations, your mind will likely wander. Whenever you notice that you've lost touch with what is happening at present, gently return your attention to what you are doing. Let yourself eat only as much as you need to feel full and then stop.

WHAT DID YOU DISCOVER?

Eating an entire meal as meditation practice usually brings up a variety of reactions. Take a moment now to jot down what you noticed.

_____

_____

Eating this way, most people find it takes longer to eat, flavors are more vivid, and they feel full sooner. While the practice can feel strange at first, it can also be very appealing. Many of us struggle with what and how much to eat—trying to balance our desires against our best judgment. You will likely find that eating mindfully helps resolve this tension.

Since eating is something we need to do in daily life, eating meditation can be either a formal or an informal practice, depending on how much time we allot to it and whether or not we are also being social. When eating alone, we can choose to eliminate the usual distractions and actually pay attention to our food. If we have enough time, we can do this very slowly, as in the formal practice just described. Of course, most of us will have the opportunity to do this only occasionally.

When we have less time, we can still try to pay attention—we may just wind up chewing and swallowing more quickly. Eating alone can become a regular opportunity for this sort of informal practice. When we're eating socially with others, our attention will naturally be divided, but we can still remind ourselves to attend to the taste of our food, put down our fork or spoon while chewing, and notice when we've had enough.

At least occasionally, try making a meal into a formal eating meditation session. It usually takes about half an hour to eat a simple meal in this way. Doing this not only sheds light on the experience of eating but also tends to rub off on our other mealtimes, helping us be more attentive during them as well.

Now that you've had a taste of several concentration practices, the next step is to see how they can be used to cultivate mindfulness further. In Chapter 4 we'll explore this process and see how you can weave together formal and informal practices to create a routine that fits your particular life.

CHAPTER 4

Building a mindful life

As we discussed in the last chapter, concentration focuses the mind, while mindfulness turns our attention to whatever is most prominent in our awareness. Concentration practices are useful for calming an agitated mind, developing mental stability, noticing the richness of life, and increasing awareness of what is happening in the mind at each moment. Mindfulness practice holds the promise of helping us see how the mind works—in particular how it creates suffering and how that suffering can be alleviated. A certain degree of concentration is necessary to practice mindfulness; without it we can't clearly observe the workings of the mind and get lost in our thoughts about what's happening rather than experiencing it directly. Because concentration is the foundation for mindfulness practice, the exercises so far have all been presented largely as concentration practices.

From concentration to mindfulness

Most concentration practices can, however, also be done as mindfulness practices. Once you find that your mind has settled during concentration meditation, you can try shifting to mindfulness practice itself. Initially, as mentioned in Chapter 3, this involves noticing where the mind has gone when it leaves an object of attention and silently labeling these departures. For example, if during breath meditation you find your mind formulating plans, you can note to yourself "planning" and then return your attention to the breath. Should you find judgmental thoughts arising, you can note to yourself "judging." If your mind wanders off to other sensations, such as a sound in the room, you can note "hearing." These notes, uttered silently, are made in the background while your attention remains primarily with the breath.

Should the mind become particularly calm, you can then try letting go of the breath entirely as an anchor and allow your attention to go to whatever objects are uppermost in awareness—whether these are sounds, sensations of contact as you sit, emotions as they manifest in the body, or other experiences. This is sometimes referred to as *choiceless awareness*, because we allow the mind to be open to whatever enters our consciousness. The mind is allowed to wander, but unlike during periods of mindlessness, we remain alert to what is in our awareness at each moment. It is even possible to allow thoughts and images to be objects of our attention, but since most of us quickly get lost in these, this is usually practical only during intensive retreat practice.

Finding an optimal balance between concentration practice, in which we return repeatedly to a preselected object of attention, and mindfulness practice, in which we allow the mind to focus on different objects as they rise to prominence, is an art. Usually you can let the strength of your concentration be your guide. When concentration is strong, you might experiment more with mindfulness. When it is weaker and your attention is more scattered, you can return more to concentration practice.

As you develop a formal practice routine, you will likely vary which types of meditation to favor. Sometimes you will emphasize sitting meditation, while other times you will mix in the body scan, walking, or eating practices—depending on what you've discovered about the effects of each of these for you. Regardless of the type you choose, you will also vary when you do each one as a concentration or mindfulness practice. It's difficult to suggest a set pattern because each person's mind and life are unique. Nonetheless, here are a few rough guidelines.

If you can dedicate only 20 minutes at a time on a less than daily basis to formal practice, you will probably favor concentration practice because your mind won't have sufficient time to settle down. If you can practice for longer periods more frequently, you may have more opportunities to include mindfulness practice because you'll notice more sessions in which the mind becomes focused.

Even with greater intensity of practice, you might stick to concentration for days or weeks at a time when your mind is busy or agitated. During other periods, however, you might begin each meditation session with concentration practice, but once the mind settles a bit, open your field of awareness to practice mindfulness—noticing where the mind goes or allowing your attention to rest on different mental objects.

The key to making these choices is using a light touch. One form of practice isn't "better" than another. Ultimately both practices help us see how our mind works and how we inadvertently create suffering for ourselves and others. There is also considerable overlap between concentration and mindfulness practices—when doing concentration practice we can notice where the mind goes when we lose focus, and when doing mindfulness practice we still concentrate on the object at hand. It's best not to worry too much about getting a perfect balance; over time you will intuitively sense which practice to emphasize when.

Cultivating acceptance

The formal meditation practices discussed so far all involve directing attention to particular bodily sensations and observing the contents of the mind without trying to change those contents. They are oriented toward cultivating *awareness of present experience with acceptance*. Often the *acceptance* part of these practices is the most challenging. Our minds can be relentlessly judgmental—condemning us for not concentrating well, thinking too much, or feeling something we shouldn't. An amusing way to see this at work is by doing a few minutes of "judgment" meditation:

Judgment Meditation

This one usually requires only 10–15 minutes to get the point. Sit down as you would for breath meditation and follow your breath for a minute or two. Then begin to watch your thoughts. Every time a judgment arises, silently label it "judging."

WHAT DID YOU DISCOVER?

Jot down your observations.

_____

_____

_____

_____

Many people notice an inner stream that goes something like this: "Hmm, I'm doing pretty well. No judgments yet. *Judging.* Uh-oh. I should've known that I wouldn't be so good at this. *Judging.* Okay, okay, I get it. None of that. I'll just follow my breath. Rising, falling, rising, falling. There, that's better. *Judging.* Damn, I sure am relentlessly judgmental. *Judging.*"

An ancient approach to working with our harsh or judgmental tendencies is loving-kindness meditation. It can take many forms, all designed to soften our hearts and help us be more accepting of ourselves and others, to develop what has been called "affectionate awareness." Ancient meditation texts describe compassion and mindfulness as two wings of a bird—emphasizing that we need an open heart to have open eyes. Loving-kindness meditation supports clear seeing by strengthening the *intention* to be accepting and compassionate—it does not paper over our real feelings of the moment with false positive sentiments. As with all mindfulness practices, the overarching guideline is to observe and accept whatever is actually happening in the moment.

The simplest loving-kindness meditation technique involves generating feelings of compassion by silently repeating evocative phrases. This usually works best if we begin with a period of concentration meditation, perhaps attending to our breath or doing some slow walking practice. Once the mind settles a little, we begin trying to generate acceptance and compassion. Sometimes this works best if we begin by focusing on ourselves; sometimes it works better when we begin with others. The exact phrases we use are not important—you can experiment with whatever words fit your cultural background and individual preferences.

To get a feel for this meditation, it's best to do it for at least 10 minutes. If you have the time now, begin with a period of concentration practice, then read these instructions and give them a try.

—————————Loving-Kindness Meditation* —————————

Begin by repeating silently to yourself, "May I be happy, may I be peaceful, may I be free from suffering." Simply repeat this phrase, wishing or intending this for yourself. Should you find that your mind is particularly "stuck" in a problematic pattern, you can address that directly. For example, you might change the phrases

*Available in audio at *www.mindfulness-solution.com.*

to "May I be happy, may I be peaceful … ," "may I learn to let go," "may I accept whatever comes," "may I have the courage to face my fears," or "may I be forgiving."

As with the other techniques, you'll probably find after a while that your mind wanders, and you need to repeatedly return your attention to the phrases (remarkably, the mind seems able to "say" these phrases silently even when we're not paying attention to the process). Here, too, the idea is to be forgiving about this and treat it all like puppy training.

Once you've had a chance to settle into one of these phrases and you've directed compassionate intentions toward yourself, you can try moving on to others (the meditation can also be done in the reverse order, starting with another person and then moving to yourself). It's usually easiest to begin with a benefactor—someone toward whom you easily feel loving and caring. This might be a friend, family member, or other loved one; or a teacher or other inspirational figure, living or not, such as Jesus, the Buddha, or the Dalai Lama. Close your eyes, imagine the other person is with you, and feel that person's presence. Then begin repeating, "May you be happy, may you be peaceful, may you be free from suffering," or similar phrases. Again the mind is likely to wander, and you'll repeatedly need to gently bring it back to your chosen image.

Once you've focused on a person who inspires feelings of loving-kindness for a while, you can shift your attention to someone else who is important to you. One by one, call to mind people who matter. Eventually, you can expand to conjure up images of small groups, such as immediate family members or close friends. Holding them in mind, continue to repeat the phrases, directing compassionate wishes toward them. The meditation continues in this fashion, expanding outward to encompass more and more people. Should you find that the feelings of compassion or loving-kindness seem to dry up, return to images of people who more readily inspire them.

Expanding the circle, you might move on to imagine all of your family and friends together and then your coworkers, clients, neighbors, or any other group of which you are a part. Eventually, we send the same good intentions to wider and wider communities, until we are encompassing our town, city, country, and eventually everyone on the planet. This exercise can even be expanded to encompass all living things. In one classic version, it eventually settles on the phrases "May all beings be happy, may all beings be peaceful, may all beings be free of suffering."

WHAT DID YOU DISCOVER?

Loving-kindness meditation brings up very different experiences for each of us. As with other practices, you will likely have varied experiences each time you try it. Take a couple of minutes now to jot down what you noticed during each phase of the exercise, as though you were telling a friend about the experience.

Loving-kindness meditation can support both concentration and mindfulness meditation. When doing concentration practice, it's all too easy to become harshly critical of our wandering mind. Loving-kindness meditation helps strengthen our ability to be kind to ourselves when our mind strays. Similarly, when practicing mindfulness meditation and observing all the noble and not-so-noble contents that arise in awareness, loving-kindness meditation helps us greet them all as welcome visitors. Loving-kindness meditation can be integrated into a session of concentration and/or mindfulness meditation, or an entire session can be dedicated to loving-kindness meditation itself.

Paradoxical Responses

Most of us are ambivalent about many things. Sometimes we're aware of our mixed feelings; sometimes we notice them only when we finally get something that we thought we wanted. Almost all of us have had the experience of pursuing someone who seems wonderfully desirable until he or she shows interest in us—and then suddenly we become uncertain of our feelings. We see this also when others are pushing us to think, feel, or behave in a certain way. Sometimes in response to pressure we feel compelled to do the opposite.

There is a story about Milton Erickson, a psychiatrist known for unconventional therapeutic techniques. He was on a horse farm. Someone was struggling to get a horse into a barn, but the harder the horse was pulled, the more he resisted. Erickson came up with a novel approach: *pull the tail*. The horse bolted right into his stall.

Given this aspect of human (and animal) nature, you may find when you try loving-kindness exercises that unloving, unkind feelings arise. You may notice judgmental thoughts toward yourself or others. They're all okay. The purpose of these exercises isn't just to generate compassionate feeling so as to be more tolerant of ourselves and others. Like mindfulness practices, they're also designed to help illuminate how the mind operates—and to help us cultivate *awareness of current experience with acceptance*. So if you become aware of the inner Scrooge, Darth Vader, or other not-so-loving part of your personality, the idea is to say "yes" to this. Loving-kindness practices can help you be aware and accepting of these feelings as well.

This is getting complicated—how do I choose what to do?

Let's look at the different forms of meditation practice we've been discussing. Concentration practices, which choose an object of awareness and return to it repeatedly, help to focus and stabilize the mind, allowing us to become less caught in the stories that occupy so much of our consciousness. Mindfulness practice requires some concentration but then opens to whatever arises in our awareness and follows that closely. By doing this, mindfulness helps us gain insight into how our minds work, see how we generate distress, and find paths to well-being. Loving-kindness meditation cultivates the intention to be kind to ourselves and others; it therefore helps us develop an accepting attitude toward what-ever happens when practicing concentration or mindfulness meditation. As we'll see later, loving-kindness meditation can also be very useful in interpersonal relationships.

As already mentioned, figuring out which form of meditation to favor at a given moment is something of an art. When the mind is particu-larly scattered, concentration is called for. When it's judgmental, loving-kindness comes in handy. When we already have some concentration going and can be reasonably accepting of what arises, mindfulness prac-tice allows us to be open to all of our experience. Some people do a mix-ture of practices each time they set aside time to meditate:

Kate had been meditating daily for the past couple of weeks, mostly doing concentration practice centered on her breath. She found that she was generally feeling calmer and more focused at work and was having more moments of feeling present and noticing her environment. Some-times, when she sat for 45 minutes, her mind became pretty quiet and she would shift to mindfulness practice. Keeping her breath in the back-ground, she allowed her attention to rest on different body sensations that seemed to be connected to emotions. One day she noticed a tightness in her chest that felt related to guilt. Self-critical thoughts arose about hav-ing let her parents down. After feeling these for a while, she began doing loving-kindness meditation toward herself and her parents. The tightness softened and transformed into sadness. She sat with the sadness for a while and began to feel a sense of peace. Kate then went back to noticing her breath and the sounds around her.

Others focus predominantly on one or another technique for a period of time:

Jonathan had been practicing meditation for a couple of years. He was a young man with a lot of free time and had been quite disciplined about developing concentration. He really enjoyed the feelings of peace that he got from being in the present moment and not paying much atten-tion to thoughts or feelings. He spent considerable time in nature enjoy-ing its ever-changing beauty.

Yet he was lonely. Now and again longings for a girlfriend would surface. He began to realize that he was being hyperdisciplined about his concentration practice in part to block these out. When he discussed this with a meditation teacher, she suggested that he shift his practice more to mindfulness and loving-kindness. Though it was difficult, he turned his attention toward the feelings that arose in his body when he medi-tated. He noticed that he had a lot of longings to feel loved but was afraid of these—they seemed very deep and painful. To make it easier to face them, he began alternating loving-kindness meditations with his mindfulness practice. This gave him a sense that he would be okay even if he were to stay with the lonely feelings for a while.

Safety versus Uncovering

While the ultimate goal of mindfulness practices is to become comfortable with all of our experience, it can be unwise to try to do this all at once. Since the earliest days of psychotherapy, therapists have realized that different people need to work at different paces. Just as our capacity to bear experience varies from day to day, it also varies during different periods in our lives. During times when we have more supports and fewer threats, our capacity to be with difficult experiences is greater. During times when supports are lacking and we face a lot of problems, our capacity is diminished.

The capacity to bear difficult experience also varies from person to person. Some of this is genetic. Certain people are born with nervous systems that are more intensely reactive to change or threats, while others are born with systems that are less reactive. Some of our capacity to bear difficulty relates to our upbringing—people who are fortunate to have had loving, emotionally attuned caregivers tend to have an easier time handling adversity than those who didn't. Human development is very complex, however, so sometimes having it too good—not being exposed to enough adversity—can actually make a person more vulnerable to being overwhelmed. He or she becomes like a plant raised in a greenhouse that can't handle a more rough-and-tumble natural environment.

Regardless of the factors that make us more or less able to handle difficult experiences, it's important when taking up mindfulness practice to be aware of your capacities and limits. Some practices, such as sitting with the breath for long periods or participating in a silent meditation retreat, tend to bring up difficult thoughts and feelings. Freud discovered that if he simply asked a patient to lie on a couch and say whatever came to mind, eventually all sorts of unwanted thoughts and feelings would emerge. Similarly, sitting in silent meditation for long periods will sooner or later bring up all sorts of pleasant and unpleasant thoughts and feelings. Some of these will inevitably be difficult to handle.

If you can tolerate these difficult mental contents without feeling totally flooded, it will be a useful, freeing practice. However, if they make you feel very overwhelmed, the experience may make you more frightened of your own mind, and hence be counterproductive.

As in psychotherapy, it is important to think about pacing in mindfulness practice. During periods in which we find ourselves readily over-whelmed, more stabilizing practices may be most helpful. These include practices with an "outer" focus, such as walking or eating meditation. Loving-kindness practices can also add to feelings of safety, by generating compassionate feelings toward ourselves and others. They can make us feel "held" the way a parent holds a child who is in distress. In later chapters we'll discuss other techniques, such as nature meditation and mountain meditation, which also add to our sense of safety and our capacity to handle difficulties.

During periods when we're not so readily overwhelmed, we can use practices that help us move toward difficult experiences. Sitting meditation that begins with a focus on the breath and then opens into mindfulness of all mental contents tends to do this. Later we'll discuss practices that involve intentionally moving toward fear, sadness, or pain so as to increase our capacity to bear these experiences, ultimately leading to more flexibility and ease. This approach is sometimes called *moving toward the sharp points*—focusing our attention on whatever is unwelcome in the mind.

Everyone is different, and each of us will find some practices to be more useful at one time than another. With some experimentation, you'll get a feel for which is most useful for you at different moments. Keeping in mind the overall goal of becoming *aware of our current experience with acceptance* will help you find the right balance among them.

Informal mindfulness practice

Informal mindfulness practice involves doing your daily routines a little differently to become more mindful. It's like taking the stairs instead of the elevator to become more physically fit. This can begin as soon as you awaken. You can take a few moments to notice your breath, how your body feels lying in bed, the appearance of the room, the temperature of the air, and the sounds around you. Like most mindfulness exercises, this is easiest to do without multitasking—so it will work best if you awaken to a simple alarm rather than starting the day with radio news.

The rest of the morning routine can be done as a form of meditation practice. When brushing your teeth, pay attention to the physical motions involved and the taste of the toothpaste. When you shower, try to focus on the intense sensual experience of thousands of droplets striking your naked body and the feeling of rubbing slippery soap all over. When you dry yourself, try to actually feel the towel. Getting dressed, notice the colors and textures of your clothes and the feeling of putting them on.

Of course, some degree of thought is also necessary when you get ready in the morning. You may have to check the weather and your schedule to decide what to wear; you may have to figure out what you need to take along. During these "thinking tasks," simply be aware that you're thinking. But once you've made your decisions, gently try to bring your attention back to the moment-to-moment sensory experience of getting ready.

You can continue practicing mindfulness when you leave the house. Walking to the car, the bus stop, or other destination, pay attention to the sensations of your feet touching the ground and your legs moving through space. This becomes an opportunity to practice walking meditation, albeit at a normal pace. Pay attention to the weather, the sounds and smells, and everything in your visual field as you head off to work, school, or the market. You can train yourself to wake up and "smell the roses" at each moment.

Ordinary meals become an opportunity for eating meditation. While you'll need to eat most meals more quickly than you ate the raisin, you can nonetheless try to actually taste your food and notice when you are full. While this is easier to do if eating alone quietly, even when enjoying a social meal you can try to periodically turn your attention to the taste of your food.

It's actually possible to maintain this sort of intention to be present throughout the day. Specific moments that were mentioned in the last chapter such as listening to the sound of the telephone or attending to the color of vehicle taillights can become reminders to pay attention. Of course, activities that you need to do quickly or that involve a lot of thought or words are more difficult to do mindfully. Nonetheless, by doing informal mindfulness practice throughout the day you can develop a continuity of awareness of where your attention is and how your mind is responding to your circumstances.

This is a wonderful antidote to boredom. Instead of fantasizing about the next moment of entertainment, you can turn your attention to the sights and sounds of standing in line, buying a cup of coffee, and walking down the street. Instead of getting frustrated because the train is late, you can study the other passengers (discreetly), notice the architecture of the station, and attend to the sensations in your body as you sit and wait. There is always something interesting to do—just pay attention to what is occurring *right now*.

As you go through the day this way, you'll become aware of which activities are more conducive to mind*ful*ness and which reinforce mind-*less*ness. The idea is not necessarily to live like a nun or monk, but rather to become increasingly aware of where your attention is at each moment, even when you're having a wild time.

Informal mindfulness practice can continue until bedtime, which becomes an opportunity for a bit of formal practice. When lying down preparing to sleep, return your attention to the sensations of the breath. One of two things will happen: either you'll get to have eight hours of uninterrupted mindfulness practice, or you'll get a good night's sleep. We'll talk more about mindfulness practice and sleep in Chapter 7.

AN INFORMAL MINDFULNESS PRACTICE PLAN

While you can hold the intention to be aware of present experience with acceptance throughout the day, it's usually helpful to identify regular life activities that lend themselves to informal practice and commit to trying to do them mindfully each day. A number of possibilities have already been mentioned: showering, commuting to work, eating breakfast or lunch, doing the dishes, walking up or down stairs, brushing your teeth, having a cup of tea.

Take a few moments now to think of your typical day. Pick a few routine activities that you'd like to use as deliberate practice periods and write them down. Make this a little contract with yourself.

1. _____

2. _____

3. _____

Conducting a mini-retreat

An excellent way to see the power of all of the practices we've been discussing is to string them together into a "mini-retreat." This means setting aside a longer period, perhaps a few hours or an entire day, during which to develop continuity of practice. While this won't be practical for everyone, if you can afford the time, it can be a moving experience. With more time the mind often settles down, making it easier to experiment with balancing concentration, mindfulness, and loving-kindness practices and to see how they all naturally support informal practice.

A typical rhythm involves doing *Breath Awareness Meditation* for 20–45 minutes, followed by *Walking Meditation* for 15–30 minutes, and then returning to breath practice. You can intersperse *Loving-Kindness Meditation* as you see fit. If your "mini-retreat" spans a meal, it's a good idea to include silent *Eating Meditation*. As you move from activity to activity, try to make all the transitions opportunities to pay attention to your moment-to-moment experience. When we string practices together in this way, the mind tends to develop more concentration than it can when meditating for a briefer period. We become able to watch the mind and body more clearly, and there is a greater likelihood that the mind will settle sufficiently to allow for mindfulness meditation in addition to concentration practices.

We discussed in the last chapter how intensive retreat practice can be a powerful way to both support our meditation practice and gain insight into the workings of our minds. As an alternative, or in addition to setting up your own mini-retreat, you may find it very useful to participate in a structured group retreat led by an experienced leader. The Resources at the back of the book include tips on how to find a retreat opportunity suited to your particular needs.

Life preservers

Sometimes we start to lose it in the thick of a crisis. Often this involves other people: your child is tantruming in the middle of a crowded supermarket; your spouse is bringing up an issue *yet again* that you thought you had finished hashing out yesterday. Or it can center on an emotion: your heart is pounding, and you can't think straight before giving a talk; you're mentally saying good-bye to your family and friends as your plane bounces about trying to land in a thunderstorm. We can also get overwhelmed by physical sensations: desperately needing a bathroom when there's none to be found; having to go back to work despite terrible back pain. And we can be overcome by cravings: compulsively buying yet another candy bar; pouring another drink even after we've definitely had enough.

While establishing a mindfulness practice that balances formal and informal practices will increase our chances of handling these situations better, we will still sometimes feel overwhelmed. This is where mindfulness-based *life preservers* come in handy. Psychotherapists and meditation teachers have adapted ancient practices so they can be used to take refuge in the present moment during these times. They help us ride intense waves of emotion or sensation in the midst of a crisis without compulsively acting on them. These practices almost all involve bringing our attention back to what is happening right now, noticing what is going on in the body, and trying to welcome, rather than resist, the experience. While any formal or informal practice can be used as a life preserver, you'll learn particular exercises suited to different problem situations in the upcoming chapters.

Putting it all together: living life mindfully

There are many ways to put together a mindfulness practice. Informal practice opportunities present themselves regularly. While the idea is to develop a continuity of mindfulness throughout the day, it can be useful to select a few routine activities to emphasize as informal practice periods.

If you choose to do 20-minute sessions of formal practice, it's probably best to stick with one type of meditation each time so as to develop some momentum with it. If, on the other hand, you can dedicate 45 minutes at a time to formal practice, you can either spend each session doing one type or split the time between a couple of different practices (for example, 30 minutes of *Breath Awareness Meditation,* followed by 15 minutes of *Loving-Kindness Meditation* or *Walking Meditation*). Most people adjust their routine depending on how calm or busy, how critical or accepting, and how alert or sleepy their mind is during a given session. Some people choose to focus periodically on loving-kindness practice exclusively for some sessions to cultivate compassion and acceptance, while others add it to the beginning or end of a session focused on other practices. Many people favor *Walking Meditation* when feeling sleepy.

Each form of practice supports the others. Informal practice enhances our concentration and reinforces the habit of paying attention to the present moment, making it easier to do formal practice. By more intensively training the mind, formal practice makes it easier to be mindful during the rest of the day. Meditation retreats (mini or otherwise) can provide a dramatic boost to both of these daily practices. Life preservers that help us through crises both support and build on our practice at calmer times.

Like most valuable things in life, living more mindfully requires some intention and effort. This, too, is like tuning a lute—you'll need to experiment to find a practice pattern that works best for you. If you set a goal that is too ambitious for your situation and can't stick to it, you may feel like a failure and wind up giving up the whole project. If you set a goal that is too light, you may not notice the fruits of the practice and lose interest as a result. While your practice pattern will undoubtedly be different, here's how one woman put hers together:

Jennifer dabbled a bit in yoga and meditation when she was in college but didn't establish a regular practice until she was in her late 20s. She had just ended a tumultuous long-term relationship, was stressed at work, and felt a need to find herself. After taking a class at a local meditation center, she dove in with a regular 45-minute-per-day practice. She started with *Breath Awareness Meditation*. It wasn't easy. Initially her mind was often agitated and she could barely find her breath. She would try to focus on the rising and falling sensations in her belly, but her attention was repeatedly hijacked into memories of both the good times and arguments with her ex-boyfriend. She found it helped somewhat to silently label these "obsessing." Some days she could barely sit still, so she'd do *Walking Meditation* for the first 15 minutes and then work with her breath. Easing into sitting this way was easier.

Not infrequently, Jennifer was so stressed that she turned on the TV instead of meditating. Initially this felt like a relief. But she tended to eat junk food while watching, and when she turned the set off she felt worse—like she had wasted her time *and* mistreated her body. As Jennifer continued trying to practice, she noticed more and more that the things she did to soothe herself—watching TV, eating comfort foods, shopping, surfing the Internet—didn't work so well in the long run.

For informal practice, Jennifer focused on her morning shower, drive to work, and dog walking. She tried to stay with the sensations of the soap and water droplets in the shower, focused on the road and kept the radio and cell phone off during her commute, and practiced brisk walking meditation when she was out with her dog. She enjoyed noticing the weather and seasons in a new way.

When she was lonely, Jennifer's mind filled with self-critical thoughts. If she wasn't seeing friends or going out on a date on a weekend night, she'd start to feel like a loser. She'd become desperate about finding a new relationship and spent lots of energy reviewing her inadequacies. At these times, she found *Loving-Kindness Meditation* particularly helpful, as it allowed her to believe a bit less in these thoughts and focus more on the present.

One weekend Jennifer participated in what her meditation center called an "urban retreat." During the days she did sitting, walking, and eating meditation, while at night she returned home. She found that her mind became relatively quiet and she was able to shift from just trying to follow her breath to a more open, mindful awareness. She could stay with sounds, emotions, and body sensations when they became prominent without getting entirely caught up in thoughts. This helped her understand better how to balance concentration and mindfulness in her daily sittings.

As her practice progressed, Jennifer noticed that she was becoming drawn to activities that made it easier to be present. She spent more time going for walks, sitting at the beach, and soaking in the tub. She became less tempted by distraction and entertainment, and more interested in activities that supported being mindful. Her urgency to find a new relationship relaxed as she increasingly enjoyed being with herself. She sensed that when the time was right this was going to make it easier to be in a relationship.

Foundational practices

These are the basic practices that you can weave together into a personal practice plan:

Formal Meditation Practices

- *Breath Awareness Meditation* (page 55) to develop concentration and mindfulness using relatively subtle objects of awareness
- *Body Scan Meditation* (page 72) to develop concentration and mindfulness using varied objects of attention—especially helpful when the mind is agitated
- *Raisin Meditation* (page 75) to prepare for formal and informal eating meditations
- *Eating Meditation* (page 79) to develop concentration and mindfulness using an everyday life activity—and to appreciate our food
- *Walking Meditation* (page 67) to develop concentration and mind-

fulness when the mind is more restless, it's difficult to sit still, or the body is stiff

- *Loving-Kindness Meditation* (page 84) when the mind is filled with judgments or self-critical thoughts

Informal Practices

- *Walking Meditation* (page 67)
- *Eating Meditation* (page 263)
- *Driving, Showering, Tooth Brushing, Shaving (etc.) Meditation* (page 90)

Life Preservers

You'll learn how to use these and other practices for particular situations and emotional states in Part II.

- *Walking Meditation* (formal or informal; page 67)
- *Eating Meditation* (formal or informal; pages 79 and 263)

Developing a Plan

You may find it useful to jot down an initial plan. The following chart can help you organize your thoughts.

PRACTICE PLAN		
Formal Practice	*When*	*How Often*
_____	_____	_____
_____	_____	_____
_____	_____	_____
Informal Practice	*When*	*How Often*
_____	_____	_____
_____	_____	_____
_____	_____	_____

Obstacles and supports

When you start to practice mindfulness regularly, you'll probably notice that both formal and informal mindfulness practices enrich your life enormously and increase your sense of basic sanity. All of the challenges we discussed in Chapter 1 become more manageable. You'll find yourself accepting uncertainty and change more easily. Financial ups and downs, illnesses, things not going according to plan, growing older, and even death become easier to work with. You become less preoccupied with self-esteem—winning and losing, praise and blame become less of a big deal. As you watch thoughts come and go, you believe less in them and become less afflicted by the "thinking disease." You move beyond pursuing pleasure and avoiding pain as you practice accepting what is happening in each moment. You become better able to help your loved ones as your ability to be wholeheartedly present and accept them as they are increases. You see how many of your particular difficulties are inherent in the human condition and stop blaming yourself so much when you feel distress.

All of these changes make it easier to deal with daily challenges at home and at work. You'll sleep better, eat more wisely, and appreciate what you have. Life feels more meaningful. Everything gets better.

Why, Then, Is It So Easy to Stop Practicing?

I want you to be prepared when the inevitable "lapse" in mindfulness meditation practice occurs. Other desires and demands will encroach on your meditation time. You'll find that when you're fatigued or upset and most need to practice, you avoid it. Like Jennifer, you may find yourself turning on the TV and eating junk food instead of meditating. Why?

One reason is because mindfulness practice challenges our defenses and makes us vividly aware of everything that is happening in our minds and bodies right now—including the uncomfortable stuff. And we humans, like other living things, instinctively withdraw from pain. So, paradoxically, even though mindfulness practices are very effective at alleviating suffering, they require that we be willing to experience pain more vividly. It's the same way that it hurts to clean out an infected wound, even though this allows the wound to heal and ultimately leaves us feeling better. In both situations, we need faith and courage to move forward, trusting that our overall well-being is worth enduring short-term discomfort.

The rest of this book will show you how mindfulness practice can help you deal effectively with many of the different types of difficulties life brings, even when they're painful. Practicing regularly is integral to these efforts. So here are some tips on how to establish a regular practice.

Choose a Regular Meditation Time

It's a cliché, but it's true—we are all creatures of habit. Most of us are pretty good at brushing our teeth and combing our hair every day, many of us even manage to floss, and almost all of us put on a seat belt when we get into the car. If we make something part of a regular routine, we're much more likely to do it. Everyone's life is different, so finding the best time of day and days of the week for mindfulness practice is an individual matter. You will be most successful at establishing a practice, however, if you make it a regular part of your schedule. This means both choosing regular times for formal practice and choosing a few routine activities to use as daily informal practice opportunities.

Do It with Others

Another true cliché—we're social creatures. Most of us will let ourselves down more readily than we will let down others. If you know any other people interested in meditation and can fit it into your life, try scheduling a regular time to practice together. You will probably be reluctant to disappoint them by not showing up—and this can help on those days when you don't feel like meditating. It's said in some Asian traditions that "a tiger doesn't last long away from its mountain." The tiger is the meditator; the mountain is his or her community of fellow meditators. Even if you can't join a regular group, staying connected with others who practice mindfulness will provide important support. It can be difficult to deal with what arises in meditation without this. As the writer Anne Lamott famously quipped, "My mind is a bad neighborhood I try not to go into alone."

Be Realistic in Your Expectations

If you are a parent of young children, a full-time graduate student, or someone working two jobs, don't expect yourself to be able to maintain a rigorous meditation schedule. Make a realistic commitment—perhaps meditating for only 20 minutes a few days each week, with longer or more frequent sessions when the opportunity arises. Again, if you create an unrealistic expectation for yourself and fail, you may give up entirely. You will likely have a better experience by setting more modest goals and feeling good about reaching them.

Surround Yourself with Reminders

Despite the enormous benefit of mindfulness practice giving us insight into how our minds create suffering and how we can free ourselves from it, we all get trapped again and again looking for happiness in the wrong places. We discussed earlier how our evolutionarily hardwired propensities to pursue pleasure and avoid pain, and enhance our social standing, regularly get us into trouble. It can be very useful to have frequent reminders about what works and what doesn't work to enhance our well-being.

These will be different for each of us, depending on our cultural background and religious or philosophical beliefs. In general books, poetry, and art that support our appreciation of the present moment and acceptance of the things we cannot change are helpful. Reminders of our place in the circle of life, the inevitability of change, and our interconnections with other people and the wider world all also support mindfulness practice. These reminders can take many forms—books about mindfulness, tips from recovery programs, writings or symbols from various wisdom traditions, or religious literature from your faith. A number of possibilities are listed in the Resources in the back of the book. It can be very useful to have these in the bathroom, on your desk, at your bedside, or anywhere else where they can serve as reminders throughout the day.

Let Every Moment Be a Practice Opportunity

During all of the moments that aren't set aside for formal or informal mindfulness practice, you can still try to be aware of your present experience with acceptance. Surround yourself with little notes to smell the roses wherever you go. Make the conscious choice to restrict your multitasking so that everything you do can be done more mindfully. This will provide continuity to your practice, while transforming previously undervalued time like waiting in line, being stuck in traffic, or getting the mail—into valued moments.

Remember What Mindfulness Practice Is and Isn't

We discussed in Chapter 2 some common misconceptions about mindfulness practice. These can come up when we're dealing with difficult thoughts, feelings, and body sensations. Remember, this practice is not about emptying the mind, getting rid of difficult emotions, escaping life's problems, being free of pain, or experiencing never-ending bliss. Mindfulness practice is about embracing our experience as it is—and sometimes what is can be unpleasant at the moment.

It is very easy to get frustrated with your unruly mind and to want to force it to become calm and peaceful. This effort almost always backfires. The Zen master Shunryu Suzuki compares the mind to a farm animal: If you had an agitated cow or sheep, what would be the best way to help it settle down? Should you put it in a small cage or give it a wide pasture? For your mind to settle, it, too, needs a wide pasture. Unpleasant experiences need to be welcome. Fear not; like all things, they too will pass.

We've had a look at some of the reasons that life is difficult for us all, seen how our evolutionary heritage predisposes us to distress, and have had an introduction to formal and informal mindfulness practices. The rest of this book will look at how these practices can help us deal effectively with the everyday challenges of living a life. Because most of our psychological difficulties have a lot in common with each other, mindfulness practices prove to be remarkably effective tools for dealing with them all. Turning toward experience—both pleasant and unpleasant—can be remarkably freeing.

The following chapters explore how to use mindfulness practices to work with moments of anxiety, depression, and physical pain as well as difficulties posed by illness, aging, and intimate relationships. We'll also see how mindfulness practice can lead beyond managing difficulties and help us to live healthy, productive, and deeply meaningful lives.

Some of these topics are likely to be more relevant to you than others. While you can best develop a good understanding of mindfulness practices by reading through the book sequentially, you may be tempted to turn first to chapters that deal directly with issues you're facing today.

If you feel stressed, tense, or restless, worry about the future, or hate uncertainty, Chapter 5 will show you ways to understand and work with all sorts of tension, fear, and anxiety—from ordinary experiences of pressure, boredom, or insecurity to moments of sheer terror.

Instead, perhaps your mind tends to review the past and wrestle with sadness, disappointment, feelings of inadequacy, depression, or just feeling dull, down, or not fully engaged. If so, Chapter 6 offers a variety of ways to put your thoughts into perspective and ground yourself in the present moment while rejuvenating and enlivening your emotional life.

Many of us are regularly visited by physical symptoms that are either caused or exacerbated by stress, including headaches, digestive disorders, back or neck pain, insomnia, and sexual difficulties. Chapter 7 explains how resisting these symptoms actually makes them worse, and how mindfulness practices can help free you from these chronic conditions.

Do you have relationships with children, parents, romantic or business partners, friends, mentors, bosses, or subordinates? Have you noticed that these aren't always smooth or fulfilling? Welcome to the club. Chapter 8 will explore how to use mindfulness practices to reduce or resolve interpersonal conflicts while making relationships richer and more rewarding.

Few of us behave exactly as we'd like. We all have habits that add to our suffering or the suffering of others. These can include eating unhealthfully, drinking or using other intoxicants unwisely, procrastinating, not getting enough sleep, managing money poorly, neglecting family or friends, or being less honest with ourselves or others than we should. Chapter 9 shows how mindfulness practice can be helpful in both seeing these patterns and changing them.

Have you noticed any changes to your body or mind as you've grown older? Have any of these been unwelcome? After a certain (rather young) age, almost all of us become concerned about aging and illness. And if our defenses aren't rock solid, we also think about death. Chapter 10 shows how to use mindfulness practice to actually accept and embrace our evolving position in the cycle of life.

While the focus of this book is on using mindfulness practices to deal with day-to-day and more serious difficulties, their potential reaches considerably beyond this. The practices were originally developed as part of a remarkable happiness project, designed to lead anyone who undertakes it to psychological awakening and liberation from suffering. In Chapter 11 we'll see how scientific research is beginning to validate ancient wisdom in outlining this path to freedom and happiness.

You may be thinking that all of these chapters apply to you (as they do to me). If this is the case, by all means turn the page and read them in order. But if one or another issue jumps out irresistibly, feel free to go there first—just be sure to return to the others later so that you can benefit from all that mindfulness practices have to offer.

PART II

Everyday Practices for Unruly Minds, Bodies, and Relationships

CHAPTER 5

Befriending fear

Working with worry and anxiety

> I am a very old man and have suffered a great
> many misfortunes, most of which never happened.
> —MARK TWAIN

*L*ife is frightening. Every day new threats arise or old ones return. Countless things could go wrong, and many of them do. On top of this our minds regularly anticipate even more misfortunes than actually befall us.

It's no wonder we feel afraid. We hear every day about terrible things—accidents, addiction, assaults, aneurysms, adultery, Alzheimer's, attacks, amputations, abductions, atherosclerosis, abandonment, AIDS—and these are just a few at the beginning of the alphabet. Some misfortunes are caused by other people, some by our own missteps, and many simply by the fact that everything changes—we age, our children grow up, economic conditions shift, storms brew, wood rots, metal rusts, everything that is born dies.

Fear is our mind and body's ancient, hardwired response to *every* perceived threat, no matter how subtle. We are therefore frightened much of the time, though we often don't think about it this way. Many days we just feel "stressed." When the threat is even less obvious, we might feel restless, bored, or antsy ("Nothing good is on TV"). Perhaps we find ourselves procrastinating to avoid a certain task or encounter ("I'll pay the bills tomorrow"). Or we find ourselves compulsively driven to finish projects, accomplish goals, or meet deadlines ("I can't relax until I get this done").

Fear can also show up as a stress-related physical symptom such as a headache, digestive distress, back pain, or insomnia (we'll discuss these in detail in Chapter 7). It can prompt us to drink too much, visit the refrigerator, or waste hours surfing the Internet (the topic of Chapter 9). And fear can lead to regrets about the things we avoid because of it—the phone call we duck, the opportunity we pass up, or the important encounter we put off. This avoidance then leads to more fear, as we worry about the trouble we'll face (from ourselves or someone else) for chickening out.

While sometimes we don't immediately recognize our fear, at other times we have no doubt that we're scared. We feel anxious, tense, uptight, or can't stop worrying. Perhaps we even develop sweaty palms, tight shoulders, a pounding heart, or panicked feelings. These sensations can get so intense that we desperately want to get rid of them.

Fear is also constantly changing. Our level of distress may be low one moment but high the next. We may feel anxious regularly or only sporadically. Whatever our particular patterns, most of us find that fear, worry, or anxiety gets in the way of enjoying life at least occasionally. After all, almost everything is more fun when we feel relaxed. (This may have something to do with the worldwide prevalence of drinking.)

When fear is strong, it can get in the way of our functioning at school, at work, with family, or in social situations. Whether we do poorly on the math test because we couldn't concentrate, falter during the big presentation because of nerves, yell at our kids because we're worried about their behavior, or hesitate to ask someone for a date, fear can interfere with everything we do.

Whether or not you think of yourself as being an anxious or fearful person, mindfulness practice can help you deal with your reactions to life's inevitable threats—both big and small. To use it this way, start by completing the inventory on the facing page to identify how fear, worry, and anxiety show up in your particular life.

If you're like most people, you might be surprised to see just how often fear and anxiety affect your life. Some people think of these as distinct experiences. They use the word *fear* to describe our reaction to immediate physical danger (the car going into a skid or our child running into the road) while *anxiety* involves worry (feeling nervous before an important talk or big test). The distinction isn't critical, however. Mindfulness practice helps us see that our minds and bodies respond simi-

A FEAR, WORRY,
AND ANXIETY INVENTORY

1–Rarely   2–Sometimes   3–Often   4–Very often   5–Most of the time

Using this scale of 1 to 5, rate how often each of the following happens:

- I feel tense. (_____)

- I feel like I can't stop until I finish a project. (_____)

- I worry about little things. (_____)

- I imagine the worst. (_____)

- I am bothered by headaches, neck or back pain, insomnia, or digestive troubles. (_____)

- I feel my heart beating quickly, have shortness of breath, or feel shaky. (_____)

- I find it hard to sit still. (_____)

- I worry about what others think of me. (_____)

- I feel insecure about my looks, intelligence, or level of success. (_____)

- I feel uptight or on edge. (_____)

- I get bored. (_____)

- I'm not fully relaxed. (_____)

- I worry about big problems such as money or health. (_____)

- I'm reluctant to ask someone out on a date or for a favor. (_____)

- I get nervous before public speaking. (_____)

- I'm uneasy flying on airplanes or being in high or confined spaces. (_____)

- I'm uncomfortable around spiders, snakes, dogs, or other animals. (_____)

- I'm uneasy around angry people. (_____)

larly in all of these situations and at least some fear or anxiety shows up quite regularly. It can help us work with both the little moments of fear and anxiety that pass through our minds all the time and the big ones that can be overwhelming. Whether you generally manage these well on your own or have struggled with fear and anxiety and perhaps are being treated with psychotherapy or medication, this chapter will show you how to use mindfulness practice to work more effectively with these inevitable parts of life.

Just doing the formal and informal mindfulness practices discussed in Chapters 3 and 4 is a great way to start. But by understanding how we respond to threats, and learning specific mindfulness techniques designed to work with frightened states, you can deal with them even more effectively.

No matter how subtle or disturbing it is, all fear and anxiety stems from the same adaptive evolutionary mechanisms. Understanding these responses and how they become a problem can reveal how and where mindfulness practice can help.

What exactly *is* anxiety?

Researchers point out that what we call "anxiety" is actually three inter-related processes: physiological, cognitive, and behavioral.

We experience the *physiological* aspect of anxiety as sensations in our body. These can include a racing heart, shallow breath, lightheadedness, clammy hands, restlessness, fatigue, trembling, muscle tension, or a "lump in the throat," as well as headaches, stomachaches, backaches, and a variety of other stress-related medical problems. These effects can be subtle—maybe you just feel a little embarrassed about repeatedly clearing your throat when you have to talk to a difficult customer, or find yourself fidgeting in the waiting room before your doctor's appointment.

The *cognitive* aspect of anxiety shows up as worried thoughts about the future—imagining disasters of all sorts and thinking about ways to avoid them. Perhaps on the phone with that customer a little tape in the back of your mind tells you that he thinks you're stupid, or you decide in the waiting room that your headache is really a brain tumor.

The third aspect of anxiety involves avoidant *behavior*. Not surprisingly, people try to avoid situations that bring on unpleasant physiological reactions and painful thoughts. So when we're anxious, we wind up limiting our lives, avoiding the activities and situations that we expect will make us more anxious. Unfortunately, this generally makes matters worse. Not only do we get into trouble by hiding from the customer or putting off medical care, but avoiding what we fear tends to reinforce the idea that it's actually dangerous.

Physiology run amok: another evolutionary accident

Let's take another look at our evolutionary heritage. As we discussed in Chapter 1, people are pretty pathetic animals. Imagine again one of us out on the African savannah a few million years ago with our puny teeth and claws, thin hide, comically useless fur, and tender feet, trying to find our way with limited sight, hearing, and sense of smell. How could we possibly survive?

You know the answer: it's basically our prehensile thumb (which allows us to pick things up) and our sophisticated cerebral cortex, which allows us to *think*. Other primates have the thumb; it's the capacity to think that has allowed us to dominate the planet.

As humans, we spend most of the day thinking. We're constantly looking for patterns in our environment, trying to figure out how to maximize pleasure and minimize pain. We jockey for rank in our primate troop and think a lot about how to enhance it. We look for ways to get both our bodily and psychological needs met. We are the thinking animal.

If you've been trying the mindfulness practices presented earlier, you've undoubtedly noticed that this propensity to think is remarkably robust. We can hardly spend more than a moment without thinking. This makes sense when we consider how vital it's been for our survival.

While our teeth and claws pale compared to the competition, we share with our fellow animals several other effective survival mechanisms. Of particular relevance here is what scientists have traditionally called the "fight-or-flight response."

Imagine that a bunny quietly munching grass in a field spies a fox in the distance. His body will have a number of predictable responses brought about by his autonomic nervous system working in tandem with his hormonal system. His ears will orient toward the fox (bunnies are cute when they do this), and his hearing will actually become more acute. He'll look at the fox, and his vision will actually improve. His body temperature will rise, his heart rate will increase, his breathing will quicken, and all of the voluntary muscles in his body will become tense, preparing to fight or flee (bunnies aren't particularly big fighters, so he's probably preparing to run away). All of this will happen within a few seconds.

Now imagine that the fox wanders off. Another predictable set of changes will unfold, reversing the processes of the fight-or-flight system. Soon the bunny will be calm, and his attention will return to munching on the grass.

But bunnies are poor, primitive creatures, with none of our sophisticated capacity for words and thought. Imagine that the bunny had the good fortune to have our cerebral cortex with its capacity for logical analysis. He'd be able to think, "I wonder where the fox went? Maybe he left to tell his friends about me? Maybe he's headed next door to the other field where my wife and kids are?" If the bunny really had sophisticated intellectual abilities, he could even start calculating whether he has enough carrots in his 401(k) to survive retirement.

You can imagine what these thoughts would do to the bunny's fight-or-flight system—they would keep it in emergency response mode. This is essentially what happens to us. All day long we imagine what our fox du jour is up to. We think about being late, getting sick, losing money, feeling rejected, missing out on a good time, not having the right food in the house for dinner—the list is truly endless. And each of these thoughts, even though they're not really emergencies, is accompanied by activation of our emergency response system. We have evolved two highly adaptive survival mechanisms—a capacity for sophisticated thought and a fight-or-flight system—both of which allowed our ancestors to deal with countless threats. The problem is that when these coexist in the same brain, they predispose it to feeling frightened much of the time, as well as to developing a host of stress-related medical problems.

Luckily our thumb, in contrast, doesn't seem to cause too many difficulties.

Our thinking disease: toppling forward

So this is our predicament. Because thinking has been so important to our survival, we've evolved to think almost all the time. When our thoughts are about the future, very often they include ideas about what might go wrong. This triggers our fight-or-flight system, making us feel anxious. If you pay attention to the pattern of your thoughts, you'll probably discover that you're often planning, trying to make choices to maximize pleasant experiences and minimize painful ones. This of course makes perfect sense much of the time: if it's supposed to rain, it makes sense to take an umbrella; if we're going to spend the night away from home, it makes sense to pack a toothbrush.

But the mind has a life of its own, and this propensity to plan can easily become counterproductive. Sometimes it just takes us away from the richness of this moment. We saw one example of this earlier. When we go out to eat with friends at a new restaurant, sooner or later the conversation turns to discussing other places we might like to try. There we are eating interesting food that someone put a lot of effort into preparing—and our minds are lost in fantasies of other nice meals we'd like to enjoy someday. Something similar happens to me when I'm in nature. I might be walking by a beautiful frozen lake in the winter and think, "I bet this would be a great place to swim in the summer." We're always looking forward to the next great thing—missing out on the opportunity to savor what is happening right now.

> Our propensity to keep looking forward makes us excellent planners—but it also creates anxiety as we imagine future pain.

Things get worse when instead of imagining another meal or season we start to imagine unpleasant events. This is at the heart of all anxiety. Anxiety is *anticipatory*—it involves imagining future pain.

We think about the future no matter what our current situation is. Emergency responders report that when they extricate people from crumpled automobiles, their patients express more concern about the future than about their current pain. They worry, "Will I be able to walk?" "Will my friend be okay?" Even though the injured person may be hurting very badly right now, his or her mental suffering involves imagining what may be coming next.

The Joy of Worry

It is also remarkably easy to be completely miserable even when things are actually fine at the moment. I happen to be very good at this. One way I do it is to *worry*:

I train other mental health professionals. Often I fly to another city the night before presenting a workshop. One afternoon I was driving to the airport when the traffic on the highway came to a complete stop. It was the kind of traffic jam where people get out of their cars to look around and try to figure out what happened. My mind immediately started to think, "What if I miss my flight? I think there's a later one, but this is a busy travel day; there might not be any seats. Maybe I could take a train, but I doubt if I could get there on time. And it's definitely too far to drive. This is really bad. A whole room full of professionals took the day off and paid money for a workshop, and I won't even show up. I wish I had left earlier. Well, there's nothing I can do now; I'll just have to try to figure it out when I get to the airport. Might as well try to be here now ... "

I followed my breath for a few moments and then began to think: "What if I miss my flight? I think there's a later one, but this is a busy travel day; there might not be any seats. Maybe I could take a train, but I doubt if I could get there on time ... "

Now why was my mind doing this? Why go over the same scenario repeatedly, only to come to the same upsetting conclusion? Of course, one reason that we obsess about problems is to find solutions. Sometimes this actually works, and we think of something we missed the first, second, or third time through the sequence. But another reason for all of this painful mental activity is that it gives us the feeling that we're taking action. Sitting in my car stuck in traffic, I wasn't just passively awaiting my fate. I was doing something active. I was *worrying*.

Making matters worse is the challenge of risk assessment. We have difficulty figuring out when our fears are justified and when they're not, and people frequently don't see eye to eye about this. You might assume that anxious people have unrealistic fears. Not necessarily.

Imagine, for example, that an anxious person is driving down the interstate. He or she might think, "I'm hurtling through space in a tin can at 65 miles per hour. One mistake on my part, one oversight on the part of my mechanic, or one moment of inattention on the part of another driver could result in my injury, disability, or death. This is really frightening."

A person who isn't predisposed to anxiety might drive down the same highway with very different thoughts: "I'm in a well-designed modern automobile. I'm confident that my mechanic is conscientious. I'm sure that the other people driving their cars around me are being fully attentive. That man over there yelling into his cell phone clearly has my welfare in mind. Substance abuse is a very rare problem, so I'm certain that none of the other drivers are intoxicated ... "

You see the situation. It turns out that people with anxiety problems often perceive risks accurately while those without anxiety refuse to see those risks. It's no wonder that psychotherapists generally fail when they try to talk anxious patients out of their fears—the patients simply

> The trouble is, anxious people's fears are not necessarily unrealistic.

assume that their therapist is denying reality. So, as we'll soon see, reassurance isn't the best path for resolving anxiety problems. Mindfulness practice offers a better route.

What are we really afraid of?

Triumph and Disaster

While the thoughts that trigger our fight-or-flight system might relate to immediate threats like missing a flight or dying in a car crash, more abstract concerns can also get us going. Much of our anxiety involves threats to who we think we are. We worry about our health, our wealth, and our self-image. We worry that we or our loved ones will experience pain or miss out on opportunities. As discussed in Chapter 1, every change in our life brings with it the threat of losing something we value—and change is both continuous and inevitable. Furthermore, we're all attached to our self-image, with concerns about our standing relative to others, and there is no way to come out on top all the time.

Mindfulness practice can help us change our view of ourselves and our expectations about life, bringing these more in line with reality. When we meditate or engage in informal mindfulness practices, we get to see how quickly our thoughts, feelings, and body sensations change. We see for ourselves that there is no way to hold on to the pleasant states and ward off the unpleasant ones. We notice how our self-image is also always changing—some moments we feel that we're great; other moments we feel like total failures. We notice ourselves winning and losing and watch our emotions soar up and plummet down.

Recognizing this can help us relax by taking our successes and failures less seriously. There is a wonderful quote from Rudyard Kipling that hangs over the entrance through which competitors enter the Wimbledon tennis courts in England. It exhorts them to "meet with triumph and disaster, and treat those two imposters just the same." To the extent that we can do this, we become less fearful.

As our mindfulness practice deepens over time we come to see our place in the cycle of life more clearly. We become more comfortable with the inevitability of sickness, aging, and death (the topic of Chapter 10). We also identify less with "me" as a separate organism and begin to experience ourselves more as a part of the larger universe. In fact, as we will see in Chapter 8, we can even observe that our sense of ourselves as separate from others and the wider world is a distortion.

Given our collective prognosis, we really have only a few choices. We can grow to experience ourselves as part of the web of life and become less concerned about our personal fate; we can live in denial about the reality of our fate; or we can be perpetually anxious. Mindfulness practice helps us take the first path.

The Tigers Within

Our thoughts about what we should and should not think and feel are another wellspring of anxiety. As children we are socialized by our parents—they help us learn right from wrong and teach us the rules for getting along with other people. It's interesting to look at how different cultures handle this. To ensure good behavior, most societies declare certain thoughts and feelings off limits or sinful. If we look at the Ten Commandments, we find that some focus on behavior ("You shall not steal"; "You shall not kill") while others focus on thoughts or impulses ("You shall not covet your neighbor's wife"). In many traditions, it's considered sinful to have thoughts or impulses toward bad behavior; so even thinking about stealing or killing would be taboo. Whether or not we were raised in a formal religious tradition, we all develop an inner list of thoughts and feelings that we consider "bad." Sometimes we don't even admit these to ourselves.

This is where the trouble comes in. Since human beings, like our animal cousins, have impulses toward both ethical and unethical behavior, most of us have thoughts and impulses lurking inside that we can't accept easily. For one person it's anger, for another sadness, for a third feelings of dependent longing. Some people are afraid to admit that they feel afraid. Many of us have issues about sexual feelings—either longing for people we're *not* supposed to desire or feeling guilty about not longing enough for someone we *are* supposed to desire. Some of us feel ashamed about wanting sex too much, others too little. All of us have memories of "bad" things we've done, or felt like doing, that we try to keep out of awareness.

The mind has an interesting reaction to these thoughts and feelings that we try to push away: *what we resist persists.* As a result, we constantly have to devote mental energy (usually unconsciously) to keeping certain contents of the mind out of our awareness. When one of these thoughts, feelings, or impulses gets close to our awareness, we become anxious. Freud called this *signal anxiety*, the fear we feel when some unwanted, potentially overwhelming inner experience threatens to surface. Our fight-or-flight system gets activated in response to the fear that these things will break through into awareness. Stress physiologists describe this as responding to the *tiger within* the way we evolved to respond to tigers in the outside world.

What we resist persists.   Peter was by all accounts a really nice guy. His friends and family marveled at his even temper. But recently when he was around his boss, he had felt oddly nervous. This didn't make sense, since he always did a good job and his boss liked him.

Then one day he had a dream. He woke up horrified, having just viciously stabbed his boss to death. That morning it dawned on him that he had been mad at his boss for weeks about a comment he had made— but Peter didn't want to admit that it bothered him. His "nervousness" had been signal anxiety—he was afraid of his own secret anger. We're all vulnerable to such mysterious symptoms whenever we hide feelings from ourselves.

Here again mindfulness practice offers us a way to work with the problem. While the practice can support us in behaving ethically by helping us be aware of our impulses before we act on them, it doesn't help us to block out unethical thoughts and feelings. Rather, when we practice mindfulness we work toward *accepting* all of the contents of the mind, good and bad.

This can be particularly challenging if we were raised in a culture that teaches even *thinking* about bad deeds is sinful. Most traditions that teach this do so to help people behave well. The idea is to cut off the bad impulse before it even reaches our awareness. The hope is that this way it'll never find its way to action.

Mindfulness practice offers an alternative approach: to be aware of our inner thoughts and feelings so that we can consciously decide whether or not to act on them. This can go a long way toward reducing signal anxiety. Over time, we make friends with more and more of the contents of our mind, until there are few internal surprises left to frighten us.

Avoidant behavior: *Diver Dan* in action

We've seen how our physiological reactions combined with our thoughts and feelings help keep us anxious. The third component of anxiety— avoidant behavior—also plays a big role.

Escape-Avoidance Learning

We discussed earlier our propensity to turn to self-medication or distraction to avoid unpleasant experiences. This certainly happens a lot with anxiety. Many people drink, take other drugs, watch TV, shop, or eat to try to reduce it. We also work hard to avoid situations that might bring it on. While in the short run these approaches seem to help, in the long run they limit our lives and actually bring on more anxiety. Here is a classic example:

Imagine that a man enters a supermarket and begins shopping for groceries. He walks by the display of Cocoa Puffs, and without noticing it happening he is unconsciously reminded of a disturbing childhood incident involving the cereal. Unaware of the reason, he begins to feel a little anxious. If this man has struggled with anxiety in the past, or is accustomed to distracting himself from feelings, he may become concerned about his physiological arousal. This concern activates his fight-or-flight system further, and he starts to experience stronger sensations. Now he really starts to worry, perhaps thinking that something is going wrong with his body ("Am I having a heart attack?") or imagining that others will soon notice his distress. Feeling very uncomfortable, he decides to leave the supermarket and finish his shopping another day.

Once outside, he gets relief. His heart slows down, his breathing mellows out—he feels a lot better. Learning theorists say that this relief leads to *negative reinforcement*—a tendency to repeat whatever behavior makes a bad feeling go away. The next time the man goes to the supermarket, what do you imagine will happen? It's likely that even if nothing new occurs to make him anxious—even if he doesn't go near the cereal aisle—he'll have the worried thought "I hope I don't feel like that again." This is all it will take to activate his fight-or-flight system and bring on some anxious arousal. Then he'll think, "Damn—it *is* happening again." This will bring on even more arousal, more symptoms, and more negative thoughts. If he decides to leave once more, he'll have another experience of relief and negative reinforcement. The third time he returns to the supermarket he can almost be guaranteed to have an anxiety episode and may decide to give up supermarket shopping entirely.

Stumbling into one of these patterns can really limit our lives. We can end up refusing to fly in an airplane, cross a bridge, stand in a crowd, swim in a pool, go to the post office, or walk in the woods—fearful that we'll get panicky again. It doesn't matter what memory or random event brought on the anxiety in the first place. By escaping from the situation in which it occurred in order to get relief, we learn to fear and avoid *that* situation. Occasionally, people start to avoid so many activities that they develop *agoraphobia*—literally fear of the marketplace—and become reluctant to leave the house. Most of us, however, develop these problems to lesser degrees in one or another area of our lives.

Perhaps you find yourself reluctant to ask people out on dates, speak in front of an audience, drive on the highway, or be around spiders or snakes. Perhaps you try to avoid dealing with angry people or have difficulty asserting yourself when someone treats you unfairly. Maybe you're uncomfortable with heights or enclosed spaces. We all have some areas in which we restrict our lives out of fear of fear. It is only natural to want to avoid activities that make us anxious.

Breaking Free

Luckily, psychologists have figured out a number of ways to undo these patterns when we become trapped in them. Most involve what is called *exposure and response prevention*. This means facing our fears—placing ourselves in the situation that brings up anxiety and remaining there until the anxiety abates by itself. When studying treatments in the laboratory, psychologists often experiment with snake phobias. While most snake phobias aren't a big deal, they can get so severe that people are reluctant to even walk in a park. This symptom was studied so extensively in the 1980s that researchers joked there wasn't a single college senior left in America at the time with an untreated snake phobia—they had all been recruited for studies in the psychology department.

Effective treatment goes like this: We begin with the subject in one room and the snake in another, locked in a cage. Once the subject settles down, the snake is brought into the subject's room, still locked in its cage. If the subject becomes anxious, he or she just stays there, looking at the snake as long as necessary until he or she begins to relax. The process continues, unlocking the cage, taking off the lid, and so forth, until the subject is actually able to handle the snake. Assuming that the researchers had the foresight to pick a nonvenomous species, just a few of these sessions can cure the snake phobia.

The same principle—approaching what we fear and staying with it until the anxiety eventually abates—works for almost all anxiety problems. It is the opposite of escape–avoidance learning and is a path toward psychological freedom. Mindfulness practice is actually an ancient form of this treatment, which is why it can be so helpful in working with anxiety. Here is how the Buddha described the process some 2,500 years ago:

Why do I dwell always expecting fear and dread? What if I subdue that fear and dread keeping the same posture that I am in when it comes upon me? While I walked, the fear and dread came upon me; I neither stood nor sat nor lay down until I had subdued that fear and dread.

This simple description is the key to using mindfulness to work with fears both big and small. We'll discuss shortly how to develop your own program for dealing with anxiety as it arises in your life. But to prepare, it will be helpful to get a feel for what approaching rather than avoiding "fear and dread" is like. One way to do this is by deliberately generating some anxiety and practicing *being with* it. This increases our capacity to bear fear.

There is a mindfulness-based exercise that can help you learn how to shift from avoiding to embracing fear. You'll want to have about 20 minutes to try it. Do it right now if you have the time, or return to this a little later when you have the chance.

--------- *Stepping into Fear** ---------

Begin with a few minutes of silent meditation, focusing on the breath. Do this with your eyes closed, and once you feel as though you've settled into your body, pick up the book again for the rest of the instructions:

Now that you've attended to your breath for a little while, begin to scan your body to see if you can detect any anxious or tense feeling. If not, try to generate these by thinking of something that is anxiety provoking for you. Do this now for a minute or two.

Once you locate some anxiety or tension in your body, see if you can make it grow. Perhaps you can do this just by focusing on the physiological arousal in your body, or you may have to conjure up more frightening images or thoughts. The idea is to create as

*Available in audio at *www.mindfulness-solution.com.*

strong a feeling of anxiety as you can, so that you can really practice bearing it. Spend a few minutes doing this before reading further.

Now that you've developed a clear experience of anxiety, try intensifying it. Make it as strong as you can while sitting here holding this book. Don't worry; this is safe. I promise it won't last forever.

Once you feel as though you've generated about as much anxiety as you can muster, see if you can hold on to it. Set a timer or look at your watch and try to keep the anxiety going at the same level for at least 10 minutes. If it starts to fade, try to intensify it again. Return to these instructions once 10 minutes or more have passed.

Now that you've practiced bearing your anxiety, you can bring your attention back to your breath for a few more minutes and feel what that is like.

What did you notice? Different people have different reactions to this exercise. Some find that their anxiety gets quite intense and stays there for a while, even when the exercise is over. Others find that it is somewhat difficult to maintain anxiety at a high level; they need to keep escalating the intensity of imagined catastrophes to keep it going. Sometimes strange physical sensations arise that themselves are alarming. Some people feel overwhelmed by the experience and are tempted to quit early (quitting early isn't recommended, because this tends to reinforce our fear).

George was skeptical when I first described *Stepping into Fear*. He had been struggling with anxiety ever since he started a new job and had been trying one relaxation technique after another. While he was sometimes able to control his fear, it often got the better of him. The idea of "bringing it on" seemed particularly foolhardy. I told him that I had never known of anyone dying during the exercise. So out of a combination of desperation and trust in me, he gave it a try.

The anxiety was there at the ready as soon as George attended to his breath. Just turning his attention inward was alarming. He found that he could easily intensify the anxiety by bringing his attention to physiological sensations—tightness in his stomach and throat, heart beating quickly, tense shoulders. Despite being tempted to turn to relaxation techniques, with encouragement George soldiered on. When asked to amplify his anxiety further, he thought of a presentation coming up at work and in no time started to feel panicky.

Even though urges to run away from his anxiety kept arising, George stayed with his tension and rapidly beating heart. After a while he found that his symptoms started to fluctuate, and he needed to imagine increasingly dire situations to keep them up. He had his boss chew him out in front of his coworkers, saw himself getting fired, and lost his house. He eventually had to imagine traffic accidents and grave medical diagnoses. After a while it started to seem funny. While he still felt some anxiety at the end of the exercise, it was less intense, and more important, it felt less serious.

Like George, many people find that when they move toward the anxiety instead of trying to reduce it, the anxiety eventually either runs out of steam or begins to fall into perspective—it requires resistance for "fuel." The challenge is to stay with it long enough. This is a key discovery. Seeing that anxiety is both approachable and self-limiting when we don't fight it gives us the courage we need to move toward anxiety when it arises in our daily life. It is at the heart of a mindfulness-based program for working with fear.

If you find yourself regularly having thoughts like "I hope I don't feel anxious when ... " or "I've got to get this to stop," practicing the *Stepping into Fear* exercise can help. You can either add it from time to time to a period of formal mindfulness meditation or try it during the day, when you notice fear-resisting thoughts arising in your mind. Just leave yourself enough time so that you don't quit as soon as the anxiety becomes intense, but can stay with it until it stabilizes or subsides.

Cognitive-behavioral therapy on steroids

In addition to counteracting the impulse toward experiential avoidance that keeps us stuck in anxiety, mindfulness practice can help us directly tackle another engine that keeps fear going—our thinking disease. Through meditation we can see that our thinking habit is very strong and our attempts to stop it are futile. Rather than trying to control it, mindfulness practice gives us new perspective on our thought process.

We notice how all of our thoughts are conditioned by our experience and how this determines what will make us anxious. If you've been abandoned in the past, you'll have fears of abandonment. If you've had a medical problem, you'll get anxious about your health. If you've had trouble in school, you'll fear appearing stupid. The list goes on and on. When you can see your thoughts arising and passing and see how your reactions to them are all conditioned by past events, you'll naturally take them less seriously.

You'll also come to see that pleasant and unpleasant thoughts and feelings will continue to arise no matter what you do. So often we fantasize that if only we could get all of our ducks in a row—arrange the perfect work and family situation—we would be stress free and happy. Mindfulness practice reveals that no matter what our circumstances, the mind continues to be restless and moods keep changing. All of our thoughts and feelings will arise and pass away, only to be replaced by new ones. Even terrible thoughts and feelings will eventually change. Knowing this makes it harder to take them so seriously.

Using mindfulness in this way can be a powerful adjunct to techniques people often learn in psychotherapy. A widely used form of treatment with considerable research support is called *cognitive-behavioral therapy* (CBT). At its heart is coming to identify which of our thoughts are rational and helpful and which ones are irrational and counterproductive. The idea is to refute the irrational thoughts and replace them with rational ones. In the case of anxiety this may involve examining *catastrophic* thinking. These are the sorts of thoughts we all have from time to time in which we assume the worst: "If I get nervous giving this presentation, everyone will think I'm an idiot, and I'll be fired." "The plane is going to crash and we'll all be killed." Ad infinitum.

In CBT people learn to challenge catastrophic thinking. Mindfulness practice takes a different tack. Instead of trying to refute unhelpful thoughts, we learn to view all thoughts as passing events, like clouds drifting in the sky or bubbles traveling on a stream. There's no need to argue with ourselves; we can avoid getting trapped by irrational or counterproductive thoughts just by letting them go. The fact that mindfulness provides practice in letting go of *all* thoughts means that the practices in this book can make CBT efforts to challenge the narrower category of irrational thoughts even more effective.

While mindfulness practices by themselves can help you deal with all sorts of anxiety, if your fears are incapacitating, outside help may also be in order—how to decide is discussed at the end of the chapter.

> Mindfulness practice helps us avoid the trap of counterproductive thoughts by learning to let them go.

Mindfulness practices for anxious times

As a first step in working mindfully with anxiety, establish a regular practice along the lines discussed in Chapters 3 and 4. This will form the foundation for specific anxiety-oriented techniques.

An important part of regular practice involves recognizing and accepting the contents of our hearts and minds during both formal practice and the rest of our day. Since one possible source of distress is the signal anxiety that arises when unwanted thoughts or feelings threaten to come into awareness, it is particularly important to try to welcome these—however unsavory or ignoble they may be.

Once you've got a regular practice going, you can modify it to suit periods when you feel a little anxious and employ special techniques during the day when anxiety is particularly acute. The exact approach you use will depend on your experience of the moment (which, of course, is always changing). Just as you can balance concentration, mindfulness, and loving-kindness practices depending on whether your mind is focused or scattered, self-critical, or accepting, you can choose different ways of working with anxiety depending on its quality, its intensity, and how overwhelmed you feel. You can use the techniques presented here either on your own or as part of a psychotherapeutic program if you're working with a therapist.

Modifying Your Regular Practice

When you're anxious but not feeling overwhelmed, a few simple modifications of your regular mindfulness practice program may be helpful. Which you choose will depend on the quality of the anxiety you're experiencing. While all anxiety has physical, cognitive, and behavioral components, sometimes one of these components predominates, and the anxiety responds best to a particular approach.

Anxiety in the Body

Sometimes fear or anxiety is particularly physiological. Acute fear of getting on stage, confronting a coworker, or hearing the results of a test can make us feel nervous, experience shallow breathing and a rapid heartbeat, or perspire. Longer-term anxiety over something like a loved one's health, a project at work, or our financial situation can lead us to develop tense shoulders, stomachaches, or restless and unsettled feelings. When our symptoms are mostly physical, bringing attention to the body is particularly helpful. The heart of this practice, as in the *Stepping into Fear* exercise described earlier, is to approach rather than avoid or fight the sensations in our body. As with any period of formal meditation practice, the following exercise will work best if you set aside at least 20 minutes for it. However, once you've had some experience, you can shift into it for shorter periods, using it as a life preserver whenever anxious feelings arise.

——————— *Mindfulness of Anxiety in the Body* ———————

Begin by focusing your breath for a few minutes as you've done before. Once you can stay with at least a few cycles, let the breath recede into the background and choose your anxiety sensations as the primary object of attention. Feel how they manifest in the body—notice the body's heart rate, breathing rhythm, perspiration, muscle tension, restlessness, and so forth. Try to approach these sensations with an attitude of interest or curiosity—not asking what they mean or where they come from, but just investigating how they feel in each instant. See if the sensations are solid or perhaps subtly changing from moment to moment. As you've done before, whenever your mind begins to wander away from the sensations, gently bring it back.

Notice too any urges to withdraw from the anxiety sensations—to get up, shift position, or make them stop. The key here is to stay with what is happening in the body rather than trying to make the sensations stop or go away.

This meditation practice, like most mindfulness-oriented approaches to anxiety, involves sitting with experiences and letting them run their course rather than trying to change them. When we do this, it interrupts an important mechanism that maintains anxiety, since we're no longer generating fear of the anxiety itself. This approach also frees us to make intelligent or skillful choices, no longer bound by concerns over whether one path will generate more fear than another—since we become confident that we can sit with whatever sensations arise. Each new wave of anxiety becomes another opportunity to practice increasing our capacity to bear it—to become stronger and freer.

This is actually a powerful way to develop courage. I once heard an actor describe a conversation he had had with one of the early astronauts. The actor was about to play him in a movie and wanted to understand what it felt like to pilot an experimental aircraft. The actor asked, "How did you do it? I wouldn't have had the courage. I would've been scared shitless." The astronaut replied, "I was scared shitless. Almost every time I went up. Nobody had ever flown these planes that high before, and we had no idea if they'd hold together. Courage isn't about not feeling fear— courage is about feeling fully afraid and doing what it makes sense to do anyway."

Working with Worry

All worry is anticipatory. Even in terrible current circumstances, our worry is about what is going to happen next, not about what is happening right now. Since mindfulness practice cultivates *awareness of present experience with acceptance*, it tends to bring our attention out of the past or future and into the current moment.

And the present is usually safe. Just as the bunny focused on eating grass isn't anxious once the fox has left, so we become much calmer when we can bring our attention to whatever is happening right now. In fact, we eventually realize through mindfulness practice that *only the present actually exists.* Everything else is a story about the past and the future. Reminding ourselves to return to our experience in the present moment can therefore be very helpful in putting our worried thoughts into perspective.

> Only the present actually exists. Everything else is just a story about the past or future.

While a general mindfulness practice program repeatedly brings your attention back to sensations in the present moment and helps you take anticipatory thoughts less seriously, some modifications are particularly helpful when you're caught up in worry. The following exercise will work best if you set aside at least 20 minutes to do it. However, like the focusing on anxiety in the body, once you've had some practice, you can try this for shorter periods whenever you find yourself getting stuck in anxious thoughts.

Thoughts Are Just Thoughts

Begin by focusing on your breath for a few minutes. See if you can follow complete cycles, from the beginning of an inhalation to the point of fullness, back to the point of relative emptiness, and then beginning again. If you're worried, it won't take long for thoughts about the future to arise. For the first few minutes, every time you notice that your attention has wandered from the breath to the thoughts, just gently bring your attention back to the breath.

After doing this for a little while, you can try introducing a little imagery. When thoughts arise in the mind, imagine them to be clouds passing through the sky. Notice that "you" are not these thoughts. Rather "you" are awareness itself—you are the sky and the thoughts are the clouds, rain, and snow that occupy it for a time. The sky remains steady throughout.

An alternative is to imagine that thoughts are like bubbles in a stream—appearing and disappearing, passing by. Here "you" are the stream bank, watching the water continually flowing while the bubbles come and go, either bursting or traveling on. If you prefer machines to nature, you can even try imagining that "you" are watching a conveyor belt, while the thoughts move along—clunk, clunk, clunk—only to fall off at the end of the line.

The idea here is not to stop or change the thoughts, but to no longer identify with and believe in each one.

Ilana had always been a worrier. As a teenager and young adult she worried about her health and success; now as a mom she mostly worried about her kids' health and success. Sometimes these worries really got out of hand, like when she fretted that her son might slip on the ice walking home from the bus stop, her daughter might get strep throat again, her son might not get off the bench in basketball, and her daughter might not finish her history paper.

Initially, mindfulness practice was very difficult. Ilana quickly saw that she had been relying on distractions to calm herself down. Spending time alone with her mind was alarming—it was a worry machine. So she was eager to try something designed to help her let go of thoughts.

Ilana began the *Thoughts Are Just Thoughts* practice by trying to follow her breath and, as usual, had difficulty staying with even one full cycle. Once she developed a little concentration, she decided to shift her attention to her thoughts. Instead of arguing with each one or adding it to her to-do list, she just let them appear and disappear, like bubbles passing on a stream:

> "I hope Jimmy has a good day at school."
> "I wonder what I should make for dinner."
> "It might snow—should I pick the kids up at the bus?"
> "How will I get everyone to their activities on Tuesday?"
> "I really should be following my breath."

The thoughts kept coming, and Ilana kept letting them go. While she was tempted to follow up on each one and make a decision, solve a problem, or add something to her schedule, she decided instead to just watch the passing show. After some practice, she began to feel less crazed.

Life Preservers for Rough Waters

Sometimes our anxiety is stronger, and sometimes it is weaker. And sometimes our capacity to be with experience is stronger, and sometimes it is weaker. While we are most free when we can fully experience whatever arises in our body and mind, there are times when we aren't ready for this. We may feel too agitated to sit still or too inundated by our fear to approach it directly.

When anxiety feels overwhelming, we may not be able to function very well, much less maintain our regular mindfulness practice routine. Luckily, there are mindfulness exercises that can increase our capacity to bear the anxiety sensations without exacerbating them. These can substitute for our usual formal mindfulness practices (some of which are tough to do when we feel overwhelmed by anxiety) or also be used as informal practices during the day when anxiety is particularly acute.

As mentioned earlier, *Mindfulness of Anxiety in the Body* can be used as a life preserver when the physical sensations of anxiety are particularly acute. Others are best suited to different circumstances and states of mind.

Meditation in Action

When we're particularly restless or agitated, walking meditation is often easier than sitting meditation. You'll recall from Chapter 3 that walking meditation is a concentration practice that involves focusing attention on the sensations of our feet making contact with the ground and our legs moving through space. There are at least two reasons that this is easier than sitting meditation when we feel very anxious.

First, moving tends to reduce muscle tension (that's why people often pace or fidget when they're nervous). This reduces the felt intensity of anxious feeling, making it easier to bear. Second, walking meditation has more of an "outer" than an "inner" focus. When we sit and follow our breath, our attention is toward the inside of our body. This tends to invite thoughts and feelings into awareness. While in the long run it's important to become aware of these and learn to accept them, when we're feeling overwhelmed it's usually better to establish a sense of safety first. Focusing on external sensations such as the feet contacting the ground and the legs moving through space tends to "ground" us in external reality, providing a sense of safety and strength.

You can include more formal walking meditation in your practice when you feel overwhelmed by anxiety. You can also experiment with walking mindfully as an informal practice, moving about your day if you feel flooded. Remember, though, that the point of this isn't to make the anxious feelings go away—but rather to increase your capacity to bear them by grounding yourself in other sensations of the present moment.

Taking Refuge in Outside Reality

Another practice that can be very useful when we feel overwhelmed involves noticing nature. This has even more of an outer focus than walking meditation, because it concentrates on things entirely outside our bodies. It can be helpful when anxiety is particularly extreme.

A patient I know well came to my office looking unusually distressed. She grew up in a very abusive household and consequently becomes easily overwhelmed when people are mean to her. She had had an encounter with someone who really bullied her and was now consumed with anxiety. It was so bad that she felt confused, imagined seeing things that weren't actually there, and could barely drive to my office. While she found it helpful to discuss what had brought her to this state, even after talking about the incident she still felt overwhelmed and disorganized.

I asked her if she'd be interested in trying a meditation practice to help her tolerate her feelings. When she agreed, I invited her to stand with me at the window and look at a tree. I asked her to start at the top of the tree and describe everything she saw in detail—the leaves, the branches, and the details of color and texture. Once she had done this, we moved on to another tree and eventually to everything else we could see out the window. I told her we weren't trying to make her anxiety go away or wipe out her feelings about the hostile encounter, but rather bring some of her attention to the reality of the external world here and now—so that she could notice that her thoughts and feelings arose against a backdrop of present reality.

After focusing on nature outside in this way for about 15 minutes, she began to feel more confident. She was less afraid of hallucinating and felt better able to function. Since our session was ending, and I had another patient scheduled, I suggested she spend the next hour walking around the neighborhood noticing all the trees and plants, bringing her attention to them as we had done at the window. She did this, and when I saw her at our next break, she felt okay about driving home and continuing with her day. While this approach may not always help a person regain confidence when in extreme distress, often it can.

———————————————*Nature Meditation*———————————————

To try this yourself, simply turn your attention fully to the world around you. If you can get to a window or go outside, use the natural world as a focus as my patient did. If you need to stay in a room and can't go to the window, you can do the same thing with the walls, floor, and objects in the room. The idea is to systematically look at everything in your visual field and describe it. If your mind wanders to thoughts or body sensations, just gently bring it back to the outside world. As with walking meditation, this can be used as a formal meditation practice, replacing breath meditation during particularly anxious times, or as an informal practice as you go about your day. If you do it as a formal practice, try to allot at least 20 minutes to give your mind time to develop some concentration.

Luckily, most of us don't feel totally overwhelmed by anxiety very often. But it's nice to know that this technique can help when we do.

Simply bringing attention to objects in the outer world and returning our attention to those objects whenever the mind drifts back to our fears can really help put things into perspective.

Cultivating Stability

There is an alternate method that you can try when feeling overwhelmed by anxiety. It is a formal practice that is inner focused, but designed nonetheless to increase your capacity to bear anxiety without heightening anxious feelings in the process.

When we are highly anxious, we can get very caught in our thoughts. It's as though we're completely focused on the clouds and don't notice the larger sky that contains them. Like the *Thoughts Are Just Thoughts* exercise, this one helps us shift our focus from the particular contents of our minds to the experience of awareness itself. Unlike other practices that focus on sensations, this one works with imagery.

Practice this first when you feel calmer so you have it available in your tool kit for more overwhelming times. You'll need to set aside 10–15 minutes. Try it now if you have the time and aren't feeling overwhelmed at the moment. In the future, if you feel agitated and have trouble sitting still, you can precede this practice with a period of walking or nature meditation.

——— *Mountain Meditation** ———

In this exercise you will imagine being a mountain going through seasonal changes. The first time you try this, it may work best to read about a season and then put aside the book and sit with its images for a few minutes. Once you feel you've settled into and explored one season, open your eyes briefly to read the next one and then close them again to explore it.

Spring

Imagine that you are a mountain. You're very large and very solid, and you've been on your spot for a long, long time. Of course, like all things, you change; but you change very slowly, in geologic time. At this moment it's springtime. There is life everywhere. The trees

—————

*Available in audio at *www.mindfulness-solution.com*.

all have new leaves, flowers are in bloom, and insects are flying about. Animals are taking care of their young, the birds are back from their migrations. Each day is different—sometimes it's cloudy, cool, and raining; other times it's sunny and warm. As night turns to day and day to night, you sit there, experiencing life unfolding everywhere. As the days go by, they gradually get longer and the nights become shorter. Each one is different. You remain solid and still, experiencing all the changes on and about you.

(Close your eyes for a few minutes now and see how it feels to be a mountain in the spring, noticing all the activity on and about you.)

Summer

The days are continuing to get longer, and now it stays light until quite late. Sometimes it is quite warm, and the animals seek shade. Insects are now everywhere, crawling and flying about. Young animals are venturing out on their own. Sometimes the air is quite still and the sun is bright. Other times violent thunderstorms rumble through, lightning strikes, and rain falls in buckets. Sometimes the streams gush and tumble down your sides; other times they are nearly dry. All this activity unfolds while you sit there, quite solid, observing it all. As the days go by you notice that they are gradually becoming shorter, though they remain quite warm. You remain massive and stable, taking it all in.

(Close your eyes for a few minutes now to experience the summer.)

Autumn

The sun is now setting noticeably earlier, and the nights are beginning to be cool. You see that leaves are starting to change color and animals are preparing for winter. Birds are starting to leave. Every day is different—some are sunny and warm, but now some are cool and crisp. As day turns to night, and night to day, the leaves continue to change—some becoming brilliant in color. Sometimes it rains gently, sometimes it is stormy, other times it is quiet and peaceful. The days continue to shorten until it really gets dark early, and the nights are actually cold. You notice now that many of the trees have dropped their leaves and plants have turned from green to brown. While everything on and about you transforms, you remain relatively still and unchanging.

(Close your eyes now to be with the autumn.)

Winter

The first snow has arrived. Everything is transformed. Streams are frozen; all is covered in white. You see the animals only occasionally—mostly you notice their tracks. Very few birds are around, and the insects seem to have disappeared. Some days are sunny and warmer; others are quite cold. Fierce storms come through with blinding snow and biting wind. You're able to sit solidly, fearlessly, taking it all in.

As night turns to day and day to night you notice that the days are beginning to get longer again. Some days it's actually warm enough that the snow begins to melt and streams start to flow, but other days it all freezes again. Eventually there are more warm days than cold and you begin to see bare ground. You notice the first shoots of young plants and realize that spring is almost here.

(Again close your eyes to be with the experience.)

Walking, nature, and mountain meditations aren't the only mindfulness-oriented techniques that can be helpful when we feel overwhelmed by anxiety. A variety of meditative physical practices such as yoga and tai chi can also be very effective in bringing our attention back to the present while increasing our sense of safety and capacity to be with experience. These practices have the added benefit of gently stretching and moving muscles, helping to release the muscular tension that is part of our fear response. Good sources for basic yoga instructions can be found in the Resources at the back of the book.

Skillful action

Until now, we've been discussing how mindfulness practice can help us work with a variety of anxiety states and how it helps counteract the mental habits that make us anxious. Sometimes, however, fear is well founded and needs to be taken as a call to action. If my patient were to complain that she gets very nervous when walking in a dangerous neighborhood at night or when her car tire starts to wobble, I might suggest that she respond to her fear not by doing meditation but by taking action. Fear obviously serves an important protective function in our lives. Just as pain can keep us from damaging tissues by teaching us not to touch a hot stove, fear can signal us to get out of danger. In fact, people who aren't fearful enough often get themselves into trouble repeatedly. (Drivers with bumper stickers that say "Shit Happens" may indeed suffer more than an average number of misfortunes.)

Many external situations can lead to anxiety. Threats to our health, safety, or economic survival can make us fearful, as can living with abusive individuals, being in stressful work environments, or participating in relationships in which we cannot be honest. Even here, though, mindfulness practice can help. It can make it easier to see the reality of our situation and notice how it frightens us moment by moment. As we become aware of this we realize that we need to do more than meditate—we need to change our living situation.

So in addition to using the practices we've been discussing to gain perspective on our anxious thoughts, we need also to ask ourselves, "Is this a thought I should listen to?" If it is, then the best strategy is actually to take action rather than simply watch worried thoughts arise and pass until disaster strikes.

Putting it all together

Fear and anxiety come in so many forms that there is no single approach that will be best for everyone. Still, there are general guidelines that you can follow that will leave you less plagued by anxious feelings and more courageous in your daily life.

As mentioned earlier, the heart of the program is your general mindfulness practice, including both regular formal meditation and daily informal practice. In addition to balancing your formal meditation among concentration, mindfulness, and loving-kindness practices, try the *Mindfulness of Anxiety in the Body* practice when you experience more physical symptoms of anxiety and *Thoughts Are Just Thoughts* practice when you are more worried. Whether your anxiety is predominately physiological or cognitive, increasing the times during the day that you do informal practice will focus your attention more on the present, thereby helping your mind to be less caught in anxious feelings and thoughts. *Loving-Kindness Meditation* (Chapter 4) can be particularly helpful if a lot of self-critical thoughts about being too anxious or too agitated to meditate arise.

Should you notice that you are getting caught in avoidant behavior— fearing your anxiety and having thoughts like "I hope this doesn't get any worse" or "I hope I don't get nervous at _____," repeating the *Stepping into Fear* exercise can be useful. Give yourself plenty of time (at least 20 minutes) to see how intensely you can feel your fear and try to hold it at its maximum level. By returning to the exercise periodically, eventually you'll feel less afraid of your anxiety states.

If you encounter periods when your anxiety is overwhelming and either making you miserable or interfering with your ability to function, you'll be best served by employing one or more *life preservers*. *Walking Meditation* is a good choice when you are just too agitated to sit still. It works well as a formal practice or as an informal practice as you move about your day. *Mindfulness of Anxiety in the Body* can also be practiced for brief periods when physical symptoms are very intense.

Nature Meditation is helpful when the waves of anxiety are particularly rough, as it tends to draw our attention out of our body and thoughts and remind us that the world still exists and all is not lost. You can practice this both formally for longer periods if you have time or informally when you have a moment in the day to notice your surroundings.

If you can sit still for 10–15 minutes, the *Mountain Meditation* is particularly useful to reinforce your ability to watch the coming and going of everything in your mind. It will help you identify less with each worry or wave of tension and develop the courage necessary to ride bigger and bigger waves.

When feelings of anxiety hit in the middle of important activities that you can't stop, the best approach is usually to turn that activity into an informal practice opportunity. Sometimes this calls for a creative modification of one of the practices we've been discussing. Even in the midst of an important meeting, you can take a few moments to just be with the sensations of anxiety in the body (a moment of *Mindfulness of Anxiety in the Body* practice) or tune in to the colors, textures, sound, and tactile feel of the room (a moment of *Nature Meditation*, albeit indoors). Practicing in this way, we discover over and over a guiding principle: by bringing our attention to the present, and not fighting our fear, fear becomes manageable.

While your experience may be different, my patient's adventure with anxiety illustrates how various mindfulness practices can fit together:

Jerry hadn't always thought of himself as an anxious person. As a kid he had been good at sports, smart, and hard working. His father pushed him, and he succeeded at almost everything he tried. He was, however, always a bit shy. Despite being capable and attractive, he didn't date very much and always felt a little awkward with girls.

After graduating from college Jerry moved up quickly in the business world, becoming a vice president in a large, successful company by the time he was 30. He had a lot of responsibility and felt confident about his analytical skills, but developed some new insecurities. He wondered if his superiors thought he was too young for the position and was concerned that his subordinates were envious, especially since many were older than him.

One day at a board meeting Jerry froze. Out of the blue his heart started racing and he couldn't think clearly. He excused himself to go to the bathroom, splashed water on his face, and returned to somehow muddle through his presentation.

Jerry worried about it happening again. He now noticed whenever he became nervous and often struggled to calm himself down. He took deep breaths and told himself not to worry. Increasingly concerned that his anxiety would interfere with his career, he came to see me for help.

Together we looked at how Jerry handled emotions (fear and sadness were taboo) and the images he had of himself (they alternated between greatness and inadequacy). We looked at his father's high expectations and how attached to succeeding he had become. While these traditional therapeutic approaches were helpful, it soon became clear that Jerry was getting totally caught up in worried thoughts and was growing more and more frightened of his anxiety symptoms. So I introduced him to mindfulness practice.

At first it did not come easily. Jerry was very action-oriented, and he wanted to *do* something about his problem—not just sit there. The idea of *being with* experiences rather than fixing them was pretty strange. Nonetheless, he trusted me, so he stayed with it.

Being very busy and wanting to also keep working out, he settled on a 20-minute, every-other-day formal practice schedule, doing informal practice during his commute. He soon realized that his mind was extremely busy and a good percentage of his thoughts were worries—including worries about his anxiety symptoms. He saw that when he wasn't anxious he often felt sad. He also noticed that he held a lot of tension in his neck and shoulders and found it painful to sit for the 20 minutes.

Because Jerry had become so afraid of anxiety sensations, I had him try the *Stepping into Fear* exercise in the office. It didn't take him long to generate a good amount of anxiety, and he asked me on several occasions if I really thought this was a good idea, since it seemed to be making matters worse. Nonetheless he stuck it out and eventually noticed that it took effort to keep his fear at full throttle. He also saw that the anxiety sensations themselves were actually "not so bad."

Having had this experience, Jerry was open to trying the *Mindfulness of Anxiety in the Body* practice during formal meditation sessions in which he felt anxious. He noticed that the sensations of anxiety changed somewhat unpredictably over the course of each sitting. He also saw that when he worried about "getting nervous" the sensations usually got worse, while they tended to calm down if he just stayed with what was happening in his body. And he felt the sadness that seemed to lurk behind the anxiety.

Jerry's anxiety never reached a level where he couldn't sit with it, so he didn't use any of the life preservers as formal practices. However, his anxiety did occasionally reach crescendos at work, so he turned to a variation on *Nature Meditation* and a little *Mindfulness of Anxiety in the Body* when this happened. Whether at a meeting, preparing a presentation, or traveling to a big event, if he began to feel overwhelmed by his anxiety Jerry practiced bringing his attention to carefully observing his physical environment. Sometimes it was nature if he could look out the window or walk outside; other times it was just the room he was in. He would allow his body to generate whatever symptoms it wanted, practice a few moments of *Mindfulness of Anxiety in the Body,* and then return his attention to the environment.

As he continued to practice mindfulness and pay attention to his emotions, Jerry became less concerned with his anxiety and more interested in finding meaning in his life. He began to look at what made intimate relationships difficult for him and discovered a deep longing for closeness. Achievement at his job became less important, he began dating more, and he grew more interested in the moment-to-moment experience of living. In retrospect he saw his anxiety problems as a sign that his values had been out of balance and that important, vulnerable feelings had been outside his awareness. Jerry was grateful for the wake-up call.

Mindfulness practices for anxiety and fear

Once you establish a regular formal and informal practice as described in Chapters 3 and 4, the following may be particularly helpful:

Formal Meditation Practices

- *Mindfulness of Anxiety in the Body* (page 123) when physical symptoms of anxiety are strong
- *Body Scan Meditation* (page 72) for learning to tolerate strong physical sensations
- *Thoughts Are Just Thoughts* (page 125) when worried thoughts prevail
- *Stepping into Fear* (page 118) when resistance to anxiety arises
- *Walking Meditation* (page 67) when it's very difficult to sit still
- *Mountain Meditation* (page 129) to increase your capacity to watch anxiety come and go
- *Loving-Kindness Meditation* (page 84) when hard on yourself about being anxious

Informal Practices

All of the following help to loosen the pull of worried thoughts about the future by bringing attention back to sensory experience in the present. They can all be done even when feeling agitated:

- *Walking Meditation* (page 67)
- *Nature Meditation* (page 128)
- *Eating Meditation* (page 263)
- *Informal Driving, Showering, Tooth Brushing, Shaving, etc., Meditation* (page 90)

Life Preservers

- *Walking Meditation* (formal or informal; page 67) when feeling overwhelmed and agitated
- *Nature Meditation* (formal or informal; page 128) when feeling overwhelmed in the midst of responsibilities
- *Mountain Meditation* (page 129) to increase your capacity to watch anxiety come and go
- *Mindfulness of Anxiety in the Body* (page 123)—practiced briefly when physical symptoms of anxiety are strong

Developing a plan

You may find it useful to jot down an action plan for working with fear and anxiety. The following chart can help you organize your thoughts:

PRACTICE PLAN

Begin by reflecting on how and when anxiety arises in your life.

Situations in Which I Most Often Feel Anxious: _____

_____

_____

_____

My Most Common Anxiety Symptoms:

Physiological (body sensations): _____

_____

Cognitive (worried thoughts): _____

_____

Behavioral (things I avoid): _____

_____

Times I Most Need a Life Preserver: _____

_____

_____

Now, based on what you've read about and experienced with the different practices, jot down an initial practice plan (you can vary this as your needs change).

Formal Practice	*When*	*How Often*
_____	_____	_____
_____	_____	_____
_____	_____	_____

(cont.)

Informal Practice	When	How Often
_____	_____	_____
_____	_____	_____
_____	_____	_____

Life Preserver	Likely Situation
_____	_____
_____	_____
_____	_____

When you need more help

While mindfulness practice can be enormously useful in working with anxiety, sometimes it makes sense to pursue other avenues as well. Jerry came to mindfulness practice through psychotherapy. Other people come to psychotherapy through mindfulness practice. If you find your anxiety is part of a vicious cycle in which you avoid activities such as going to work or socializing and this in turn creates new problems that bring on more anxiety, professional treatment is probably in order. This should include consulting with a mental health professional to understand what is creating and maintaining the anxiety and to explore your options for dealing with it. In some cases prescription medication can be of use to break cycles of fear and avoidance. Professional help can supplement mindfulness practice in helping you identify other, perhaps hidden emotions that lie beneath and fuel your anxiety. This can be done in psychodynamic psychotherapy and other exploratory approaches that look at the roots of your current reactions in past experiences, and revisiting those that may have been difficult to fully embrace at the time. Cognitive behavioral approaches of the type described earlier can be particularly helpful when obsessive thinking or compulsive actions are part of an anxiety problem. This can help you identify thought patterns that bring on anxiety and develop a plan for systematically facing fears. Tips on finding a therapist, along with the resources for working with anxiety, can be found in the Resources at the back of this book.

The ultimate goal of psychotherapy should be the same as the aim of mindfulness practice—to be able to live freely and accept the contents of our minds and the events of our lives. In the long run, increasing our capacity to feel our feelings, accept our thoughts, and bear anxiety rather than fight it is the best path to a full and rich life.

Now that you've thoroughly mastered your reactions to living in a terrifying world, perhaps you're ready to tackle some other colorful emotions. The next chapter will show how mindfulness practices can help us work effectively with two other regular visitors: sadness and depression.

CHAPTER 6

Entering
the dark places

Seeing sadness and
depression in a new light

*H*ave you ever thought about the difference between sadness and depression? I've posed this question to psychotherapists, and they come up with a variety of answers. Sometimes they suggest that depression lasts longer than sadness. But I point out that it's perfectly possible to feel sad for days in a row and yet be quite depressed for just a few hours. Then they suggest that sadness arises in response to external events, while depression comes from the inside and has a life of its own. But I remind them that we can get very depressed after a misfortune such as the loss of a job or relationship and yet can feel sad without apparent cause. Finally, after some discussion, they come to the conclusion that *sadness feels alive and fluid* and is an essential part of living a full life, while *depression feels dead and stuck* and gets in the way of living. This realization leads to another surprise: by helping us really be with sadness (and other emotions), mindfulness practice can keep us from getting stuck in depression.

Varieties of depression

Depression comes in many forms. It can be mild or severe, brief or long-lasting. It can arise mostly from environmental circumstances or come mostly from a biological predisposition. When severe, it can be crippling. It sucks the joy out of everything, ruins relationships, interferes with work, and leaves us wishing that our life would just be over. Even when mild, depression makes it hard to really enjoy and appreciate living.

It may seem strange, then, that it's not uncommon to be depressed without knowing it. Many of us expect depression to feel like deep melancholy, but instead it can appear as a mysterious loss of energy or interest. We may feel agitated by little annoyances, guilty about our thoughts or actions, indecisive, pessimistic, or plagued by self-critical thoughts. Sometimes depression brings physical symptoms such as insomnia, sleeping too much, restlessness, loss of sexual interest, or either over- or undereating. The effects of depression can also be subtle, so that all we notice is feeling a bit bored, restless, or disengaged.

Even if you don't think of yourself as a particularly depressed person, mindfulness practice can help you work constructively with negative moods when they visit. To see why this might make sense, take a moment to reflect on how depression may be affecting you (please use the inventory on the following page).

What did you discover? Most people find they have some of these experiences at least occasionally. While many of them can also stem from physical disease, poor health habits, anxiety, or attention problems, depression is often the culprit when several cluster together.

The rest of this chapter will look at some ways that depression comes about and how mindfulness practice can help us work with it no matter how it appears. Embracing sadness and other emotions through mindfulness practice helps keep us from getting stuck in depression. And you might be surprised to find that depression can even be an opportunity for psychological or spiritual awakening when approached mindfully.

There may be times when a given practice makes matters worse and may not be appropriate for your current situation. I'll give you some ideas for when you might try each one, but everybody is different, so you'll do best to experiment and trust your judgment about what fits your needs at the moment. Especially if depression is interfering with your daily life, you might also benefit from other ways of working with it, such as psychotherapy, medication, or a more detailed self-help program. I'll describe how you can determine what kind of help you might need and where you can find assistance at the end of the chapter.

A DEPRESSION INVENTORY

1–Rarely   2–Sometimes   3–Often   4–Very often   5–Most of the time

Using this scale of 1 to 5, rate how often each of the following happens:

- I feel sad, down, or unhappy. (_____)
- I find myself losing or gaining weight without dieting. (_____)
- I lose interest in things that used to matter to me. (_____)
- I feel a lack of energy or strength. (_____)
- I either have trouble sleeping at night or sleep more than I think I should. (_____)
- I feel guilty or have a bad conscience. (_____)
- Even when good things happen, I don't really feel cheerful. (_____)
- It's hard for me to concentrate on things like reading, TV, or hobbies. (_____)
- I feel stuck, trapped, or caught. (_____)
- I feel restless or agitated and find it hard to really relax. (_____)
- I feel like a failure. (_____)
- I have difficulty making decisions. (_____)
- Sex just doesn't interest me very much anymore. (_____)
- I don't feel very alive or engaged in my life. (_____)
- I find myself crying even when nothing particularly bad happens. (_____)
- I don't like myself very much. (_____)
- It's hard for me to get motivated. (_____)
- I feel subdued. (_____)
- I don't feel very confident. (_____)
- I either don't have much of an appetite or can't seem to stop eating. (_____)
- The future doesn't look very good to me. (_____)
- I find other people irritating. (_____)
- I feel tired of living. (_____)

All or nothing

Sadness and depression have a curious relationship. We can feel sad as part of a depressed mood, we can be depressed about feeling sad too often, and we can even become sad about being depressed and missing out on life. The way we deal with sadness can also have a lot to do with how depressed we get.

Most of us aren't big fans of sadness. As with anxiety, our usual approach is to try to get rid of it. We may distract ourselves, hoping to work up some positive feeling by turning our attention to other things. We may try to cheer ourselves up by thinking happy thoughts. (As Maria sings in *The Sound of Music*, "I simply remember my favorite things, and then I don't feel so bad.") And then of course there are the old standbys of alcohol, other drugs, eating, gambling, shopping, and sex.

But maybe we should be careful what we wish for. Without sadness as part of our emotional life, would we even be able to recognize joy? The fact is, we're aware of negative states partly by their contrast with positive ones. We know fear by contrast with safety; we know anger by contrast with love, affection, or acceptance; and we know sadness by contrast with joy or happiness. In fact, we recognize everything by comparing it with its opposite: big versus small, full versus empty, wet versus dry, hot versus cold.

And having sadness in our lives doesn't just make it possible to recognize joy. It may make it possible to *feel* joy. Something curious happens whenever we try to cut out one side of our emotional experience: we dampen the other side as well. Emotions are like waves in the physical world. Picture a wave either in water or depicted on an oscilloscope. (It looks like an *s* lying on its side.) What happens if you dampen the bottom of the wave? The top of the wave also flattens out. Cutting off one pole of a sensory or emotional experience compresses the other pole. Take the edge off your appetite by filling up with too much bread at a restaurant and the rest of the meal isn't as enjoyable. And who hasn't held back from a romantic relationship to avoid getting hurt only to miss out on the joys of love?

Trying to eliminate painful feelings flattens out our emotional life, leading to a general deadness. This is one aspect of what happens in depression. In our attempts to avoid feeling sadness, we cut ourselves off from joy and interest. It turns out that we can either have it all—the ups and the downs of life—or nothing.

> Without sadness, we might not be able to recognize—or feel—*joy*.

It turns out that squelching almost any feeling—excitement, sexual arousal, fear, or anger—can contribute to depression. There seem to be several mechanisms afoot here. In the last chapter we discussed *signal anxiety*—the fear experienced when an unwanted thought or emotion threatens to break into our awareness. When this persists over time, we can feel its effects in the form of exhaustion, sleep difficulties, trouble concentrating, and other depression symptoms. The mind and body get tired out, and we lose our vitality. Furthering the problem, to keep thoughts and feelings out of awareness, the mind may detach or shut down, adding to our sense of deadness.

Squelching anger seems to be particularly problematic in this regard. Freud hypothesized that depression can be caused by anger turned against the self and called suicide *murder in the 180th degree*. The anger toward others that we can't acknowledge gets directed at ourselves and shows up in the form of guilt, feelings of inadequacy, and self-critical thoughts. While we don't all become suicidal, unacknowledged anger often plays a big role in depression.

Mindfulness practice can help us stay more aware of these underlying feelings, thereby helping us either stave off depression or work through bouts when they arise. I saw this vividly during my first intensive silent meditation retreat.

I had recently graduated from college and separated from my girlfriend. While the full story is complicated, the net result was that she moved far away and was now living with her old boyfriend—leaving me lonely and depressed. I was able to function, but I felt little joy and was preoccupied with my longing for her. Feeling like I had to do *something*, I signed up for a 10-day silent meditation retreat. I thought it would help me be more present and think less about my ex-girlfriend.

For the first day or two of the retreat my mind was busy and restless, but I was encouraged to notice that my concentration was strengthening. As time went on, my mind became more peaceful and I had sweet moments of enjoying the natural surroundings.

Then the demons arrived. Vivid images of my girlfriend appeared. First there were the images of how beautiful she was and memories of our lovemaking, full of longing and sexual arousal. Then waves of sadness washed over me as the images unfolded like film on a movie screen, and I realized how intensely I missed her. With no available distractions, the scenes played over and over for hours at a time.

Then the thoughts of her with her old boyfriend arrived and broke my heart. After this came the anger. It was not ordinary anger, but volcanic rage. I imagined violently attacking them, literally tearing off their limbs. Not a pretty sight—and it was replayed repeatedly. While I knew that meditation practice could bring a person in touch with underlying feelings, I hadn't expected *this*.

As the retreat continued, these images and their attendant feelings came and went. Other emotions arose also, including moments of deep joy and peace. When the retreat was over and I reentered "normal" life, I was still lonely and missed my ex-girlfriend, but my mood was transformed. Instead of feeling depressed, I now felt very alive—experiencing moments of sadness and anger interspersed with interest and joy.

Mindfulness of Emotion

By allowing us to fully experience our feelings in this way, mindfulness practice helps keep us from getting stuck in depression. While this can happen during an intensive retreat, it can also occur in daily meditation or through informal mindfulness practice. We come alive by attending to feelings right now—by attending to *what* is happening at the moment, rather than speculating as to *why* it is happening. You can begin to see this for yourself by doing a brief, simple exercise. Later you can use this exercise both as a way to "come home" to your feelings throughout the day and as a formal meditation practice for times when you sense that you're not fully in touch with your emotional experience. This takes only a few minutes, so perhaps you can try it now:

———— *Noting Emotions in the Body* ————

After reading these instructions, close your eyes and connect with your breath for a few minutes. Next see if you can identify what emotions are occurring. How do they manifest in your body? Do you feel them in your throat, eyes, chest, or belly? Try to stay with these emotions and sensations and breathe with them. Notice whatever takes you away from the feelings and how you can come back to them.

In depression we exacerbate our suffering by turning away from pain. We become less aware of our feelings and are left feeling lifeless in the bargain. In mindfulness practice we turn toward the experience at hand, challenging the depressive stance. A key to being able to do this is noticing emotions as they appear in the body. We see that all emotions are actually sets of bodily sensations accompanied by thoughts and images. Using the skill of being with and attending to pleasant and unpleasant bodily sensations that you develop in meditation, you can learn to explore emotions as they arise in the body. This makes them much easier to bear and increases your capacity to be with them.

If you just had trouble connecting to feelings in the *Noting Emotions in the Body* practice, there is a variation that may help you observe emotions on a physical level more clearly and systematically. You may wish to try the exercise on the facing page on a few occasions until you get the hang of it. If locating different emotions in the body remains challenging, keep trying it periodically until noticing emotions in the body becomes second nature. The exercise will require about 10 minutes to complete each time.

In mindfulness practice we can also attend to our reactions to emotions. Which ones do you usually turn away from? Which ones do you judge, thinking "I really shouldn't feel this"? Mindfulness practice allows us to see judgmental thoughts about feelings just like any other thoughts—coming and going like clouds in the sky. This makes it easier to accept and be with all of our emotions.

Miriam had often struggled with depression. Her mother never made a secret of her preference for Miriam's brother, and her father was emotionally absent. No wonder Miriam felt insecure and had difficulty connecting to people.

Recently she had run into trouble with Marty, one of her few friends. Their long-standing platonic relationship had never felt balanced, but lately Marty was being particularly self-centered. One day after he canceled plans at the last minute, Miriam became really depressed.

She started thinking that her life had always been the same: other people had love, but she didn't. She was awkward, unattractive, and unequipped to fend for herself in this competitive world. She felt hopeless.

Having practiced meditation on and off, she sensed that meditating might help. She knew the incident with Marty had triggered her depression but was confused about her feelings. She started by focusing on her breath and then expanded her awareness to do the *Noting Emotions in the Body* practice. First she noticed a lump in her throat, soft tears, and an

SURVEYING EMOTIONS IN THE BODY

Take a moment to close your eyes and breathe, tuning in to the sensations in your body. Once your mind has settled a bit, imagine something has happened that brings you great joy. Notice how you feel joy in your body. What happens in your face, your chest, and other areas? Take a moment to jot these down next to "Joy" on the lines below.

Now close your eyes again, settle into your body and breath, and imagine something has happened that brings you great sadness. Notice what happens in your face, throat, chest, belly, and other areas. Take a moment to jot these down next to "Sadness."

Continue filling in the lines below in this manner, taking time with each of the other emotions—fear, anger, disgust, shame, and guilt—to notice exactly how they feel. Jot down which areas of your body are affected by each and exactly what you experience in that area.

Joy: _____

Sadness: _____

Fear: _____

Anger: _____

Disgust: _____

Shame: _____

Guilt: _____

empty feeling around her heart—familiar feelings of sadness and being unlovable. As she stayed with these for a number of minutes, the sensations shifted and she began to feel pressure in her chest and tension in her shoulders, along with thoughts of what a jerk Marty was. She realized that she was really pissed off at him but had been afraid to feel this—not wanting to lose one of her only friends. Miriam recalled the other times that he had hurt her but she had said nothing. As she resolved to tell him what she was feeling and demand better treatment, her depression started to lift a little.

Finding Missing Emotions

We all find it easier to connect with some feelings than others. Miriam had a direct line to sadness and feeling unlovable, but anger tended to stay buried. Another way to become aware of our emotional experience is to look for the feelings we neglect. You can do this by filling in the chart on the facing page over the course of several days. Review each category at the end of the day and note the triggering event, which emotion arose, how strong it was, and how you reacted to it.

At the end of a few days, look at your chart. Do some emotions show up repeatedly? Are others missing? Are there some emotions that you notice you always try to get rid of? It is the missing or unwanted emotions that deserve particular attention. Every time you notice them arising in the future, whether during formal mindfulness practice or during your normal routine, make a point to notice them as they appear in the body and try to attend to them until they pass by themselves.

The thinking disease strikes again

Thinking plays a huge role in depression. When we're depressed, we get lost in negative ideas about ourselves and our situation. Thoughts like "I'm a failure," "No one cares about me," and "There must be something wrong with me" repeat like broken records. Psychologists call this *ruminating*—going over and over the same thought like a cow chewing its cud. We ruminate about our losses, failures, mistakes, shortcomings, and poor prospects.

Just as anxiety is perpetuated by worried thoughts about future misfortune, depression is often fueled by negative thoughts about the past. Because thinking is so important for our survival, we turn to it repeatedly—even when it's not the least bit helpful. When we're anxious, each worried thought reviews the same scenario, complete with a disaster at the end, creating yet more anxiety. In depression, we brood or ruminate for the same reason we worry when anxious—using our analytical mind makes us feel as though we're working to solve the problem. We review what has gone wrong to prepare for what will come next. Unfortunately, depressed moods generate negative thoughts, so our conclusions are almost always depressing.

OBSERVING EMOTIONS
THROUGHOUT THE DAY

Triggering Event and Emotion That Arose (joy, sadness, fear, worry, anger, frustration, disgust, shame, guilt, etc.)	Strength of Feeling 1 = mild 2 = moderate 3 = strong	Reaction to Feeling (push away, hold on, ignore, express, turn into action, etc.)
Family		
Friends/Social		
Work/School		
Hobby/Recreation/Leisure		
Other		

Adapted from Ronald D. Siegel, Michael H. Urdang, & Douglas R. Johnson, *Back Sense: A Revolutionary Approach to Halting the Cycle of Chronic Back Pain.* New York: Broadway Books (2001, pp. 123–124). Copyright 2001 by Ronald D. Siegel, Michael H. Urdang, & Douglas R. Johnson. Adapted by permission.

From Sadness to Depression

Cognitive scientists describe a mechanism by which we can get particularly stuck in negative thoughts. Working with people who had experienced repeated bouts of serious depression, researchers discovered that they react to sadness differently than people who have never been very depressed. This happens because of a peculiar quirk of our memory system.

Memory is highly dependent on contextual cues. Think about a time when you visited your old elementary school or college. Hundreds of memories probably came to mind—things you may not have thought about for years. A girl or boy you liked, a kind or mean teacher, a place you used to sit and think. Contexts activate memories.

By the same token, when we learn something new, our chances of remembering it are much greater if we try to recall it in the same environment in which we first learned it. In a fascinating study, British psychologists showed divers lists of words both under water and on the beach. When the divers' memory was later tested in both locations, they were best able to recall words in the environment in which they were first learned.

This principle can cause big problems when the "context" for our thoughts is a mood. If we were depressed the last time we felt sad or discouraged, our low mood was probably accompanied by self-critical, negative thoughts. So the next time we get sad or discouraged our mind is going to recall those negative thoughts. If we don't have perspective on this process, we'll likely believe in these thoughts and get depressed again. We won't realize

> Once depression has filled our heads with negative thoughts, the same self-critical tapes are likely to pop up whenever we feel sad or discouraged in the future, leading to a new episode of depression.

that we're reexperiencing past thoughts—hearing old tapes playing—but will take them as reality. Each time we go through a period of depression, a deeper connection builds between low mood and negative thoughts, making it more likely that the cycle will repeat.

Emotional Meteorology

In working with depression, cognitive behavioral therapists traditionally encourage their patients to separate rational from irrational thoughts and to favor the rational ones. They help patients identify automatic negative thoughts—repetitive tapes—and refute their messages. While this can be useful, it runs up against the problem that depressed moods color our thinking. There is a simple exercise that you can do from time to time to see this at work. Take a moment to give it a try.

NOTING HOW THOUGHTS CHANGE

If you're feeling at all depressed right now, think back to the last time you felt good. Remember your thoughts at the time? The sense of optimism, imagining pleasant things to come? Close your eyes and take a minute to recall how your life looked and what you imagined for your future.

If you're feeling good right now, think back to the last time that you felt depressed. Remember the negative thoughts? Imagining things will never get better, feeling bad about yourself? Close your eyes for a minute and recall that experience.

Our moods can change like the weather, and with each change comes a different set of thoughts. When we're in a particular mood, we tend to believe the thoughts that accompany it. So when we try to argue with ourselves and see the other side of things, it's very difficult to believe in a point of view that doesn't match our mood. When people are depressed, they think, "Oh yeah, I used to think I was all right. But now I realize I was just fooling myself."

The Mindfulness Alternative

Just as mindfulness practice can loosen our belief in anxious thoughts, it can help us take depressive thoughts more lightly. Instead of arguing with the negative thoughts, we work to see them as passing phenomena—dark clouds passing through the sky. This is at the heart of a treatment system developed in Canada by Zindel Segal and in Great Britain by Mark Williams and John Teasdale called *mindfulness-based cognitive therapy* (MBCT), which has proven to be remarkably effective at helping people avoid relapsing into serious depressive episodes. The approach teaches people mindfulness practices with a particular emphasis on not taking any thoughts too seriously but rather staying grounded in sensual reality here and now.

A major research study using this approach gave scientific credibility to the use of mindfulness practice in psychotherapy. Psychologists taught mindfulness practice to patients who had had serious episodes of depression in the past but were not currently stuck in one. They also educated the patients about how negative thoughts are triggered by low moods and how they might become more aware of their emotions. The results were startling. For people who had had three or more depressive episodes in the past, the chances of relapsing over the course of a year were cut in half by participating in at least four sessions of the program. In another, more recent study, MBCT was shown to be as effective as antidepressants in preventing relapses of depression and allowed many subjects to discontinue their medication.

Thoughts Are Not Reality

Mindfulness practice can help us take our thoughts less seriously in other ways too, ways that help not just with serious bouts of depression but also with the brief or mild episodes that many of us experience regularly. Mindfulness practice brings all sorts of insights into the workings of the mind. Perhaps the hardest to grasp is the idea that thoughts are not reality. We're so accustomed to providing a narrative track to our lives and believing in our story that to see things otherwise is a real challenge.

It can be fascinating to see the different stories we generate during different moods. Imagine walking down the street and spying an acquaintance. You wave to say hi. She continues walking, seeming to ignore you. What just happened? In one mood you might think, "I guess she's preoccupied with something and didn't notice me." In another, "I guess I'm not too important to her—she didn't seem to notice me." If you're really depressed, you might assume "She thinks I'm not even worth acknowledging."

Usually we have no way to determine the truth. Our conclusions are shaped by our moods and are as a consequence terribly unreliable. The designers of the MBCT program put it this way: "Our life is like a silent film on which we each write our own commentary." A famous Zen master, trying to communicate that our thoughts are not reality, used to say, "A finger pointing to the moon is not the moon." Unfortunately, most of the time we just believe in our stories.

Because we get so stuck in our thoughts when depressed and those thoughts tend to be so negative, meditative techniques that help us identify less with thoughts can be particularly helpful. There are two basic approaches we can try.

Coming to Our Senses

One method calls for strengthening our connection to moment-to-moment sensual reality in the present to draw our attention away from inner narratives. You might try this for a few moments whenever you find yourself stuck in a depressive chain of thought:

———————*Taking Refuge in Present Sensations*———————

Right now, bring your attention to the sensations in your right hand. Notice how the skin feels as it contacts the air: warm, cool, or neutral? Feel any tingling or feelings of pressure coming from the inside of your hand. See if you can sense the space between your fingers, the points of contact between your hand and this book. Just focus on these sensations for a few moments.

Now slowly and attentively slide your hand up and down the edge of the book, and notice how it feels. See how the sensations of contact are different from thoughts or images of holding the book? Try this both with your eyes open, so that you can see your hand moving, and with your eyes closed. Observe what a difference vision makes.

You may notice that this exercise feels similar to the *Body Scan Meditation* described in Chapter 3, except that there we didn't move, and we explored not just the right hand but every part of the body. In the MBCT program, therapists ask patients to do the *Body Scan* for 45 minutes a day, six days a week, to reinforce the habit of being with bodily sensations rather than getting lost in thought. If you find yourself ruminating regularly, you may find it helpful to adopt this "high dose" of attending to body sensations. If not, you can just return to the *Taking Refuge in Present Sensations* practice when depressive thoughts come up.

Grounding our awareness in the body in these ways is a potent antidote to being lost in thought. Another alternative that also helps increase body awareness is gentle yoga practice. Good sources of introductory instructions for this can be found in the Resources at the back of this book.

Mindfulness of Thinking

Complementing these body-focused techniques are cognitive exercises designed to help us listen less to our thoughts. One ancient practice involves labeling the kind of thought that arises in the mind. You might try this either for a few minutes now or the next time you do formal mindfulness practice:

———————————— *Thought Labeling** ————————————

Begin by settling into your seat. Feel your body make contact with the chair or cushion. Notice your breath and begin to focus on the sensations of your belly rising and falling or the sensations of the air as it enters and leaves your nostrils with each inhalation and exhalation. Once the body and mind have settled somewhat, you'll probably find that thoughts appear. When the thoughts arise, label them silently before letting them go. You don't need very many categories. You might choose labels such as "planning," "doubting," "judging," "fantasizing," obsessing," or "criticizing." The particular labels aren't crucial; what matters is using them to avoid being captured by stories or repetitive tapes. Once you label a thought, gently bring your attention back to the breath.

If you find that your attention is repeatedly carried away by particular stories, try making up a humorous label for them. Give these *greatest hits* their own names, such as your "I blew it again" tape, "I can't get no respect" tape, "I never get what I want" tape, and so on.

You can make this a consistent part of your meditation practice if you find that your mind regularly gets swept away by depressive thoughts. It also works well to gain perspective on the obsessive, anxious thoughts that sometimes accompany agitated moods.

The next time Miriam saw Marty, she confronted him with how hurt and angry she felt. He did not respond well. He got defensive and angry,

---

*Available in audio at *www.mindfulness-solution.com*.

telling her she was too demanding and that's why she had hardly any friends.

Miriam was crushed. Negative thoughts came rushing in: "He's right." "Nobody likes to be around me." "It's hopeless." "I'll never have any real friends." Feeling herself sinking, she tried meditating some more.

Initially she returned to the *Noting Emotions in the Body* practice. She again felt her sadness, but found it harder to connect with anger at Marty. The negative thoughts really captured her attention. She saw herself being carried away by a very dark river.

To get her bearings and keep from drowning, Miriam started taking time throughout the day to do the *Taking Refuge in Present Sensations* practice. Periodically noticing that her thoughts weren't the only reality—that there was also the reality of touch, sight, sound, and smell—kept her afloat. She also did more formal meditation practice, emphasizing *Thought Labeling*. This helped her believe a little less in her self-doubting and self-critical thoughts. She realized that the cascade of negativity had been triggered by Marty's reaction and the thoughts arose most when her rage at him diminished. This prompted her to examine more carefully her reluctance to be with the anger.

Thought Labeling is only one of several ways to gain perspective on our thinking. In the last chapter you practiced letting thoughts come and go like clouds in the sky or bubbles in a stream using the *Thoughts Are Just Thoughts* practice. Yet another way to support this attitude is through *Listening Meditation*. (We did a few minutes of this at the end of the first breath meditation.) You might try this exercise too, either right now or as part of your regular meditation sessions, as another way to lighten the grip of depressive thoughts:

Listening Meditation*

Begin again with settling into your seat and focusing on your breath. Once the body and mind have calmed down, start to shift your attention from the breath to the sounds around you. Allow the sensations of breath to be in the background, while bringing your attention to whatever strikes your ears. Try to just hear the sound vibrations as you might listen to a symphony or the sounds of the ocean. You're

---

*Available in audio at *www.mindfulness-solution.com*.

not trying to identify what you hear (a bird, the heating system, etc.) but rather to take it in as a sensual experience, like music.

Listening meditation can have an interesting effect on our relationship to thoughts. Some cognitive scientists have long speculated that what we call "thinking" is actually a relatively new human acquisition. Examining ancient writing, they hypothesize that until Homer's time most people described what we call "thinking" as hearing voices from gods or spirits. If we take a moment to examine how we experience "thought," we realize that it involves words forming silently in our minds. Count to five silently right now and you'll see what I mean. Really, close your eyes and try it. Notice how the numbers appear as a voice "speaking" inside your head? Young children often describe their thoughts as "voices"—as though coming from a cartoon angel or devil standing on their shoulders that tells them to do something good or bad.

When we practice listening meditation, we identify with awareness itself in the hearing realm. This transfers nicely to "listening" to thoughts as though they were just sounds—like voices from the outside that we needn't heed. We come to see thoughts and their attendant emotions as passing events like sounds, sights, smells, tastes, and touch sensations. This helps to keep them from drowning out other experiences.

Loving the Demons to Death

Sometimes, despite trying to ground ourselves in sensual reality and let thoughts come and go, we still find ourselves caught up in harsh and judgmental thoughts about ourselves. After all, the judging mind is especially frisky when we're depressed. Good/bad, adequate/inadequate, lovable/unlovable, smart/stupid: every action invites an evaluation—and we usually give ourselves bad grades.

When this tendency is particularly strong, you may find it useful to do some *Loving-Kindness Meditation* to generate some compassion toward yourself and your emotional predicament. As described in Chapter 4, this can be done in different ways. You can begin by generating kind feelings toward another person first or begin with yourself. You can modify the phrases to fit your current situation. For example, to deal with a judgmental mind you might repeat, "May I be happy, may I be peaceful, may I be free from suffering ... may I be kind to myself" or "may I accept myself just as I am." The idea is to gently challenge a harsh stance toward ourselves by generating some self-compassion. Of course, as we discussed earlier, paradoxical effects may arise in which you find yourself arguing that you really don't deserve kindness. Should that happen, just accept those thoughts as well and return your attention to directing caring intentions toward yourself. (For additional techniques to develop self-compassion, you might wish to look at my friend and colleague Christopher Germer's book, *The Mindful Path to Self-Compassion: Freeing Yourself from Destructive Thoughts and Emotions.*)

Taking refuge in the present moment

Becoming aware of your emotional states, seeing how they influence your thinking, learning to take your thoughts more lightly, and developing self-compassion can go a long way toward keeping depression at bay. There are times, however, when you may still get totally caught in a mind storm of negative thought. These are the moments when mindfulness would be most useful. They are also the moments when it's typically most difficult to set aside time to meditate formally or even use routine activities as opportunities for informal practice.

The developers of MBCT teach their patients a brief, simple exercise designed to boost perspective in these moments. Many people find that it works well as an anchor in stormy times—including when we're in danger of doing something impulsive out of desperation. It can also help when we feel confused or sense that something is bothering us but we're not sure what it is. The exercise is designed to help us identify less with our thoughts, experience directly whatever is happening right now in our mind and body, and face whatever is difficult. The idea is first to practice the technique on a schedule, perhaps a few times a day, and then to have it handy whenever needed. Since it is a very brief formal practice, you can use it as a "time-out" from difficult situations. The technique has three parts:

--------------- *Three-Minute Breathing Space* ---------------

Step 1: Becoming Aware

Begin by deliberately adopting an erect and dignified posture, either sitting or standing. If possible, close your eyes. Then, bringing your awareness to your inner experience, ask: What is my experience right now?

- What *thoughts* are going through the mind? Notice them as passing mental events.
- What *feelings* are here? Turn your attention in particular toward any emotional discomfort or unpleasant feelings.
- What *body sensations* are here right now? Scan the body quickly to notice any tightness or bracing.

Step 2: Gathering

Bring your attention to the breath—notice that if all is well, you are already breathing. Notice the belly rising on an in-breath and falling on the out-breath. Try to follow it closely for a few cycles to further bring your attention into the present.

Step 3: Expanding

Now expand your awareness beyond your breath to take in a sense of your body as a whole, including your posture and facial expression. Notice and breathe into any areas of tension, as you did during the *Body Scan Meditation*. Allow your body to soften and open. You might suggest to yourself, "It's okay … whatever it is, it's already here: let me feel it."

As best you can, bring this accepting awareness into the next moments of your day.

Adapted from Mark Williams, John Teasdale, Zindel Segal, & Jon Kabat-Zinn, *The Mindful Way through Depression: Freeing Yourself from Chronic Unhappiness*. New York: The Guilford Press (2007, pp. 183–184). Copyright 2007 by The Guilford Press. Adapted by permission.

The idea of this exercise is not to make unpleasant feelings go away, but to increase our capacity to bear them. It does this by shifting our attention from the story about our experience to the reality of the present moment and using a short break from activity to remind us we can be aware of our present experience with acceptance. It is a brief opportunity to take refuge in the present moment. The *Three-Minute Breathing Space* combines elements of the other practices into a life preserver that can be very handy when we feel desperate.

Entering the dark places

Our attempts to avoid anxiety can actually trap us in it. Trying to avoid difficult emotions can also contribute to depression. These are good reasons to want to open to unpleasant feelings. But another compelling reason to venture into our most difficult emotions is to become fully alive and experience the joys and wonder of life—to live all the ups along with the downs. If you do enough formal mindfulness practice (as the story of my first retreat illustrates), difficult feelings are likely to start to arise on their own. But when you feel prepared explore further, you can also intentionally invite these feelings into your daily practice.

For a variety of reasons, it's not easy to face painful emotions. Most of us learn to hide negative moods from a very young age. Your parents may have tried to cheer you up when you were sad or angry, inadvertently sending the message that something was very wrong if you felt down. Or perhaps they were concerned about appearances and made it clear that moping or expressing anger was unattractive or impolite. Among peers, too, most of us get the message that only losers have bad moods. After all, if you were successful, you'd feel good. If you had a hot boyfriend or girlfriend, were good at sports and academics, and were popular, why would you be sad or angry? This brings out our hardwired desire to look good in the eyes of others—to try to raise our rank in the primate troop. Almost everyone fakes happiness at times to keep up an image. "How are you?" people ask. "Fine, thank you," we answer. (Again, some people go further and give that really obnoxious reply designed to make everyone else feel bad: "*Awesome!*")

Emotional freedom—freedom from the fear of loneliness, despair, rage, or self-hate—depends on overcoming this conditioning. Here, deliberately approaching difficult emotions can really make a difference. As with the *Stepping into Fear* exercise in the last chapter, however, you need to figure out whether you feel safe enough at the moment to take this on. It probably doesn't make sense to do when particularly depressed or isolated. But if you're ready to further tackle increasing your capacity to bear difficult feelings, set aside about 20 minutes for the following meditation. You can try it instead of one of your regular formal practice sessions. The exercise is especially helpful when you sense some sadness in the background to which you haven't fully connected—perhaps because you've been keeping busy to avoid it:

*Stepping into Sadness**

Begin with a few minutes of silent meditation, focusing on the breath. Do this first with your eyes closed. Once you feel as though you've settled into your body, pick up the book again and read the rest of the instructions:

Now that you've attended to your breath for a little while, if your mind can focus somewhat, scan the body for sensations associated with sadness. If you can't find any, try thinking of something that usually makes you sad. Bring your attention to the sensations and see if you can notice them in detail—sensing their form and texture. Do this for a minute or two.

Once you've located the sensations of sadness, see if you can make them grow. You can do this either by just continuing to focus on them in the body or by generating sad images or thoughts. The idea is to ramp the feelings up to their maximum intensity so you can work on increasing your capacity to bear them. Spend several minutes doing this before reading on.

Now that you've developed a clear experience of sadness, try intensifying it further. Try to make it as strong as you can while sitting here holding this book. Fear not; this is safe. If tears come, just let them flow. It's only a feeling, and it won't last forever.

---

*Available in audio at *www.mindfulness-solution.com*.

Once the feeling of sadness reaches its maximum intensity, try to stay with it. Do this for another 10 minutes. Note when impulses arise to move away from the sadness and how you respond to these.

Now that you've practiced being with sadness, you can bring your attention back to your breath for a few more minutes and feel what this is like before you open your eyes.

What did you notice? Like the *Stepping into Fear* exercise, this one usually brings up different reactions in different people at different times. Sometimes it's hard to generate sad feelings; other times they come readily. Sometimes an impulse to pull away from the sadness arises. Many people feel afraid that the feelings will be too deep or last too long. But staying with the exercise usually reveals that sadness, like fear, is self-limiting. In fact, it can be difficult to maintain sadness at its peak throughout the whole exercise. Practicing this from time to time, especially when we sense ourselves avoiding sadness, can make it easier to approach.

A related practice can help you get over an aversion to anger. On another occasion, if you're feeling ready to explore other intense feelings, try the *Stepping into Anger* exercise. This, too, can be done in place of a regular formal mindfulness practice period. It's done in exactly the same way, only substituting anger for sadness. The exercise can be useful if you sense anger or annoyance in the background to which you haven't fully connected. Like the other *Stepping Into* practices, it demonstrates that angry feelings are not actually dangerous. While they can be intense, they, too, are self-limiting—especially when welcomed.

Once you've had opportunities to try both *Stepping into Sadness* and *Stepping into Anger*, notice how they are different for you. Was one easier? Was one more unnerving? We tend to vary in our comfort with different feelings, and trying these practices is another way to gain insight into this.

A variation on these exercises, designed to cultivate compassion for others while increasing our own capacity to open to psychological pain, is called *Tonglen Practice*. It is an ancient form of meditation developed in Tibet. Like *Loving-Kindness Meditation*, this can be practiced with a focus on either other people or ourselves initially. Also like loving-kindness practice, you may find it helpful to integrate this regularly into a period of formal practice. While loving-kindness practice is a good antidote to excessively critical thoughts, this practice can be particularly useful when we are feeling sad or angry.

Tonglen Practice*

Begin by finding a meditative posture, settling into your seat, and breathing. Next generate in your mind an image of someone you know is suffering right now—if you are working with sadness, anger, or depression, you might focus on someone who is particularly sad, angry, or despairing. With every in-breath, imagine breathing in the pain of the suffering person, and with every out-breath send the person peace, happiness, or whatever you imagine would alleviate his or her suffering. The idea is to fully take in the pain of the other and to practice being with it while sending out a loving intention toward him or her.

Like the *Stepping Into* exercises, this practice goes against our usual instinct. Instead of trying to get away from negative emotions, we practice taking them in, being with them wholeheartedly. It has the added advantage of connecting us with other people, which can help us feel "held" in difficult moments.

During times when you're feeling a lot of psychological pain, you may find a variation of this practice easier: Imagine breathing in your own difficult feelings while simultaneously breathing in the pain of the millions of others on the planet who are feeling the same stuckness or discomfort at this very moment. As you breathe out, send yourself and all the others peace, happiness, or whatever else you and they might need.

While Miriam felt her meditation was helping her get some perspective on her negative thoughts, she was feeling very isolated after her encounter with Marty. His comments made her feel like a reject. She had done *Tonglen Practice* before and hoped that it might help her feel less

---

*Available in audio at *www.mindfulness-solution.com*.

alone with her pain. Still feeling pretty fragile, she tried breathing in her own suffering along with that of others and breathing out love and care. She imagined all of the people who felt isolated and rejected at this very moment, including those who were worse off than her. Images of abandoned children, widows and widowers, invalids in nursing homes, and refugees came to mind. They were joined by jilted lovers, laid-off workers, and failing students. She breathed in their pain along with her own and breathed out kindness, care, and love. It was painful. Tears came to her eyes. But it also felt somehow "right." The practice seemed to loosen the grip of her self-critical patter while making her feel less alone.

In *Tonglen* and the other practices, the idea is to welcome and make friends with all emotions, including the painful ones. A classic poem from the 13th-century Persian poet Rumi captures the attitude beautifully:

The Guest House

This being human is a guest house.
Every morning a new arrival.

A joy, a depression, a meanness,
some momentary awareness comes
as an unexpected visitor.

Welcome and entertain them all!
Even if they're a crowd of sorrows,
who violently sweep your house
empty of its furniture,
still, treat each guest honorably.
He may be clearing you out
for some new delight.

The dark thought, the shame, the malice,
meet them at the door laughing,
and invite them in.

Be grateful for whoever comes,
because each has been sent
as a guide from beyond.

From Coleman Barks and John Moyne, *The Essential Rumi* (San Francisco: Harper, 1997). Originally published by Threshold Books. Copyright 1995 by Coleman Barks and John Moyne. Reprinted with permission from Coleman Barks (trans.).

As we are able to welcome emotions—including negative ones—everything becomes workable. The very act of turning our attention toward difficult experiences gives us a sense that we'll be able to deal with them. We shift from striving to feel good to trying to awaken to whatever we're actually feeling in the moment. Ironically, it can be a real relief to be liberated from the tyranny of needing to be in a good mood.

Depression as an opportunity

Emotional freedom is a pretty compelling reason to want to explore our most difficult feelings. But being more mindful of sadness and depression can open another door—one that leads to a more meaningful life. As you know, the disconnection that comes with depression can make existence feel pretty empty. It's only natural as depression deepens to ask, "What really matters?" Cut off from feeling alive, our first answer is often "Nothing." If, however, we investigate further, we have the opportunity to reconnect with our most deeply held values.

In the hubbub of daily life, most of us overlook the question. Much of the time we're so busy trying to get to the next moment of pleasure and avoid the next moment of pain that we don't think about what really matters. When we're depressed, these pursuits don't work so well—we're not so easily entertained. Depression also tends to slow us down, to disengage us from our frenetic pace. As a result, depression can open us to the possibility of reflection and redirection.

Exploring depression can help us find out what really matters to us.

When we're depressed, we also notice a lot of things that we otherwise ignore. We see the reality of loss. We realize that we can't really hold on to anything, that our attempts to do so are like grasping at Jell-O. We notice ourselves aging, our lives slipping by. We recognize that we are actually going to die.

These realizations can be powerful motivators to turn our attention toward what matters. Because our energy is usually low when we are depressed, we might think, "I'll start to live differently once I feel better." An alternative, however, is to use our greater awareness of life's brevity to engage right now, to orient our attention toward what matters most.

My friend and colleague Stephanie Morgan points out that asking ourselves fundamental questions can help with depressed moods. Take a moment right now to think about where you find meaning in life. You may find it helpful to jot down your answers.

WHAT REALLY MATTERS?

What is your heart's desire?

_____

_____

_____

What truly matters to you?

_____

_____

_____

Given whatever time you have left on this planet, how would you most like to live it?

_____

_____

_____

Adapted from Stephanie P. Morgan, "Depression: Turning toward Life," in Christopher K. Germer, Ronald D. Siegel, and Paul R. Fulton (Eds.), *Mindfulness and Psychotherapy* (New York: Guilford Press, 2005). Copyright 2005 by The Guilford Press. Adapted by permission.

What came to mind? For most people, the answers lie in connection—connection to other people, connection to nature, or connection to some talent or interest. Sometimes this is expressed in religious terms as connection to God, soul, or spirit. It almost always includes moving beyond preoccupation with "me." We spend an inordinate amount of energy concerned with "me," but in the long run this doesn't give life much meaning—especially given our unfortunate prognosis.

Mindfulness practice can provide a way to focus our attention on what gives our life meaning. Attending to what is actually happening, including its pleasant and unpleasant aspects, helps us reconnect to the world outside of ourselves. We also see firsthand how our attempts at distraction only leave us feeling more disconnected, and we taste the alternative of connecting to what is happening in the moment. As we'll see in Chapter 8, mindfulness can also help us see the futility of being preoccupied with "me," making it easier to connect to others.

The Dark Night of the Soul

Most of the world's psychological and spiritual traditions describe a phase in development when things fall apart. Our views about our identity and our plans for the future get disrupted and we no longer know who we are or where we're going. We resist these crises, since they're both painful and disorienting. But they almost always open the door for greater flexibility and awareness.

The first challenge in entering such a state is dealing with our fear of it. For reasons mentioned earlier, most of us resist dark moods not just because they're painful, but also because we associate them with failure. We don't want others to know about them and fear that they wouldn't want to be near us if they knew how bad we felt. We can feel toxic and contagious, afraid that our bad mood will bring others down.

Mindfulness practice allows us instead to approach our negative moods with interest and curiosity. It can help us not fear despair. Instead, we can turn toward our distress and ask, "What is this? What can I observe about the workings of the mind while in this mood?" Sometimes this leads to important insights into who we are.

The thoughts that go through our minds all day define who we think we are, who others are, and what life is about. They are shaped by our personal and cultural history—and tend to limit our flexibility. For example, if I think of myself as an intelligent, kind, generous man, I'll have difficulty acknowledging the parts of me that are confused, angry, and greedy. I'll also be judgmental about those attributes when I see them in you. During a moment of psychological crisis, however, I may notice just how confused, angry, and greedy I am too. While this may initially be disruptive and depressing, it also offers me the opportunity to develop a broader sense of who I am. I might actually come to realize that I'm an intelligent, kind, generous man sometimes, but sometimes not. In the long run, this will make me a wiser person and better able to connect to others.

If we can open to our depressive crisis as an interesting development—an opportunity to see how our mind works and how we generate beliefs—it can contribute to our awakening. My experience on an

Mindfulness during a psychological crisis can help us accept the parts of ourselves we may not like—and thereby make us less judgmental toward others.

intensive retreat after losing my girlfriend taught me a lot about how I managed emotions and who I really was. Miriam's struggle to deal with her reactions to Marty helped her connect with important feelings, gain perspective on her thoughts, and sense her common ground with others. These were not isolated experiences. Taking the time to really be with and explore difficult feelings can be freeing for anyone.

Putting it all together

Because sadness and depression visit us in so many forms for so many different reasons, there is no single best way to work with them. Nonetheless, certain broad principles can guide us. All of the exercises presented in this chapter assume that you've established a regular mindfulness practice of the sort described in Chapters 3 and 4. Depending on your commitments, hopefully you can do informal mindfulness practice daily and formal practice at least a few times each week.

Next, attend to the difference between sadness and depression in your own experience. Sadness tends to be fluid, alive, and poignant—if we have the good sense to embrace it. Depression, on the other hand, usually feels dead, static, and alienating. Because our attempts to avoid or banish sadness and other emotions can trap us in depression, it's important to systematically make friends with all feelings.

Try to pay attention when they naturally arise throughout your day. The simplest way is with the *Noting Emotions in the Body* practice. Periodically sense whatever emotions are present and observe their effects on your body. Allow yourself in particular to experience how they feel in your face, throat, chest, and belly. Focusing on the sensations in the body connected with emotions will counteract any tendency to pull away from them. If you have difficulty with this, you might return to the *Surveying Emotions in the Body* chart to practice observing the body sensations that correspond to each emotion. This will make it easier to identify feelings as they arise.

Sometimes feelings are so blocked that we are completely unaware of them. Completing the *Observing Emotions throughout the Day* chart over the course of several days can provide important clues about where to look. Any emotion that doesn't appear is worthy of exploration.

Should you notice feelings that are absent or that you tend to ignore or resist, you might try the *Stepping Into* exercises to become more comfortable with them. Since these practices purposely amplify negative emotions, it's best to use them when feeling supported or otherwise ready for a challenge rather than when feeling overwhelmed. The *Stepping into Sadness* exercise can help when you sense yourself avoiding sad feelings (perhaps by staying busy) or cutting off tears (perhaps trying to be "strong"). You can try it in place of one or more of your formal practice periods.

Unacknowledged anger is a big problem for many people. Because anger threatens to disrupt relationships and get us into trouble, many of us try not to feel (much less express) it. If you sense that this is the case for you, try the *Stepping into Anger* exercise. Don't be alarmed if you notice a reservoir of rage like the one I discovered during my first meditation retreat—these are more common than most of us expect. As you become more comfortable with anger, you can connect with it and other emotions during the day using the *Noting Emotions in the Body* practice.

Some people only use the *Stepping Into* exercises once or twice just to see for themselves that sadness and anger are bearable and self-limiting. Others find them helpful to revisit periodically to re-welcome these feelings. With a little experimentation, you'll discover for yourself how to best use them.

Countering the Thinking Disease

While getting comfortable with your emotions is almost always helpful, depending on your history and circumstances, you may still fall into depression from time to time. Unlike sadness, depression usually includes self-critical, pessimistic thinking. If you find yourself caught in such negative rumination, there are several techniques to try. Begin with the *Noting How Thoughts Change* exercise to remind yourself that thoughts really can't be trusted—they vary with our emotional weather. Then periodically throughout your day do the *Taking Refuge in Present Sensations* practice to shift your attention out of your thoughts and into sensory reality. During formal practice periods, experiment with *Thought Labeling* and *Listening Meditation*. Both of these help us not take our thoughts so seriously and gain perspective on how they arise and pass. Finally, if your thoughts are particularly self-critical, be sure to include *Loving-Kindness Meditation* as part of your formal practice to cultivate self-acceptance.

Throw Yourself a Life Preserver

Becoming aware and accepting of emotions and putting thoughts into perspective can go a long way toward lessening the overall grip of depressive moods. Nonetheless, there may still be moments when they overwhelm you. The *Three-Minute Breathing Space* can be used when these occur. It's best to practice this first when you're not overwhelmed so that you can have it handy when you need it. Remember—the idea is not to get rid of difficult feelings, but rather to notice your thoughts, connect to your emotions as they appear in the body, and remind yourself that you can open to and accept whatever is happening in the moment.

In addition to using the *Three-Minute Breathing Space* during overwhelming moments throughout the day, you might also try the *Tonglen Practice* in place of your usual formal meditation. During rough periods it helps to include yourself in the breathing out of peace, healing, or whatever you and others suffering with you may need at the moment. *Nature Meditation* (Chapter 5) and *Taking Refuge in Present Sensations* can also help to draw you out of your thought stream when you are feeling overwhelmed—into the safety of the moment and the wider world.

Finally, to take advantage of the potential of depression for psychological or spiritual growth, allow yourself to reflect on what really matters to you and what old beliefs, self-images, or attachments you might relinquish. Indeed, your troubles might, as Rumi suggested, be "clearing you out for some new delight"—even if it doesn't feel like this at the moment.

Think of all these exercises as parts of a tool kit. By experimenting, you'll discover how each affects you at different times. As long as you're working to allow yourself to feel a full range of emotion and not believe too strongly in your thoughts, mindfulness practice can help you find your way through both sadness and depression.

While your own path will undoubtedly be different, here is how this unfolded for Gail:

On the outside, Gail had a good childhood. She grew up in a nice suburb with two successful parents, a younger brother, and an older sister. Her conservative, churchgoing family was well respected in the community. She dressed nicely, went to a good school, and got good grades.

Beneath the surface, however, all was not well. Her sister, Paula, was a year older, very pretty, and very popular. Gail looked up to her and wanted to play with Paula and her friends. But Paula would have none of it. In fact, she took every opportunity she could to reject Gail, call her ugly and stupid, and persuade her friends to join in the fun.

Things got particularly bad when they got to middle school. Time and again Paula and her friends went out of their way to humiliate Gail.

Desperate for friendship, Gail gravitated to an older girl in the neighborhood who was also something of an outsider. Their relationship eventually became sexual—bringing Gail great comfort but, because of her religious background, great shame.

One day Gail's world imploded. Paula walked in on her kissing her friend. Disgusted (and secretly delighted), Paula told their parents, who got predictably upset and barred Gail from ever seeing the girl again.

Gail remained a loner during both high school and college. She felt like a "reject" and was secretly ashamed of her early sexual relationship. While she continued to do well in school, she was slow to date and insecure about her looks, and assumed that other kids wouldn't like her.

These feelings lasted into her 20s, when she came to see me. She wasn't sleeping well, got little joy from her work, felt agitated, and still had few friends. Gail was now interested in men but remained conflicted about romance and sex. Despite being bright, thoughtful, and physically attractive, she couldn't believe that any men really liked her. She had casual sex, thinking it was the only way to keep them interested. Relationships ended painfully.

Gail sought me out because she was interested in mindfulness meditation. It had made her feel more relaxed, and she was impressed by the kindness of the teacher who taught her meditation class. When we met, she had already begun noticing how emotions can be observed in the body and was hopeful that this might make them less overwhelming to her.

After getting a sense of her history and current situation, we began looking at her relationship to different emotions. She became aware that after a relationship ended she quickly "put it out of my mind" so as not to sink into depression. We discussed how, by blocking out feelings, she might be contributing to her depression.

Once she began to trust me, we tried the *Stepping into Sadness* exercise. At first Gail didn't feel much, but after staying with it for a while, she found that her sadness felt like "a deep lake" that she was afraid to enter. I encouraged her to risk it, and while plenty of tears came, she discovered that the sadness was bearable.

On another occasion we tried the *Stepping into Anger* exercise. This was even more frightening, since despite her disappointments Gail wanted to think of herself as a "good girl"—not an angry woman. It didn't take long to discover that the image of Paula worked beautifully to bring up anger. As she started to amplify it, memories of middle school returned, and a feeling of rage "like a nuclear bomb" welled up.

After experimenting with these emotions in the office, Gail found it easier to notice them the rest of the time. She realized that she was very often either sad or angry—but didn't want to be.

Because her mind was filled with self-critical, insecure thoughts, I encouraged her to notice how different her thoughts about herself were on "good" days than on "bad" ones using the *How Thoughts Change* exercise. I suggested she try the *Taking Refuge in Present Sensations* practice when negative thoughts intruded. Since she was already grounded in meditation, this came easily to her. She had already been exposed to *Thought Labeling, Listening Meditation,* and *Loving-Kindness Meditation* (Chapter 4) in her meditation class, so it was also easy for her to integrate these into her daily practice.

Not surprisingly, Gail noticed that her depressive moods were triggered whenever she felt rejected. Often she would react impulsively, saying or doing things she later regretted. I suggested that she try the *Three-Minute Breathing Space* when she felt overwhelmed and compelled to act. This helped her tune in to her thoughts and feelings and feel "held" for a few moments before she said or did anything rash.

Gail's general mindfulness practice along with these exercises helped. She began to see that it wasn't external events that were making her so miserable, but her thoughts about them. She saw how she had come to really believe distorted ideas about herself that were established in childhood and began to appreciate that they might not represent "reality." She also became freer to cry and express her anger when hurt.

In the process, Gail also explored what really mattered to her. She saw that above all she wanted to be able to love and be loved without so much fear. She became aware of many ways that she'd been dishonest— trying to sound cool, acting sophisticated, or exaggerating accomplishments—so that people would like her. She grew interested instead in being forthright with others and forming genuine connections.

Gail's depression makes a lot of sense given her history. So far, her story has not ended happily ever after. But she now sees her situation as workable, feels like she is on a good path, and is grateful to her mindfulness practice for helping her walk along it.

Mindfulness practices for depression

Once you establish a regular formal and informal practice as described in Chapters 3 and 4, you can try the following:

Formal Meditation Practices

- *Noting Emotions in the Body* (page 145) to bring unacknowledged emotions into awareness
- *Stepping into Sadness* (page 160) when you notice resistance to sadness
- *Stepping into Anger* (page 161) when you notice resistance to anger
- *Taking Refuge in Present Sensations* (page 153) to anchor attention in the world outside of depressive thoughts
- *Thought Labeling* (page 154) to gain perspective on streams of depressive thoughts
- *Listening Meditation* (page 155) or *Thoughts Are Just Thoughts* (page 125) to practice letting go of depressive thoughts
- *Loving-Kindness Meditation* (page 84) to soothe self-critical chatter
- *Tonglen Practice* (page 162) when feeling isolated with sadness or disappointment

Informal Practices

All of these help to loosen the pull of depressive rumination by bringing attention back to sensory experience in the present:

- *Walking Meditation* (page 67)
- *Nature Meditation* (page 128)
- *Eating Meditation* (page 263)
- *Driving, Showering, Tooth Brushing, Shaving (etc.) Meditation* (page 90)

Life Preservers

- *Three-Minute Breathing Space* (page 162) when feeling overwhelmed by depressive thoughts and feelings, particularly if tempted to do something impulsive
- *Taking Refuge in Present Sensations* (page 153) to bring attention to the safety of the world outside of depressive thoughts
- *Tonglen Practice* (page 162) when feeling isolated by sadness or disappointment
- *Nature Meditation* (formal or informal; page 128) when feeling isolated or overwhelmed

Developing a plan

You may find it useful to jot down an action plan for working with depressive thoughts and feelings. The following chart can help you organize your thoughts:

PRACTICE PLAN

Begin by reflecting on how and when depression arises in your life.

Situations in Which I Most Often Feel Depressed: _____

_____

_____

_____

My Most Common Depression Symptoms:

Physical: _____

_____

Cognitive (negative thoughts): _____

_____

Behavioral (things I do or avoid compulsively): _____

_____

Times I Most Need a Life Preserver: _____

_____

_____

Now, based on what you've read about and experienced with the different practices, jot down an initial practice plan (you can vary this as your needs change).

(cont.)

Formal Practice	When	How Often
_____	_____	_____
_____	_____	_____
_____	_____	_____

Informal Practice	When	How Often
_____	_____	_____
_____	_____	_____
_____	_____	_____

Life Preserver	Likely Situation
_____	_____
_____	_____
_____	_____

Might I benefit from psychotherapy, medication, or other approaches?

When depression becomes either long-lasting or severe, additional help is a good idea. This is especially true when the symptoms of depression cause more depression. When a depressed mood keeps you from functioning at work or school or cuts you off from friends or family, you can get stuck in a vicious cycle. Life will indeed be depressing if you are unemployed and friendless. It's important to interrupt this cycle. Depression can even be dangerous if you become suicidal or otherwise self-destructive. These are times when no one should try to go it alone.

While psychotherapy comes in a number of forms, just having the opportunity to talk honestly with someone about your situation usually helps. You can feel so isolated when depressed; connecting with someone who is actively trying to understand your experience can be enormously useful. You may wish to find a therapist who is familiar with mindfulness practice and mindfulness-oriented treatment. Don't be afraid to ask about this. Some therapists will tend to work more in the present, helping you observe your thinking and moods. Others will look more into your past, to understand why your current circumstances are bringing up particular feelings. As Gail's story illustrates, both approaches can be useful. Most important is that you feel as though you can be honest with a therapist and can share your observation about what is helpful in your work together. Further suggestions for finding a therapist can be found in the Resources at the back of this book.

Medication can also play a useful role in working with depression. If you have a family history of the problem, it can help to offset any biological predisposition you may have toward becoming depressed. Even if you don't have this history, medication tends to provide a "floor" under your mood so that you don't sink too deep. This can help you continue to function while learning to work with your thoughts and feelings.

Though the thrust of this chapter has been about learning to approach and *be with* difficult experience, balance and common sense are important. In one interesting study, meditators taking antidepressant medication felt that it supported their meditation practice, making it easier not to get completely caught in self-critical thought streams. The goal in using medication along with mindfulness practice and psychotherapy is to help you function fully and maintain perspective while still having access to a full range of emotion. In this way all of your efforts support one another and contribute to living a rich and rewarding life.

If you are currently struggling with significant depression, or have in the past, you might also want to get a copy of a self-treatment book written by the designers of MBCT, *The Mindful Way through Depression*. This book expands on some of what we've been discussing here and presents a program that has been shown to be effective in reducing the likelihood of recurrent bouts of serious depression. It can be used alone or as an adjunct to both psychotherapy and medication. Other helpful guides are listed in the Resources at the back of this book.

The approaches described in the last two chapters can help you work effectively with all sorts of distressing states of mind. But of course it's not just our minds that are unruly—our bodies give us trouble as well. In the next chapter we'll look at how to use mindfulness practices to deal with a colorful assortment of common physical ailments.

CHAPTER 7

Beyond managing
symptoms

*Transforming pain
and stress-related medical problems*

I t's a beautiful summer evening. You're sitting on the porch watching the sunset, getting ready to enjoy a glass of wine. Everything is bathed in a wonderful light. Looking forward to relaxing, you wonder if you might have just heard a faint sound. "Nah—it was just my imagination." A minute later it becomes more distinct: "zzzzzzzzzzzzzzzzzzzz." And then louder: "ZZZZZZZZZZZZZZZZZZ." Damn. They're here. In no time at all you're quixotically swatting at the air, becoming more and more agitated. Defeated, you give up and go inside.

Now, mosquito bites aren't really that painful and aren't that dangerous either (except for regional outbreaks of West Nile virus or eastern equine encephalitis, and a few exotic tropical diseases). But concern about being bitten can still ruin an evening. Have you ever gone camping and had a mosquito join you in the tent? One very small insect can cause a lot of suffering.

Once, when on a silent meditation retreat, we were instructed to experiment with mosquitoes. If one landed on us, we were invited to just allow it to feast. There was very little sensation when my first guest touched down. I could hardly even feel when the mosquito stuck its proboscis into my skin, injected anticoagulant to keep my blood from clotting, and filled its belly. It was actually very interesting to see it swell up, turn red, and fly away. A few minutes later the itching began, but even that wasn't disturbing as long as I just attended to the sensations without resisting them. While I didn't realize it at the time, watching a mosquito eat held the key to dealing successfully with a host of medical problems.

One cause, many ailments

Nobody likes pain or illness. Throughout history people have gone to great lengths to avoid them—by performing rituals, gathering medicinal plants, praying to gods, or more recently developing modern hygiene and medicine. Despite our best efforts, we're still visited regularly by both.

Some pain and illness is unavoidable, and some can be prevented with thought and care. A remarkable amount of pain and illness, however, is actually caused by our attempts to get rid of it. Like the psychological difficulties we've been discussing, a lot of physical disorders result unwittingly from our efforts to avoid unpleasant experience—in essence, from swatting at mosquitoes. Stress—our reaction to things we don't like—is at the heart of all of these problems.

The range of medical conditions that are either caused or exacerbated by stress is remarkable. Depending on the criteria used, some 60–90% of all physician visits are for stress-related disorders. Take a moment to see how many of these have afflicted you at one time or another (please use the inventory on the following page).

While each of these conditions can have many causes, they all can result from or be exacerbated by psychological processes. Foremost among those processes is our tendency to reject unpleasant experiences. Because this propensity is often central to the ailments listed above, mindfulness can help resolve them.

The strange case of chronic back pain

Chronic back pain offers a good example of how this works. I got involved in treating this condition through a personal encounter that shed light on both what causes the problem and how mindfulness practice can help resolve it. As we'll see, it turns out that the principles involved in understanding and treating chronic back pain can also help us deal with a wide range of other pain problems and stress-related medical disorders.

In the late 1980s I spent four miserable months flat on my back with

A STRESS-RELATED MEDICAL INVENTORY

Place a check mark next to each of these symptoms you have experienced.

- Recurrent headaches (_____)
- Heartburn or sour stomach (_____)
- Intestinal cramping (_____)
- Unexplained diarrhea or constipation (_____)
- Chronic neck pain (_____)
- Chronic back pain (_____)
- Chronic pelvic pain (_____)
- Difficulty sleeping (_____)
- Sexual difficulties: lost erections, premature ejaculation, lack of interest, or difficulty reaching orgasm (_____)
- Persistent itching (_____)
- Eczema or hives (_____)
- Ringing in the ears (tinnitus) (_____)
- Tooth grinding at night (bruxism) (_____)
- Nail biting (_____)
- Jaw pain or tension (TMJ) (_____)
- Unexplained fatigue (_____)
- Frequent colds and sore throats (_____)
- Asthma (_____)

a herniated disk. After working out on a cross-country ski machine, I developed pain and numbness running down my left leg. When it got worse, I sought medical advice and eventually found myself in an orthopedist's office. He did a CT scan, diagnosed the problem as a herniated L5-S1 disk, and recommended bed rest.

Since I was on the faculty of a medical school, I had access to orthopedic texts. I kept these on my nightstand next to my radiology report.

I read repeatedly that the disk might heal with rest—but if it didn't I'd need surgery, which was often unsuccessful. As the days went on, I saw no improvement.

Desperate for a more active approach, I saw a sports medicine specialist. He took a look at my CT scan and told me that if I didn't stay off my feet and avoid sitting, I'd be "begging for surgery" in six months. Not what I wanted to hear.

I was getting so depressed and anxious that I felt I couldn't stay in bed any longer. So I decided to build a platform in my office. Thus began a bizarre parody of the classical psychoanalytic scene—I'd be lying down on a makeshift couch as my patients sat up and wondered about my pathology and prognosis. Driving to work, I'd lean my car seat as far back as I could, barely seeing over the steering wheel, trying to take weight off my spine. It's a miracle that I didn't kill myself or someone else.

After a couple of months my wife, who is also a clinical psychologist, made an observation: "You know, sweetheart, you seem to complain more about the pain whenever we have an argument." You can imagine how much I appreciated her insight. Now not only did I have to suffer with this horrible pain, but I had to endure her psychological theories. I knew better. My pain was due to the disk—after all, I reread my radiology report nightly.

Still trying to be helpful, my wife brought home Norman Cousins's book *Anatomy of an Illness*. Cousins was a famous journalist who had cured himself of degenerative arthritis by taking high doses of vitamin C, watching Marx brothers films, and laughing. It was a very inspirational story but didn't seem relevant. "That's very nice for *Norman*," I told my wife, "but I have a *herniated disk!*"

Around the same time, a friend had been urging me to speak with a mutual professional acquaintance. She had supposedly cured her back problem by treating it as a muscle tension disorder—a reaction to stress. "Here we go again," I thought. "This is my punishment for hanging out with psychotherapists."

Partly out of desperation, partly to get everyone to stop bugging me, I called her.

"What are you doing right now?" she asked.

"Lying down—that's all I ever do."

"Why don't you go out and buy groceries for the family—your wife will appreciate it."

"Great, a feminist conspiracy," I thought. She went on to describe how she had recovered fully from chronic back pain by getting physically active and treating the pain as a muscle tension syndrome rather than an orthopedic problem.

I wasn't about to get groceries, but I was so desperate, I thought I'd try an experiment. At that point, I couldn't walk for more than a block before the pain became intense. So I set out to challenge myself. I walked a block. Right on cue, I felt pain down my left leg. Determined to persevere, I walked another two blocks. To my utter surprise, now not only did I have pain going down my left leg, but I felt it in my right leg also. "That was a brilliant idea," I thought.

Hobbling home, I realized that it actually may have been a good idea after all. According to my radiology report, I should only have pain running down my left leg. If I felt it on the right too, either I'd shattered my spine completely (a hypothesis I entertained), or the pain might be due to something else. Maybe muscle tension *was* at least part of the problem.

I was desperate to get better. I started reading everything I could about stress, muscle tension, and chronic back pain and began moving more even though it hurt. Within a couple of weeks I had removed the platform from my office and was driving more or less normally. Soon I was exercising and doing yoga again. I felt like I had awakened from a very bad dream.

I was so impressed by this experience that I set about to learn what I could about mind–body interactions and the potential of using psychological interventions to help with medical problems. I soon realized that mindfulness practice could be enormously useful in these efforts and began collaborating with area physicians and incorporating it into my work. What I learned studying and treating back pain held the key to using mindfulness practice to work effectively with a surprisingly wide range of stress-related disorders.

Bad Back?

It turns out that the vast majority of chronic back pain is, as in my case, caused by muscle tension, and this tension is maintained by psychological stress. It's necessary to understand this in order to get better. If we believe instead that our pain is due to a damaged disk or other spinal structure, it will be very difficult for us to relax about it and move normally.

While there isn't room here for all the details, let me mention a few of the most compelling pieces of evidence supporting this idea. First, it turns out that the condition of the spine usually has little bearing on whether or not a person is in pain:

- Approximately two-thirds of people who have never suffered serious back pain have the same sorts of "abnormal" back structures, like herniated disks, that are often blamed for chronic back pain.
- Millions of people who suffer chronic back pain show no "abnormalities" in their backs whatsoever, even after extensive testing.
- Many people continue to have pain after "successful" surgical repair. There is little relation between the mechanical success of repairs and whether the patient is still in pain.

Other studies give us clues to the role of psychological stress and muscle tension:

- The worldwide epidemic of chronic back pain is limited mostly to industrialized nations. Remarkably, there is little chronic back pain in developing countries, where people do "backbreaking" labor, use primitive furniture and tools, don't sleep on top-of-the-line Posturepedic mattresses, and drive long distances over rutted roads sitting in the backs of old pickup trucks.
- Psychological stress, and particularly job dissatisfaction, predicts who will develop disabling back pain more reliably than do physical measures or the physical demands of one's job.
- Rapidly returning to full, vigorous, physical activity is usually both safe and the most effective way to resolve back pain episodes.

None of this would make sense if most back pain were caused by herniated disks and other structural problems, but it all makes a lot of sense if back pain is caused by stress and muscle tension.

The Chronic Back Pain Cycle

Emotional stress turns into back pain through a process that my colleagues and I call the *chronic back pain cycle*. It can begin with either an emotional or a physical event. Imagine, for example, that you do some unusually heavy lifting, perhaps putting in an air conditioner in the early summer or shoveling snow at the start of winter. You strain your back, and it begins to hurt. If you happen to live in an industrialized culture with an epidemic of back problems, you might begin to have some worried thoughts: "I hope I didn't injure my back like my cousin did." "I hope I'll be able to go to work tomorrow." If the pain is intense or persistent, these thoughts will begin to make you anxious.

Try a little experiment right now (this will require a bit of dramatic acting—don't be shy). In pantomime, demonstrate with your face and body what fear looks like. Really ham it up. (Don't worry; nobody is watching.) Hold the pose for a few seconds. What do you feel in your body? Which muscles become tense?

You can see here for yourself that fear produces muscle tension. And you know from other experience that muscle tension increases pain. Just think about how much neck muscles can hurt after a stressful day or how painful a charley horse in the calf can be.

So this is how the chronic back pain cycle works. Our initial pain causes worried thoughts, these thoughts create anxiety, and this anxiety causes muscles to tighten. Tight muscles cause increased pain, and increased pain triggers even more dire worried thoughts. Once the cycle sets in, other emotions, such as frustration and anger, get into the act.

Take a moment to do a little more dramatic acting. In pantomime, show first frustration and then anger with your face and body. Really ham it up again. (Nobody is watching now either.) Hold each pose for a few seconds. Notice how these secondary emotions produce even more muscle tension?

The *Back Sense* program

My colleagues and I developed *Back Sense*, a step-by-step treatment program incorporating mindfulness meditation that helps people interrupt this cycle. The program has three basic elements, all of which work best in tandem with mindfulness practice: (1) *understand the problem*, (2) *resume full physical activity*, and (3) *work with negative emotions*. I'll review the program and then show how the same steps along with mindfulness techniques can help with other pain and stress-related physical problems.*

---

*Before beginning the program, it is important to have a thorough physical examination to rule out rare but potentially serious medical causes for pain and to receive a doctor's permission to resume normal activities. Without such permission, it will be very difficult to overcome your fears. Physiatrists (rehabilitation physicians) are good sources for such evaluations, as they are most likely to encourage your return to full movement. The good news is that these rare medical disorders, which include tumors, infections, injuries, and unusual structural abnormalities, are the cause of only about one in 200 cases of chronic back pain.

Step 1: Understand the Problem

As we saw when discussing anxiety and depression, understanding a problem is an important first step in overcoming it. In the case of chronic back pain, we all need to see for ourselves the role that muscle tension is playing. As long as you believe your back is damaged, you'll be afraid to move normally and you'll restrict your movements accordingly. This will make your muscles stiff and weak. It will also keep your fear elevated, which will keep the pain cycle going.

While you can read about back pain and get explanations from doctors, direct observation of the role your mind plays in the problem is really the only way to alter your view. If you're currently suffering from back pain or pain in another part of your body, try this exercise:

MONITORING YOUR WORRIED THOUGHTS

Keep a small notebook with you during the day. Each time you have a worried thought about your back (or other area of concern), put a hash mark in the book. See how many times in the course of each hour one of these thoughts appears.

If you're really struggling, you may find that these thoughts arise every few minutes—or even more frequently when doing things that you fear will aggravate your condition. Noticing this, you can begin to observe the role that fear of pain or discomfort may be playing in the problem. (Similar worried thoughts usually surround other stress-related conditions.)

Mindfulness practice reveals that we can't really trust our thoughts, because they are so strongly colored by both our history and our mood of the moment. Just as our minds fill with self-critical thoughts when we're depressed or fearful thoughts when we're anxious, we have frightened, frustrated, and angry thoughts when in chronic pain. When the pain is more intense, we tend to believe we must have a serious injury; when we hurt less, we can entertain the possibility that our condition may be more workable—it might actually be

> When pain is intense, we tend to believe we're seriously injured. When pain is mild, we're more likely to consider that the problem may be caused by stress.

a muscle tension problem. With mindfulness practice, we come to observe these changes in thought patterns unfolding moment by moment and to see how the negative beliefs increase tension throughout our bodies.

Step 2: Resume Normal Activity

It's essential to resume a normal life to overcome chronic back pain. When you don't move normally, your muscles get weak and you lose flexibility. Also, keeping yourself from moving normally can make you increasingly fearful—anxious whenever you venture outside your comfort range. You may eventually develop *kinesiophobia*, or fear of movement. Just as you could get overwhelmed with anxiety every time you enter a supermarket and therefore start avoiding shopping, you can also be conditioned to get anxious every time you bend, twist, sit, or stand—and restrict your movement accordingly. Should you dare to move, you'll tense up from the fear and naturally experience more pain as a result. You'll then conclude, "This is bad for me—I shouldn't do it," and a pattern of avoidance will set in. In the same way that a person can go from fearing the supermarket to becoming agoraphobic and never leaving the house, a back pain sufferer can progress from avoiding some movements to living as though his or her spine were made of glass.

An important step in overcoming kinesiophobia is taking stock of what you fear. If you are struggling with back or other chronic pain, take a moment now to list on the facing page any activities that you currently avoid or limit because of it.

Chapter 5 explained that the antidote to avoidance patterns is to face our fears and use mindfulness practice to be with the experience that ensues—even if it's unpleasant. The same approach works with chronic back pain and related problems. If you have activities on the list, mindfulness practice can help you reclaim them. We'll return to your list shortly.

The Story of the Two Arrows

A famous sermon given by the Buddha some 2,500 years ago addresses how we can approach pain mindfully. It's as useful today as it was then.

The Two Arrows

When touched with a feeling of pain, the uninstructed run-of-the-mill person sorrows, grieves, and laments, beats his breast, becomes distraught. So

LOST ACTIVITIES

List daily routines and any work, social, sports, family, travel, or other activities that you limit out of concern about your pain. Rate your feeling about each one as **P**leasant, **U**npleasant, or **N**eutral.

Activity	Feeling (P, U, or N)	Activity	Feeling (P, U, or N)
_____	( )	_____	( )
_____	( )	_____	( )
_____	( )	_____	( )
_____	( )	_____	( )

Adapted from Ronald D. Siegel, Michael H. Urdang, & Douglas R. Johnson, *Back Sense: A Revolutionary Approach to Halting the Cycle of Chronic Back Pain.* New York: Broadway Books (2001, pp. 86–87). Copyright 2001 by Ronald D. Siegel, Michael H. Urdang, & Douglas R. Johnson. Adapted by permission.

he feels two pains, physical and mental. Just as if they were to shoot a man with an arrow and, right afterward, were to shoot him with another one, so that he would feel the pains of two arrows.

Let's look at this carefully. The first arrow in the story refers to raw pain sensations—the moment-to-moment throbbing, burning, aching, or stabbing that we call "pain." These are body sensations unadorned by commentary—they are what is happening in the body right now.

The second arrow refers to our responses to these pain sensations. This is where things get interesting. With a little mindfulness, we see that we have all sorts of aversion responses to pain. Some of these are physical, such as tensing our muscles to "brace" or "guard" against the pain, or holding our bodies in particular positions to avoid triggering it. Other reactions are emotional, such as feeling angry at ourselves or others for bringing it on ("I never should have shoveled all that snow"; "You should never have asked me to put in the air conditioner") or feeling frightened ("What if this never gets better?"). Mindfulness practice allows us to see the two arrows as distinct. As we'll see, the first arrow (pain sensations) is inevitable, but we can choose whether or not to impale ourselves with the second arrow (our aversion responses).

Mind Moments

The best way to distinguish between the two arrows is with concentration practice. This helps us develop the mental precision we need to see the pain sensations and notice that our aversion responses to them are actually distinct from the pain. You'll need 20–25 minutes to see how this works. If you have the time now, please give it a try. If not, return to this exercise later. It's easiest to do when you're experiencing some pain, but you can get a feel for the practice even when you're not:

———————— *Separating the Two Arrows** ————————

Begin by settling into your meditation seat and finding your breath. For the first 10–15 minutes, simply practice following your breath as you've done before, focusing on either the rising and falling sensations of your belly or the sensations of air entering and leaving the nostrils at the tip of your nose. Every time your mind wanders from the breath, gently bring it back. Remember this is like puppy training: the mind wanders; you lovingly bring it back. It wanders again; you lovingly bring it back again.

As you meditate, try to observe the breath with as much precision as possible. Notice the texture of each breath and examine its complex and varied qualities. See if you can develop an attitude of interest or curiosity toward all of these sensations. Begin meditating now and return to the rest of the instructions in 10–15 minutes.

Now that your mind has settled a bit, begin to shift your focus to wherever you feel the most discomfort in your body. These may be mild sensations or strong ones. The idea is to allow your breath to settle into the background and to bring the painful or uncomfortable sensations to the foreground.

Begin by just bringing your attention to the general area of the pain. Relax and settle into the physical sensations. Try to carefully observe their nature—burning, tight, piercing, dull, sharp, etc.

*Available in audio at *www.mindfulness-solution.com*.

Once you've identified what's happening, narrow your attention to zero in on the particular spot in your body that hurts the most.

Try to bring the same attitude of precision, interest, and curiosity to the discomfort that you brought to the breath. You're not trying to change it, but rather to really see it clearly. Notice how the sensations vary subtly from moment to moment. Perhaps one moment they throb, while the next they burn or ache. See if you can observe that "pain" is actually a series of momentary sensations strung together like frames in a movie, providing an illusion of continuity.

If your pain is intense, you may find that you start to feel overwhelmed or that your mind recoils from the pain sensations. Should this happen, experiment with bringing your attention back to the general area of the pain or even back to the breath for a while, before returning your attention to its precise source. Shifting your focus in this way will probably help you stay with the experience longer.

As you sit with the pain sensations, notice any thoughts that arise in the mind. You might experiment with labeling them: fearing, hating, worrying, etc. The idea is to notice that the thoughts come and go independent of the pain sensations.

Continue being with the pain sensations for the next 10 minutes or so.

If you're dealing with chronic pain, you'll find it helpful to integrate *Separating the Two Arrows* into your regular formal practice. You'll then also be able to use it as a life preserver to deal with moments during the day when you struggle with pain sensations.

Monks and nuns who devote many hours to meditation practice report that the mind becomes capable of discerning very minute sensations. In ancient times, before they could measure milliseconds or nanoseconds, the monks and nuns described the shortest observable moment of consciousness as a *mind moment*. It was defined as "one ten thousandth of the time it takes a bubble to burst." While in daily meditation most of us won't reach this level of refinement, we are nonetheless heading in this direction with the *Separating the Two Arrows* exercise. When we experience pain sensations this way—as a set of ever-changing momentary blips in consciousness—they become much easier to bear.

A Mathematical Formula

The story of the two arrows points toward the principle outlined in Chapter 2: a great deal of suffering is generated by resistance to experience. We've seen how this operates in anxiety and depression, where our efforts to feel better trap us into feeling worse. The same thing happens with physical pain. The good news is that *awareness of present experience with acceptance* can help us deal effectively with physical pain just as it helps us work with difficult emotions.

I was describing this mechanism one day to a patient from MIT. He said, as people from MIT often do, "I think there's a mathematical formula for that." I asked him what it might be. He said, "Pain times resistance equals suffering." Here's how this works. When pain sensations are extremely intense (such as when an elephant steps on our foot), we are likely to suffer unless we can manage to have virtually no resistance (which is very improbable). When pain is mild or moderate, if our resistance to it is low, suffering will also be limited—but if our resistance to the same pain is high, we will still suffer a lot. Put differently, to the extent that we can accept our pain, we won't suffer. This is the Buddha's story of the two arrows expressed mathematically. We see it vividly with mosquitoes—even though the pain of a bite is very mild, resisting being bitten can make us miserable.

$$\text{Pain} \times \text{Resistance} = \text{Suffering}$$

I'm not suggesting that it's as easy to be with intense pain as it is to be with a mosquito bite. But the approach can be the same. By intentionally bringing our attention to the pain sensations and adopting an accepting attitude, we can tolerate far more pain than we may have thought possible. This is vital for reclaiming lost activities.

Relativity

One of the most important insights gleaned from mindfulness practice is the fact that everything changes. Much of the time this is distressing. (As mentioned in Chapter 1, an awful lot of our psychological difficulty comes from trying to deal with our inevitable losses throughout the life cycle.)

When we're in pain, however, the reality of constant change can be a relief. One of the biggest obstacles to accepting pain is the fear that it will be unremitting. And when we're in pain, time slows down. Albert Einstein was once asked for a tangible way to understand relativity. He said, "When a man sits with a pretty girl for an hour, it seems like a minute. But let him sit on a hot stove for a minute and it's longer than any hour. That's relativity."

There is an interesting experiment that demonstrates the importance of time and expectations in pain perception. To induce pain without getting sued, researchers insert a subject's hand in ice water (it's harmless, but it can really hurt). If they tell people they'll have to keep their hand in the water for 10 minutes and ask them to rate their pain after 20 seconds, most subjects report that the pain is already intense and they don't think they'll be able to complete the experiment. If, on the other hand, the researchers tell subjects that they will have to keep their hand in the water for only 30 seconds and ask them to rate their pain after 20 seconds, most report that the pain is quite mild. Anxiety about being subjected to unremitting pain actually *increases the intensity of the pain sensations.*

Worrying that pain will never end increases the intensity of the pain we feel.

In the case of back and other musculoskeletal pain, worry about not getting better traps us in the pain cycle in two ways. First, anxiety tightens muscles, which directly increases pain. Second, anxiety increases the intensity with which we experience the pain sensations coming from those tightened muscles.

This helps us see why mindfulness practice can be so useful in working with bodily discomfort. By bringing our attention back to the pain sensations in the present, our future-oriented anxiety is reduced. Furthermore, by cultivating acceptance of the pain sensations, we don't amplify them with resistance.

By practicing mindfulness with pain, we learn to separate the two arrows. We come to accept that pain is inevitable but free ourselves from much of the usual suffering: the aversive thoughts, wishes for relief, catastrophic fantasies about our future, self-critical judgments, and all of the fear, anger, and frustration about our condition. And this frees us to do things even though they hurt, as long as we know they're not damaging.

Urge Surfing

Most people with chronic back pain and similar disorders are more disturbed by being disabled or limited in their activities than they are by the pain itself. If you can see that it's possible to live a full life despite having pain, you'll feel less fear and anger about it—and hence suffer less. We've seen how approaching pain sensations mindfully, rather than trying to banish them, can help interrupt chronic pain cycles. But what can you do when some activities just seem to hurt too much?

Mindfulness can help us deal with not only the pain sensations but also the feeling that they are too much to bear. Let me give you an example:

Sarah was a police officer who loved her work. Her back pain began when her cruiser was totaled after being hit by a drunk driver. MRIs and other tests were all negative. She had been through an active physical therapy program but was still in pain and couldn't do her regular job. During the past year she had held an administrative position, but the funding for this assignment was ending, and she either needed to get back into a cruiser or leave the force. The prospect of becoming an unemployed single mother was intolerable.

Sarah was understandably both anxious and angry. I asked her what stood in the way of her returning to regular duty. "I need to be able to sit in that cruiser," she said.

I proposed that we practice sitting together. I invited her to sit and try the *Separating the Two Arrows* meditation. At first, when she shifted her attention from her breath to the sensations of back pain, she was okay with the pain. The sensations weren't too bad, and she was able to observe how the pain itself was distinct from her distress about it. After about 20 minutes, however, she announced, "I have to get up. The pain is too intense." I asked her, "Where in your body do you feel 'I have to get up'?" At first she was puzzled by the question and said that she had to get up because her back hurt. But when I asked her to sit a little longer and see if she could locate the urge to get up, she found it. She said there was a pressure in her chest and neck, an urgency to get relief.

I suggested that she bring her attention to this urge to get up. Notice its texture, its detail. See if, like the pain, it was really made up of a series of momentary sensations strung together. She described it as a kind of pressure or tightness, and as she continued to follow it she saw that it came in waves. It would increase, reach a crescendo, and then subside for a bit, until the next wave began.

Sarah was able to remain in the chair longer than she had expected by *urge surfing*—riding the waves of discomfort. The pain sensations remained, but she felt less compelled to fix them once she saw that the urge to get up was distinct from the pain. This gave her confidence for the first time that she might be able to return to the cruiser.

You can use urge surfing as a life preserver when you feel compelled to stop an activity because of pain. It can help you separate feelings of desperation from the pain itself. Allow at least 10 minutes to try this the first time:

──────────── *Urge Surfing for Pain** ────────────

Close your eyes and bring your attention first to your breath for a few minutes. Next allow yourself to be with the pain sensations, attending to them with curiosity and interest. See how they change from moment to moment.

If the urge to get up or stop your activity arises, notice exactly where in your body you feel the urge. Bring your full attention to it, noticing its intensity and texture. See how the urge to get up or stop is distinct from the pain sensations themselves.

Now return your attention partially to your breath. Using your breath as a surfboard, ride each wave of urgency from its beginning as a small wavelet to the point where it crests. Allow each wave to rise up as high as it wants, trusting that it will reach a crescendo and then subside again.

We'll see in Chapter 9 how urge surfing can also help with other difficulties, including substance use problems and compulsive behaviors.

Relinquishing Control

As is the case with anxiety and depression, attempts to control pain are often at the heart of our difficulties. We're like children growing their first seedling. Wanting to speed the process, little kids pull on the tender shoot—killing the plant in the process. Mindfulness practice helps us differentiate what we can fruitfully control from what we cannot. In the case of back pain and other stress-related disorders, we can control our behavior but not our symptoms. I often suggest to my patients that symptoms are in the hands of nature, fate, or God. They're like the weather—we can't meaningfully influence them. Our actions, on the other hand, are

─────────────────
*Available in audio at *www.mindfulness-solution.com*.

very much under our control. We can choose to move normally and systematically resume a full life.

Even after getting a doctor's permission to move normally, many people remain trapped in chronic pain cycles because they think they need to eliminate pain *before* resuming activity. Unfortunately, they can wind up waiting forever, because normal movement is usually necessary to interrupt pain cycles. With mindfulness practice we can learn to deal effectively with the fear and discomfort that arise when we start moving again—an important step toward resolving our problem.

Step 3: Work with Negative Emotions

For many sufferers understanding that their pain is due to muscle tension rather than structural damage and using mindfulness techniques to support a return to full normal movement is all it takes to break free from chronic back pain. The pain–worry–fear–pain cycle is interrupted and they're done. For others, though, additional processes also keep muscles tight. Mindfulness can help with these too.

Chapter 5 explained how our evolutionary heritage sets us up for anxiety. Our fight-or-flight system, so well suited to dealing with emergencies, becomes stuck on "on" because of our nonstop thinking. You'll recall that one aspect of this arousal system involves muscle tension. We (and other animals) tense the muscles in our body when we perceive danger, preparing to fight, freeze, or flee.

You may also recall that this tensing occurs not only in response to external threats, such as the tiger in the jungle, but also to internal threats—the tigers within. This is Freud's signal anxiety, the tension we feel when an unwanted thought or emotion threatens to surface.

Sometimes chronic back pain starts with a muscle strain or moment of overuse. Other times, however, there is no plausible physical trigger. In these cases it's often a threatening emotion, which may be outside our immediate awareness, that starts the pain cycle. There is actually a lot of evidence that resisting these unwanted feelings plays a role in pain and stress-related disorders. Mindfulness practice can help us recognize and feel them.

John was an unusually nice guy. He was a loyal friend and a hard worker. He grew up in a stable family but always had trouble with his older brother. John was sensitive and artistic; his brother tough and athletic. While John put up with a lot of teasing and bullying from his brother and other tough kids when he was young, he eventually found love and companionship among artistic types. He now had a good job and a good marriage and had been pretty happy until his back went out.

John couldn't figure out what caused it. He had had backaches before, but this one just wouldn't go away. He tried the usual treatments, but nothing worked. The doctors found a bulging disk but said they didn't think this was causing the pain.

When I started working with him, I found John to be shy, soft-spoken, and wary of confrontation. I taught him the *Separating the Two Arrows* technique to work with the pain as he started returning to normal activities. As we discussed the history of his problem, he realized that it had begun when his mother became terminally ill. This was a particularly difficult time, as his older brother took charge of her care and ignored John's wishes.

As John started to meditate, he was flooded with emotion. He discovered that he was frightened about his back, sad about his mother's death, and enraged with his brother. This last emotion was particularly challenging since he had always tried to avoid conflict.

With continued mindfulness meditation, he became more and more comfortable with all of his feelings—fear, sadness, and even anger. He wasn't quite so nice anymore, but in the process his back pain receded.

By waking us up to the full range of our emotional experience, mindfulness practice helps us stop fearing the tigers within, allowing our muscles to relax and the pain to diminish.

Putting it all together

As with anxiety and depression, chronic back pain comes in many forms, so no single approach is going to be optimal for everyone. Still, most people should start by getting a thorough medical evaluation to rule out problems that would make a return to normal activity unwise. The important question to ask the doctor is "Do you have good reason to believe that exercising and otherwise living my life normally will actually damage my back?" If the answer is "No, exercise may be painful but probably won't cause any permanent damage," you're ready to go.

Next, you'll need to see how fear and worry play a part in the problem—to notice all the anxious thoughts that come up when the pain increases. You can use the *Monitoring Your Worried Thoughts* exercise to do this. The more clearly you can see your pain as a stress-related rather than orthopedic problem, the faster you'll recover.

Once you have permission to use your body normally and have looked at your fears, start resuming normal activities that you may have given up out of concern for your back. Look at your *Lost Activities* list on page 185. Pick an activity to resume that (1) you believe is not damaging (although it might be painful); (2) you rated as *pleasant* (this will enhance your motivation); (3) wouldn't be too intimidating to resume (to keep your fear manageable); and (4) you could do three or more times per week. This last criterion is important so that you get to see your pain level fluctuate while you do the activity regularly (to help break the association between the activity and the pain). You can write out your plan here:

ACTIVITY PLAN

Activity: _____

Frequency: _____
    (How often you'll do it—times a day or week)

Duration: _____
    (How long you'll do it—time, distance, number of repetitions)

Intensity: _____
    (How hard you'll do it—weight, speed, etc.)

Adapted from Ronald D. Siegel, Michael H. Urdang, & Douglas R. Johnson, *Back Sense: A Revolutionary Approach to Halting the Cycle of Chronic Back Pain*. New York: Broadway Books (2001, p. 91). Copyright 2001 by Ronald D. Siegel, Michael H. Urdang, & Douglas R. Johnson. Adapted by permission.

The idea is to stick with your plan long enough to stop fearing that the activity is making your condition worse. A structured, vigorous exercise program to develop strength, flexibility, and endurance can also be very helpful both in getting over fears of movement and in returning your muscles to normal functioning.

During this phase more anxiety will probably arise. The regular practice program described in Chapters 3 and 4 will provide a good foundation for working with this, perhaps emphasizing the *Body Scan Meditation* (Chapter 3) to practice *being with* a wide range of physical sensations. It will also be helpful to refer to Chapter 5 and review various mindfulness techniques for working with anxiety, choosing one or another depending on how overwhelmed you feel. If you're plagued by worried thoughts about your back, the *Thought Labeling* practice described in Chapter 6 can also be useful.

This is also the time to use the *Separating the Two Arrows* meditation periodically to help you relax into your pain, rather than fear and fight it. Practicing this will increase your capacity to bear discomfort. Should the pain become particularly intense, so that you feel compelled to stop an activity, try *Urge Surfing*. Just as Sarah did, notice where in your body you feel the urge to get up from sitting, to stop walking, to stop lifting, and so forth. Bring your attention to that urge just as you did to the pain in the *Separating the Two Arrows* meditation—notice its texture, intensity, and other qualities. You'll probably find, like Sarah, that the urge to stop builds and then subsides.

If you still have pain once you've been using your body normally, it's time to look at other emotional forces that may be contributing to your continuing tension. The exercises and practices outlined in Chapter 6, especially *Noting Emotions in the Body, Surveying Emotions in the Body*, and *Observing Emotions throughout the Day* can help you become more aware of these.

For further guidance on following the *Back Sense* program, including a thorough discussion of chronic back pain diagnoses and treatment along with detailed, step-by-step instructions on getting a good medical workup, resuming normal activities, establishing a structured exercise program, and working with negative emotions, you can visit *www.backsense.org* or read the self-treatment guide *Back Sense: A Revolutionary Approach to Halting the Cycle of Chronic Back Pain*.

Other pain disorders

A remarkable variety of pain disorders follow the same pattern as chronic back pain. Neck, jaw, wrist, knee, foot, shoulder, pelvic, and headache pain are the most common. Of course any one of these could be caused by an injury, infection, or other medical condition. But they can all also be caused or maintained by chronic tension cycles in which fear of the symptom and attempts to avoid discomfort keep us trapped.

The first step in addressing these symptoms is getting a good medical workup, preferably from a physician who understands the complex interactions among the mind, behavior, and pain. You'll need to find out if you can move freely without damaging your body. Physiatrists (rehabilitation physicians) are often good sources of advice.

Once physical causes other than tension are ruled out, the same three steps—understand the problem, resume full physical activity, and work with negative emotions—can often be used successfully to resolve the problem. The research evidence pointing to muscle tension as the cause of most chronic back pain is very compelling. Evidence is just beginning to accumulate suggesting that pain in these other areas follows a similar pattern.

Digestive difficulties

Ever experience a "nervous stomach"? Recall the story in Chapter 5 of the astronaut feeling "scared *shitless*" when he flew in untested aircraft. The gastrointestinal system is remarkably sensitive to our emotional state. I remember learning early in my training that the two most widely prescribed drugs at the time were Valium (a tranquilizer) and Tagamet (a then-new stomach acid controller). This was not an accident.

Stress physiologists tell us that our digestive system reacts to perceived danger in complex ways. When an animal is threatened and its fight-or-flight system is activated, its digestive system shuts down (scientists say there is no need to digest your own lunch when you are about to become somebody else's lunch). When the threat is over, the system can rebound, overshoot its normal activity level, and become hyperactive. Scientists have also known for many years that the stomach secretes more acid when an animal repeatedly feels threatened, leading (in humans at least) to heartburn, bloating, and other symptoms of indigestion.

These digestive events often escape our attention. However, if they become particularly intense or long-lasting, they can develop into disruptive cycles. As in the case of back pain, these cycles may begin with an external stressor, such as a viral infection or food poisoning. But they can also begin with the cumulative effects of emotional upset.

The trouble really starts once we become concerned with a symptom. For example, irritable bowel syndrome, in which diarrhea can alternate with constipation, creates fear about not being able to get to a bathroom on time. Heartburn creates worry about being unable to eat a normal diet or, worse, developing cancer because of continued irritation. As in the back pain cycle, these concerns generate fear and other emotions, which in turn bring on more symptoms.

Most medical interventions attempt to control the symptoms with drugs or dietary changes. While these measures can be helpful, they can also keep us preoccupied with our symptoms, with micromanaging our diet or bathroom habits in an effort to get things under control.

Just as in muscle tension disorders, often (1) understanding the problem, (2) resuming full normal activity, and (3) working with negative emotions turns out to be a better strategy—and mindfulness can support it. Again, serious diseases that might be causing the symptoms need to be ruled out first. After that, you can use mindfulness to observe all the worried thoughts that arise about your digestive system. You can use meditation practices to label the thoughts and increase your capacity to fully experience and tolerate your symptoms. As you relax into the various sensations, it becomes easier to return to normal eating and bathroom habits. New gurgles, bubbles, cramps, and aches are no longer cause for alarm, but rather interesting sensations to explore. You practice letting go—relinquishing control over the symptoms, allowing them to come and go like the weather. At the same time, you turn your attention to living normally.

Mindfulness practice facilitates this shift in attitude. It can also help us work with underlying stressful emotions that may be contributing to digestive distress. Here is how one of my patients used mindfulness practice to recover from her chronic gastrointestinal problems:

Maria was a successful professional in her mid-40s. She managed to stay on top of the demands of a busy career, a marriage, and three children. The only problem was her stomach.

For several years she had struggled with heartburn, bloating, embarrassing gas, and alternating diarrhea and constipation. She regularly consulted doctors and alternative healers and took medicines and dietary supplements to control her symptoms. Wanting to get to the bottom of her problem, she systematically studied which foods seemed to bring it on and had as a result given up dairy products, tomatoes, chocolate, caffeine, peppers, and spicy foods. Each time she gave up another food her symptoms improved for a while but then returned. Most recently a doctor had speculated that she was suffering from "leaky gut syndrome," in which her food wasn't being digested normally. He suggested that she follow an even more restrictive diet, which was making eating a nightmare.

Shortly after I met Maria it became clear that she was very tightly wound. Between all of her responsibilities and micromanaging her diet, she was perpetually tense. It also became clear that she had long ago learned to push disturbing emotions out of her mind in an effort to tend to all of her responsibilities.

Maria made several important observations during her first few attempts at mindfulness meditation. She realized that she was indeed very anxious—her mind was regularly reeling with worried thoughts about her work, her family, and her digestive system. She also became aware that she had become obsessed with food and digestion. Every few seconds she would turn her attention to her belly to see whether it felt "normal."

After a bit more mindfulness practice, Maria noticed that upsetting thoughts kept arising despite her efforts to ignore them. When she began to explore these, she realized she was sad about her life—she had everything she had thought she wanted but felt alienated from her husband and unfulfilled at work.

Together these observations helped Maria entertain the possibility that perhaps her digestive difficulties were caused more by her mind than by her diet. She decided to risk eating a normal, healthy diet and attend to her emotions instead of her menu. Maria began to see that sometimes her digestive distress followed an emotional upset. As she added back foods, she realized this didn't necessarily make her symptoms worse— they were actually more reactive to her moods. Eventually she worked her way back to eating normally, using mindfulness practice to deal with both her anxiety about symptoms and the other emotions in her life. After a couple of months, her digestive system settled down and she was able to turn her attention to improving her job and marriage.

Mindfulness Practices for Digestive Difficulties

Here again there is no single approach that will suit everyone, but Maria's experience suggests some guidelines. As with muscle tension pain, you can begin by just noticing how often worried or anxious thoughts about your symptoms arise—the *Monitoring Your Worried Thoughts* exercise can help. If the anxiety is strong, try using some of the practices in Chapter 5 to work with it. Techniques such as *Thought Labeling* (described in Chapter 6) and *Thoughts Are Just Thoughts* (Chapter 5) can be used to identify and let go of persistent worried thoughts about your digestive system.

After receiving reassurance from a trusted medical professional that you can eat a normal, healthy diet, begin eating normally (some people have bona fide food allergies or other conditions that preclude this). You can then use the *Separating the Two Arrows* and *Urge Surfing* practices discussed earlier in this chapter both to cultivate an accepting attitude toward the various sensations that occur in your digestive system and to stick with your normal diet plan. When concerns about digestion arise, simply note the worried thoughts and return your attention to your sensory experience of the moment.

If this approach doesn't take care of the problem, as with chronic back pain, it can be helpful to attend more carefully to your emotional experience—particularly those feelings that you may habitually ignore or try to avoid (the tigers within). Here the exercises and practices in Chapter 6, particularly *Noting Emotions in the Body*, *Surveying Emotions in the Body*, and *Observing Emotions throughout the Day*, can be very useful.

To understand the role of stress and anxiety in digestive disorders better, you can also consult *Irritable Bowel Syndrome and the Mind-BodySpirit Connection: 7 Steps for Living a Healthy Life with a Functional Bowel Disorder, Crohn's Disease, or Colitis.*

Sexual problems

Judging from the contents of spam filters and TV commercials, we are in the midst of an epidemic of erectile dysfunction and other sexual disorders. Why is this? Other animals don't appear to have much difficulty having sex. If they can find a willing mate, the plumbing generally works just fine.

There is an amusing little story about this that helps explain our difficulties. A novice monk was instructed to meditate and try to empty his mind of thoughts. Not surprisingly, all day long he was plagued by incessant thinking. His teacher praised his efforts and told him the next day to go and think continuously—to allow no gaps. The young monk thought this would be easy. But when he tried, he became so anxious about keeping his thoughts flowing that he couldn't get another one to come.

Our troubles in bed stem from the fact that our sexual organs have something in common with our minds—when we try to get them to do one thing, they often do the opposite. Add to this the confusing values we're taught, our intense desire to succeed in this arena, and our difficulties getting along with one another, and we have a setup for problems.

Let's take erectile dysfunction as an example. Most men have had the experience at some point of wanting to perform sexually but finding that they just couldn't get or maintain an erection. It typically starts in a situation where the man is anxious to please or impress his partner. This little bit of anxiety may be enough to interfere with a full erection. He then has the thought "I hope I don't have trouble," which of course only increases his anxiety. This further interferes with the erection, leading to additional anxious thoughts—sometimes killing his arousal entirely. Assuming he gets upset by this, the next time he's in a sexual situation the thought "I hope I don't have trouble like the last time" will arise, which is enough to start another fear–dysfunction–fear cycle.

You'll recognize parallels between this pattern and the cycles that create other anxiety disorders and stress-related medical problems such as chronic back pain and digestive distress. It's therefore no surprise that a similar approach, relying on practicing awareness of present experience with acceptance, can help resolve it. Indeed, before we had modern pharmaceutical miracles like Viagra and Cialis, the most effective treatments for these sorts of problems involved mindfulness.

In the 1970s, sex researchers William Masters and Virginia E. Johnson developed what they called *sensate focus*, a technique that is basically mindfulness meditation for sex. It eventually became a cornerstone of most sex therapy. Here are the instructions:

—————————*Sensate Focus* —————————

Begin by touching each other's bodies, but not touching your partner's breasts or genitals. Enjoy and pay attention to the texture, temperature, and other qualities of your partner's skin. Refrain from talking or having intercourse. Just bring your attention to the moment-to-moment sensations of touching your partner and of being touched by him or her. Concentrate on what you find interesting in your partner's skin—ignore for right now what you think your partner may enjoy. If an erection or vaginal lubrication occurs, so be it. If not, that's okay too.

Once you and your partner have had some success touching one another mindfully and letting go of the usual goal-orientated concerns, you're ready to move on to the next phase:

This time, begin again by touching one another's skin, paying attention to its texture, temperature, and other qualities. Again, you're not trying to please or arouse your partner, but rather are practicing being aware of the sensations of touching and being touched. This time you can include his or her entire body, including sexual organs. Just notice what it feels like to touch and be touched. Try to allow erections, vaginal lubrication, and arousal sensations to come and go as they wish.

Once you and your partner have become comfortable with this, move on to the third stage, where you begin to communicate to one another about what you find pleasurable:

Begin again by touching each other mindfully for a few minutes. Once you become comfortable with this, place your hand over your partner's hand and guide him or her as he or she touches your body. Communicate how you most like to be touched in different places—let him or her know the pace or degree of pressure that feels best. When you are being guided by your partner, focus your attention on what it feels like to touch him or her and use this as an opportunity to learn about his or her likes and dislikes. After a few minutes, switch roles. Even at this stage there's no need to get or maintain an erection, to have vaginal lubrication, or to feel aroused. Just enjoy touching and learning about your partner's body.

You'll find it most effective to practice *Sensate Focus* initially as a systematic program, devoting as many sessions to each phase as necessary. Once you and your partner have become more comfortable sexually, you can use *Sensate Focus* as a life preserver whenever anxiety about sexual performance recurs. Feel free to return to earlier steps whenever this happens.

Relationships

In addition to learning to touch and be touched mindfully, Masters and Johnson found that it was important to explore emotional issues that might contribute to sexual problems. Couples are therefore encouraged to discuss their feelings about sexuality, including messages they received growing up and the effects that past sexual experiences might have had on them. They are also asked to recognize and discuss what makes them feel closer to or more distant from each other and to pay attention to how it feels to hug, kiss, and talk. Touching one another mindfully makes it much easier to notice the role that these emotional factors play in our sexual responses.

Relationships are not easy. Even a five-minute interaction with a loved one can ruin our entire day (if it goes poorly). We are exquisitely sensitive to one another, and there is nothing quite like unresolved tensions in a couple to ruin their sex life. We'll discuss how to use mindfulness to work with these issues and to help us sustain intimate relationships in Chapter 8.

In *Sensate Focus*, once you and your partner are comfortable with mindful sensual contact and have had a chance to explore other issues that may make it difficult to be close, you're invited to include intercourse in your lovemaking. Letting go of the quest to get rid of the symptom, practicing sensual mindfulness, and attending to other emotional factors succeeds in resolving erectile dysfunction in the vast majority of cases.

Many other sexual difficulties follow a parallel pattern. Premature ejaculation is usually similar, except instead of worrying about not getting or losing an erection, the man worries about orgasming too soon. Women frequently complain of difficulty becoming lubricated or reaching orgasm, which is often caused by—you guessed it—focusing on the goal of becoming lubricated or reaching orgasm. In all of these circumstances, shifting attention from concern about performance to practicing awareness of present experience with acceptance is usually the key to resolving the difficulty.

Mindful sex feels better.

For some people, all of this is of historical interest only. Nowadays, many people turn to Viagra, Cialis, or other medications at the first sign of trouble. While these may be medically necessary, and can sometimes head off or interrupt a fear–dysfunction–fear cycle, they can also rob people of the opportunity to learn how to be really present during sex. Like eating, sex *feels better* when we are more fully mindful of it.

Sexual difficulties are also often symptoms of relationship issues. When we override these problems with medications, they may never be addressed. Because of advances in psychopharmacology, there are now many couples who can't communicate, who hate and fear each other, and who don't pay attention in bed—but who can have successful sexual intercourse on a regular basis.

Optimizing Your Sex Life

While many sexual difficulties emerge from the patterns we've been discussing, they can also be caused by medications, hormonal changes, or other medical issues. If you're experiencing a new difficulty, begin with a medical evaluation to rule out these causes. Even if medical issues are playing a role, however, a mindfulness approach can help.

Sensate Focus can optimize any sexual relationship, whether or not you're experiencing difficulties. If both you and your partner are open to it, you can even begin lovemaking with *Breath Awareness Meditation*, the *Body Scan Meditation*, or another of the concentration practices described in Chapter 3. Just as with *Eating Meditation*, this makes it easier to tune in to the moment-to-moment sensations of sensual contact while being less caught in evaluative judgments about the experience.

If you're experiencing difficulties with sexual functioning, you and your partner can explore sequentially the three *Sensate Focus* stages presented above. The key is restraining yourself from rushing into the next step before becoming fully comfortable with the one you are on— remember the goal is not to "succeed" but to be present.

Throughout the process, communication is also very important. If you (and ideally your partner) have been practicing mindfulness, you'll probably be more aware of the different thoughts and feelings that arise during sexual experiences. While perhaps initially embarrassing, sharing these can go a long way toward making you feel more relaxed with one another. This will also allow you to return together to *Sensate Focus* as a life preserver whenever performance anxiety becomes a problem. The practices designed to enhance intimate relationships that are outlined in Chapter 8 will also support your efforts to feel comfortable and connected with your partner emotionally as well as sexually.

Insomnia

Ever have difficulty sleeping? Most of us do. Here again we seem to be very different from other animals. Dogs and cats seem to sleep easily everywhere, while we buy fancy mattresses and take all sorts of drugs to try to knock ourselves out.

It doesn't take much introspection to see that our thinking disease plays a role. When we can't sleep, our minds buzz with thoughts of the past or the future. We're busy solving problems, anticipating disasters, or reviewing misfortunes when we might be resting. Many of our thoughts are frightening, activating our fight-or-flight system. It's no surprise that one function of this system is to keep us awake—we wouldn't want to start drifting off when being stalked by a tiger. Our problem is that the tigers within can stalk us all night long.

One of these tigers is usually anxiety about not getting enough sleep. That's why it's often easier to get to sleep on Friday or Saturday night than on Sunday. On Friday or Saturday we think, "It's okay if I don't get to sleep right now; I can always sleep later in the morning." On Sunday we're more likely to think, "If I don't get to sleep soon, I'll be a basket case tomorrow, and I have so much to do." Anxiety about getting to sleep can be the biggest threat we face when tossing and turning. Other inner tigers include our full assortment of fears and regrets—all of which have a way of visiting when our guard goes down at night.

Since insomnia, like other stress-related problems, is fed both by our fight against the symptom and by other disturbing emotional issues, it's no sur-

> Mindfulness can put the "tigers within" to bed so we can sleep.

prise that practicing mindfulness can be helpful. This works best when combined with other techniques.

Conventional nondrug treatments for insomnia focus on three broad strategies: *stimulus control, sleep hygiene,* and *relaxation.* Stimulus control is designed to teach us to associate the bed with sleep. To do this, you are advised not to read, watch TV, or eat in bed. Most approaches instruct patients to reserve the bed for only sleep and sex.* Furthermore, they suggest that if you are not sleeping, after around 20 minutes you should get up and read or have some (caffeine-free) tea, returning to bed when you feel tired (the idea is not to associate the bed with tossing and turning).

The second approach, sleep hygiene, is designed to establish a regular pattern of nighttime sleep. This is done by getting into bed at the same time each night, getting out of bed at the same time each morning, and avoiding naps—regardless of how long you've slept. This way you won't fall into the pattern of napping during the day to catch up on sleep, only to feel wide awake at night.

---

*You may wonder why you would reserve the bed for sleep and sex if you're trying to create an association in your mind between the bed and sleep. The answer is that health professionals are too prudish to suggest that you sleep in the bed and have sex in the living room, though this would be the better strategy.

The third approach is relaxation training. The idea here is that by practicing relaxation you can reverse the arousal of the fight-or-flight response and more readily get to sleep.

Experiences gathered during mindfulness meditation retreats have led to the development of another approach, based on three observations. First, when we practice mindfulness intensively, we find that we have a reduced need for sleep—we feel refreshed and alert with fewer hours in bed. This suggests that either some of the restorative function of sleep is met by mindfulness meditation or it helps us sleep more deeply. Second, fighting insomnia just keeps us awake. Mindfulness, with its emphasis on accepting whatever is happening in the moment, tends to defuse this battle. Third, mindfulness practice helps us let go of goal-oriented thoughts and work with difficult emotions—so it's an effective way to deal with the tigers within that keep us up at night.

Together, these observations suggest that you might try practicing mindfulness meditation when you go to bed. One of two things will happen—either you'll have an opportunity for eight hours of uninterrupted mindfulness practice or you may fail and fall asleep. Either way it's okay. If you don't sleep, you'll still get some rest and have an opportunity to work with what keeps you up at night. If you do sleep, your insomnia is resolved for the evening. In either case, the fight against the symptom, which is central to the condition, is over.

Lisa was never a very good sleeper. As a little girl she was disturbed by her noisy older brother. In high school she stayed up worrying about papers and tests, and in college she was kept awake by her roommate's studying. Even though she could get by on five or six hours of sleep, she didn't really feel alert and refreshed with less than seven or eight.

When she finally got her own apartment, Lisa made sure it would be restful. She was on the top floor facing the back. She got blackout shades and a good mattress. These all helped, and many nights she slept well.

But when things got difficult at work, or she had problems with her boyfriend or family, her sleep suffered. She'd get into ruts where she had trouble falling asleep, was tired at work the next day, and then worried even more about sleeping the next night. She hated the hours spent tossing and turning, looking at the clock, feeling more distressed the later it got. Sometimes in desperation she took Benadryl or Ambien, but she didn't like the groggy feeling the drugs gave her the next morning.

Lisa's sleep pattern transformed after her first mindfulness meditation retreat. After a week of intensive practice she became accustomed to using her downtime as an informal practice opportunity. With nothing else in particular to do, she naturally followed her breath when she got into bed.

Lisa still didn't sleep deeply every night. But restless nights were no longer such a big deal. She would stay with her breath and allow thoughts of being tired to come and go. Usually other concerns would pop into her head, but she would let these arise and pass also. Even when she didn't sleep her full seven or eight hours, she felt more rested than she had in the old days of tossing and turning, trying to doze off.

Mindfulness Practice for Sleep

If your insomnia has developed suddenly, particularly if accompanied by other new symptoms, you'll want to see your doctor to rule out any unusual illness. After this, many commonsense, conventional approaches to insomnia are good ideas: don't drink caffeinated beverages in the evening; sleep in a darkened room; avoid strenuous exercise and upsetting books or TV shows right before bed. Many people also find it helpful to practice stimulus control, in which you reserve the bed primarily for sleep, and sleep hygiene, in which you try to get to bed at the same time each night and get up at the same time each morning.

In addition to these steps, you can use mindfulness practice as Lisa did—to give up the whole battle with wakefulness. Many different practices are suitable for bedtime. If you are agitated or excited, the concentration practices presented in Chapter 3 can be helpful. *Breath Awareness Meditation*, whether focused on the belly or the tip of the nose, perhaps including labeling or counting the breath, tends to be calming. The *Body Scan Meditation* also increases mental stability and works well when lying down. Should you find yourself having difficulty accepting your current state of mind, the *Loving-Kindness Meditation* practice presented in Chapter 4 can help you cultivate soothing self-compassion.

If you're being visited by anxious thoughts, the *Thoughts Are Just Thoughts* and *Mountain Meditation* practices in Chapter 5 can also be helpful. If difficulties with sadness, anger, or other emotions seem to be interrupting your sleep, you can experiment with the exercises in Chapter 6 designed to work with these states of mind.

However, bedtime is usually not the best time to try to do more exploratory practices such as the *Stepping into Fear* practice in Chapter 5 or *Stepping into Sadness* or *Stepping into Anger* in Chapter 6, as these tend to be more energizing.

The most important principle is to use your time in bed until you fall asleep to practice *awareness of present experience with acceptance.* Say *yes* to whatever arises. Your mind and body will benefit from whatever happens—whether meditation or sleep.

Mindfulness practices for pain and stress-related medical disorders

All of the following rest on a foundation of regular formal and informal practice as described in Chapters 3 and 4. They can be adapted to most stress-related medical problems in the ways just described.

Formal Meditation Practices

- *Body Scan Meditation* (page 72) to practice being with pleasant and unpleasant physical sensations
- *Separating the Two Arrows* (page 186) to relax into pain and increase your capacity to bear it
- *Urge Surfing* (page 191) to persist with an uncomfortable activity despite the urge to stop
- *Noting Emotions in the Body* (page 145) to bring unacknowledged emotions into awareness
- *Thought Labeling* (page 154) to identify and let go of worried thoughts about your condition
- *Listening Meditation* (page 155) or *Thoughts Are Just Thoughts* (page 125) to allow worried thoughts about your condition to arise and pass
- *Sensate Focus* (page 200) to cultivate awareness and acceptance and to let go of goals during sex
- *Breath Awareness Meditation* (page 55) while lying in bed at night
- *Loving-Kindness Meditation* (page 84) to soothe self-critical chatter

Informal Practices

All of these can help bring attention to sensory experience throughout the day and away from worried thoughts about medical conditions:

- *Walking Meditation* (page 67)
- *Nature Meditation* (page 128)
- *Eating Meditation* (page 263)
- *Driving, Showering, Tooth Brushing, Shaving (etc.) Meditation* (page 90)

Life Preservers

- *Separating the Two Arrows* (page 186) for moments when you're struggling against pain
- *Urge Surfing* (page 191) for moments when you're feeling desperate to make pain go away
- *Sensate Focus* (page 200) when anxieties about sexual performance recur
- *Nature Meditation* (formal or informal; page 128) to anchor your attention in the world outside your worried thoughts and distressing body sensations

Developing a plan

You may find it useful to jot down an action plan for working with your pain or stress-related condition. The chart on the facing page can help you organize your thoughts.

When you need more help

While you may well be able to work your way through the problems discussed in this chapter by using mindfulness practices and related approaches, professional help can sometimes also be a good idea. We've discussed the importance of ruling out non-stress-related causes for various conditions. Your primary-care physician can help you do this for difficulties with sleep, digestion, and sex. A physiatrist (specialist in rehabilitation medicine) may be better equipped to clarify your diagnosis and give you permission to resume full activity in the case of back or other musculoskeletal pain.

Sometimes the fear, anger, sadness, or other emotions surrounding a medical condition are difficult to manage. Here a mental health professional may be helpful. Clinicians trained in *behavioral medicine*

PRACTICE PLAN

Begin by reflecting on how the condition is affecting your life.

Distressing Condition: _____

Situations in Which the Condition Occurs: _____

_____

Components of My Condition:

Physical: _____

_____

Cognitive (worried thoughts): _____

_____

Behavioral (things I do or avoid because of it) (use the *Lost Activities* chart in this chapter for pain conditions): _____

_____

Times I Most Need a Life Preserver: _____

_____

Now, based on what you've read about and experienced with the different practices, jot down an initial practice plan (you can vary this as your needs change).

Formal Practice	*When*	*How Often*
_____	_____	_____
_____	_____	_____
_____	_____	_____

(cont.)

Informal Practice	When	How Often
_____	_____	_____
_____	_____	_____
_____	_____	_____

Life Preserver	Likely Situation
_____	_____
_____	_____
_____	_____

For chronic pain conditions, it may help to also complete the *Activity Plan* in this chapter to support you in resuming normal activity.

specialize in working with the psychological and behavioral aspects of stress-related medical disorders. These days many of them are also familiar with mindfulness practice—so you should ask about this. Together with your medical provider, a mental health professional can help you decide when medication for sleep, digestive troubles, or pain may or may not be a good idea.

If you run into difficulties using *Sensate Focus* to deal with a sexual problem, a sex therapist can help. These mental health professionals specialize in working with couples and can help you and your partner work through both performance and relationship issues that may be contributing to your sexual difficulty. They can also help you decide whether performance-enhancing drugs such as Viagra or Cialis would be helpful or harmful.

Suggestions for finding a therapist to work with stress-related conditions along with other resources can be found at the back of the book.

One problem, many faces

It's amazing how many stress-related medical problems are caused or exacerbated by the same emotional and mental patterns. It's also remarkable to see how mindfulness practice can, therefore, help us deal with all of them. Of course this doesn't mean any of us can entirely escape pain or illness. Fortunately, mindfulness practice can also help us with those unbidden developments in our bodies that a change in attitude and behavior cannot cure—the subject of Chapter 10.

But before we get to that, let's look at how mindfulness can help us with another unavoidable challenge—the problem of getting along with other people.

CHAPTER 8

Living the full catastrophe

Mindfulness for romance, parenting, and other intimate relationships

*H*ave you ever wondered why it can be so hard to get along with other people? Why do they insist on being so difficult? The trouble seems to stem from misunderstandings about who we are—combined with the results of our misguided attempts to feel good.

Most of the world's problems have to do with our trouble cooperating. It may have always been this way. Remember Fred and Wilma's difficulties 40,000 years ago? A lot of them involved personal conflicts. There were the arguments with each other over who should haul the water on hot days. And while Fred thought it was perfectly natural to look at the sexy cavewomen on the other side of the hill, Wilma didn't see it this way at all. When she got angry about it, Fred just thought she was being cold and withholding by refusing to have sex with him. They always agreed about one thing, though—their anger at those annoyingly haughty neighbors with the big cave. They lay awake at night discussing what jerks they were. This led to regular tensions—and occasional fights—over which family got to gather berries near the stream, dig up the choicest roots, and eat the plumpest larvae.

If only Fred and Wilma had known about mindfulness practices. While these practices were originally refined by monks, nuns, and hermits, people are discovering that they have enormous potential for helping ordinary folks get along with each other. They do this in several ways. First, they change our view of who we think we are. Mindfulness practices help each of us feel less like a separate "me" and more like a part of the wider world. This creates a shift in emphasis from "me" to "us" that can go a long way toward reducing conflict. Second, mindfulness practices can help us appreciate how arbitrary our identity, beliefs, and values actually are. This can make us much more flexible. Third, they can help us actually *be with* others—through both their joys and sorrows. Really listening to other people, without immediately trying to fix or otherwise change things, can do a lot to enhance mutual understanding. Finally, mindfulness practices help us recognize our feelings and choose whether or not to act on them. This helps us respond skillfully rather than reflexively to others—which is particularly useful during tense moments. You'll see in this chapter how to use the practices you've already learned, along with some new ones, to get along better with everyone—even when everyone else is being difficult.

Who am I?

We're so accustomed to thinking about "me" that we rarely inquire deeply into who we really are. Take five minutes right now to see how central thoughts about yourself are to your stream of consciousness:

—————————— *Me, Myself, and I* ——————————

Begin by following your breath, as you've done before, for a minute or two. Then begin to take note of the content of the thoughts that occur. Just watch how often thoughts of "I want," "I think," "I feel," "I hope," "I like," or "I don't like" arise. Keep making mental notes of this for another few minutes.

Most of us take our identity for granted and don't notice how it's constructed. Anthropologists point out that our sense of self is determined by the culture in which we grow up. In the West we view individuals as separate entities more than as members of groups such as a family, a community, or the natural world. Healthy psychological maturation in the West is assumed to require that we develop a clear identity and sense of self, good boundaries, and knowledge of our personal needs. Psychologists have traditionally called this accomplishment being *well individuated*.

Other cultures, including many African, Asian, and indigenous societies, construct their identities differently. Desmond Tutu, the South African spiritual leader, says that in traditional African societies identity always involves the group. If you ask someone, "How are you?" he or she will answer, "We are fine" or "We're not doing very well." It just doesn't make sense in these cultures for an individual to feel good if the rest of his or her group is suffering.

Narcissism

Of course, even within a society, people vary in how much they're focused on themselves versus other people. Western mental health professionals diagnose individuals as having a narcissistic personality disorder when they are so preoccupied with their rank in the group that they can't get along with others (despite being the *smart monkeys*, we act a lot like other primates). These are people whose self-esteem always seems to be on the line. They worry about how they compare and how much respect others show them. Often they treat other people disrespectfully in their attempts to buttress their own self-esteem.

We all know men and women who are like this to varying degrees. We usually start to feel inadequate or competitive around them. Sometimes it's very subtle. These folks just happen to mention things that make us envious. They drop names, mention promotions, talk about their new dress or car, describe their fantastic vacation, or tell us about their child's accomplishments.

But even among healthier people, preoccupation with building up identity and maintaining self-esteem causes repeated envy, hurt, and conflict. Mindfulness practice helps us see how our view of ourselves as fundamentally separate from one another is at the heart of the problem.

When Albert Einstein developed his theory of relativity, he did much of his work through "thought experiments." He didn't have access to modern particle accelerators and had to figure things out using his imagination. We can perform a thought experiment to see how our usual sense of self is actually based on a misunderstanding. Try answering the following questions one at a time before reading the next:

A THOUGHT EXPERIMENT

Imagine you're holding an apple. If you take a bite and begin to chew it but then notice half of a worm left in the remainder of the apple, you'll probably spit out the partially chewed fruit. At this point, is that partially chewed material *you* or the *apple*? (Choose one.)

Let's now imagine that there was no worm, you continued chewing the apple, and it's now in your stomach, mixed up with digestive juices. Of course, if you're having a bad day, the stuff in your stomach could still come back up. Is that material now *you* or the *apple*? (Again, choose one.)

Imagine next that your digestive system is working well and the apple has passed from your stomach to your intestines, where the sugars in the apple have been absorbed. The sugars travel through your bloodstream and are taken up by cells in your body. The cells use the energy in the sugars to build proteins out of amino acids and create new cellular structures. Are those new cellular structures *you* or the *apple*? (Choose again.)

Finally, the fiber in the apple continues its journey through your digestive system. It enters your colon, loses its moisture, and solidifies—getting ready to be deposited in a familiar white porcelain receptacle. Is this material now *you* or *something else*? (Most of us don't like to identify with our feces, so we know the answer to this one.)

Do you see the challenge of this thought experiment? Where is the line of demarcation between "you" and "the apple"? There is no clear line. Rather, there is an apple/human system in which molecules of the apple are transformed into parts of a human being. We can perform the same thought experiment with everything we eat and every atom of oxygen we breathe. At this very moment billions of oxygen atoms are changing identity from being "the air" to being "you."

Biologists have given these matters considerable thought. They conclude that our concepts of separate organisms are arbitrary. We see this clearly when looking at an ant colony. Where is the organism—is it the individual ant or the colony? The so-called individuals each have their own roles, but all are needed for the survival of the community. In many ways the whole colony is the organism. Just as we don't consider the individual cells in our body to be separate individuals, since they all require one another for survival, we might see all the ants as interrelated parts of one colony. Unless we're subsistence farmers, we're all like the ant or body cell—totally dependent on the larger organism for survival.

.

Why don't we see it?

Despite understanding this interdependence intellectually, we have trouble living as if it were true. When I'm late for an appointment and the man ahead of me in the convenience store is purchasing twenty-six meticulously chosen lottery numbers, I don't see him as part of "me." In fact, I don't think of us as even vaguely related. I see him as in *my* way. Why?

It's one thing to intellectually recognize our interdependence with others, but another to live as if it is real.

You probably know René Descartes' famous saying "I think; therefore I am." There is more truth to this than we often realize. We construct our sense of separate identity largely through thoughts— thoughts of who I am and who you are. While this is of course necessary for everyday life (and is why all languages have words for "me" and "you"), it creates a fundamentally distorted view of the world. In fact, all of our concepts are in some ways misleading, for they draw arbitrary distinctions between things that are actually interrelated and interdependent. And as we've seen before, because thinking has been so useful for our survival, we humans think all the time.

By allowing us to gain perspective on our thoughts—to see them coming and going like clouds in the sky—mindfulness practice helps us see the arbitrary nature of the distinctions we draw. Many of the world's religious and philosophical traditions also describe this—it's our penchant for thinking in words that keeps us from seeing our connection to one another and the wider world.

Some people interpret the biblical story of Genesis this way. Adam and Eve were expelled from the Garden of Eden for eating of the Tree of Knowledge of Good and Evil. In this view, the tree represents our human proclivity for thought, for drawing distinctions between things, which is fundamental to how we accumulate knowledge and form judgments. When Adam and Eve ate the fruit, they left paradise and entered into the painful human world, becoming "aware of their nakedness." This might be seen as the onset of our thinking disease, the propensity to live in thoughts and fantasies that sets us up for so much psychological suffering.

Eastern traditions also remind us that words distort reality by creating arbitrary separations and distinctions. The central text of Taoism, the *Tao Te Ching*, begins with a line often translated as "The Way that can be described is not the absolute (true, eternal) Way." It goes on to describe how we create our understanding of reality out of opposing concepts:

> When the people of the world all know beauty as beauty,
> there arises the recognition of ugliness.
> When they all know the good as good,
> there arises the recognition of bad;
> Therefore being and non-being produce each other;
> difficult and easy complete each other;
> long and short contrast each other;
> high and low distinguish each other ...
> Therefore the wise manage affairs without interfering and teach beyond the words.

Interbeing

Mindfulness practice can help us become wise in this way. By no longer identifying so much with our thoughts and concepts, we're better able to see the interrelated nature of all things—what biologists call *ecological systems* and physicists call *fields of matter and energy*. In meditation practice we can actually observe how our thoughts create a sense of separateness. Once we develop a bit of concentration, the whole world begins to feel more alive, more interconnected. Plants, animals, and *even other people* are experienced as part of a vibrant, interactive whole. If we have a theistic perspective, mindfulness helps us connect directly with God or the Divine. Everything becomes numinous, infused with the spirit of life. From a scientific perspective, we feel ourselves to be part of nature—which is no less magical.

It is said that the first teaching that the Buddha offered was a lesson on mindfulness presented to a group of children. The Zen teacher Thich Nhat Hanh presents this story as an eating meditation that shows how mindfulness can help us appreciate this sense of interconnectedness. Here is an excerpt:

> You are all intelligent children and I am sure you will be able to understand and practice the things I will share with you.... When you children peel a tangerine, you can eat it with awareness or without awareness. What does it mean to eat a tangerine in awareness? When you are eating the tangerine, you are aware that you are eating the tangerine. You fully experience its lovely fragrance and sweet taste. When you peel the tangerine, you know that you are peeling the tangerine; when you remove a slice and put it in your mouth, you know that you are removing a slice and putting it in your

mouth; when you experience the lovely fragrance and sweet taste of the tangerine, you are aware that you are experiencing the lovely fragrance and sweet taste of the tangerine....

A person who practices mindfulness can see things in the tangerine that others are unable to see. An aware person can see the tangerine tree, the tangerine blossom in the spring, the sunlight and rain which nourished the tangerine. Looking deeply, one can see ten thousand things which have made the tangerine possible. Looking at a tangerine, a person who practices awareness can see all the wonders of the universe and how all things interact with one another....

Thich Nhat Hanh calls the reality of the interconnected nature of all things *interbeing*. As we'll soon see, awakening to this reality can do a lot to help us get along with one another.

Constructing an identity and a self

Developmental psychologists have long studied how we develop a sense of self and what can go wrong in the process. Mostly, we create our sense of who we are out of the responses we get from others. It's no surprise that people who are routinely ignored or criticized by their parents or peers typically develop negative self-images, while those who are loved and appreciated develop positive ones. Our history of success and failure when we tackle challenges—whether academic, artistic, athletic, or social—also shapes how we see ourselves. If I've always gotten A's, never got beyond drawing stick figures, regularly dropped the basketball, but still had a lot of friends, I'd view myself as a smart, artistically challenged, uncoordinated, but likable guy. It's as though we are sponges with memories. We absorb all the feedback we receive from others and create a sense of self out of this.

To see this process in action, try the exercise on the facing page, designed to illuminate our particular sense of self. It works best after a period of concentration practice, so you'll want to devote 20–30 minutes to the whole experience.

What did you notice? Often people find that the mind goes through familial roles (such as son, daughter, brother, sister, father, mother, wife, husband), social roles (friend, lover, companion), and occupational roles. Sometimes it moves on to more individual categories (man, woman) or qualities (smart person, generous person, anxious person, funny person). Sometimes images of our bodies come to mind. There is no right

WHO AM I?

Begin with 10–20 minutes of focusing your attention on your breath either at the tip of your nose or in your belly. As you've done before, try to develop a sense of interest or curiosity in the breath. Whenever your mind wanders and you get caught in a chain of narrative thoughts, gently return your attention to the breath. Try to remain with the breath for full cycles—from the beginning of an inhalation, through the point of fullness, back down to where the lungs are relatively empty and the cycle begins again.

Once your mind is reasonably settled, begin to ask yourself, "Who am I?" Notice whatever words arise in the mind in response and then repeat the question "Who am I?" Continue this process for at least several minutes, until your mind seems to run out of answers. Jot down a few of the responses that came to mind.

_____

_____

At this point, try varying the question slightly. Ask, "What am I?" Again welcome whatever thoughts arise in the mind in response. Continue asking this question until the mind seems to have run out of replies. Again, jot down a few responses.

_____

_____

response. The idea is to simply see some of the elements you use to create this sense of self.

Observing the Mind Objectively

Through mindfulness practice we come to see that all of these roles and attributes are really just concepts. We might even notice that our sense of self is actually being created each instant out of sensory experiences. To really understand this, it helps to take an objective look at how our minds work from moment to moment. By observing the mind carefully during meditation, you can notice how your awareness is built from a series of steps all unfolding very rapidly.

First there is contact between a sense organ and a sensory stimulus—awareness of seeing, hearing, touching, tasting, or smelling—as well as awareness of other mental events, such as thoughts, feelings, and images that arise. But the mind doesn't stay at this level.

Moments of sensation are immediately organized into perceptions. When we see a pattern of shape, color, and texture in the world that we associate with a "chair," the mind instantaneously moves from the level of sense contact to the perception of a "chair." This movement is of course conditioned by our past experiences and the culture in which we live—if we had never seen a chair before, we would not recognize it as such.

There's a classical psychological experiment that illustrates this movement of the mind from sensation to perception. Take a moment to look at this figure:

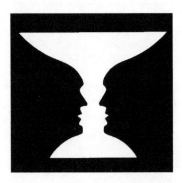

Soon you'll probably see both two faces looking at one another and a goblet. Stare at it a little longer and see if you can observe the faces and goblet simultaneously or if you actually can only see them rapidly oscillating from one to the other. (Do this for about 30 seconds before reading on.) What did you notice? Most people find that they oscillate—we have difficulty actually holding two different perceptions simultaneously. Of course, as with the chair, if you had never seen a goblet before you would probably have noticed only the faces.

Once we learn to perceive things one way, it's hard to see them otherwise. For example, look at this pattern of light and dark shapes:

PERCEPTION

Are you able to look at it and take it in as a sensory experience without reading the word? (I can't.) But if it were written in a different language, it would be easy to take in at a sensory level as a pattern of light and dark shapes and squiggles (unless, of course, you read Arabic):

إدراك

Every act of perception involves omitting some details that don't fit our expectations and filling in others. When we look at the faces and goblet, there isn't much information telling us that these are faces, but the mind has no difficulty filling in the missing information. Similarly, if you look at these words—m__ther and f__ther—the mind has no problem filling in the gaps. (As we'll soon see, knowing that our minds do this can help us avoid a lot of interpersonal difficulties.)

As we organize our sensory experience into perceptions, our minds immediately add a feeling reaction. As we've discussed before, we experience everything as pleasant, unpleasant, or neutral. A sweet taste may be pleasant, a loud sound unpleasant, while the image of this book in your hands might be neutral. These feeling reactions are immediately accompanied by intentions—we want to hold on to the pleasant, get away from the unpleasant, and ignore the neutral. You can see this for yourself with the little experiment on the following page.

When we have the same feeling reactions over and over, they solidify into our dispositions, conditioned responses, or personality characteristics—important building blocks for our identities. This is easiest to see in teenagers. They will readily tell you, "I'm really into _____ music." "I like _____ and would never wear _____." "She's such a jerk; she likes _____." Teenage identity categories—nerd, jock, stoner, emo—reflect their habitual likes and dislikes. We may imagine that as adults our identities are based on something more profound than preferences and images. Indeed, our identity categories may be more complex and varied than those of the average high school student. But if you drive a Toyota Prius, I can probably guess your feelings about national parks, cigarette smoking, and Chevy Hummers—not to mention whom you voted for in the last election.

NOTICING FEELINGS AND INTENTIONS

Take a moment to conjure up images of the following people, one by one, and note your reaction to each. Do you find the image pleasant, unpleasant, or neutral? What impulse or intention do you feel toward the image? Sense how each of these reactions feels in your body as you hold the image in mind for a few moments.

Image	Impulse or Intention Toward the Image (Attraction, Repulsion, Neutral, etc.) and Physical Reaction:
Adolf Hitler	_____
Martin Luther King, Jr.	_____
Marilyn Monroe	_____
Your first girlfriend or boyfriend	_____
Osama bin Laden	_____
George W. Bush	_____
The Dalai Lama	_____
A really sexy man	_____
A really sexy woman	_____

So where is the *self* in all of this? Careful observation reveals that it's a process. As my friend the Buddhist scholar Andrew Olendzki points out, we don't so much *exist* as we *occur*. In each moment that we experience sense contact, perceptions, feeling reactions, and habitual responses, our sense of self is born again. When we add words and describe ourselves in terms of our social roles, strengths, weaknesses, and preferences, we turn this fluid process into a sense of something solid and stable. This is how *selfing occurs*. Our mind creates an illusion of continuity out of moment-to-moment experiences,

> We don't so much *exist* as we *occur*.

much as it strings together the separate frames of a motion picture to create the illusion of continuous movement. Mindfulness meditation can help us see this in action—and become more relationally flexible as a result.

Understanding me to get along with you

When we begin to see that our identity is actually a set of patterns formed by experiences over time and our sense of self is re-created in each moment, we can take ourselves more lightly. Combined with the realization of our interdependence or lack of separateness, this shift in attitude can create far more flexibility in relating to others.

TENSE MOMENTS REFLECTION

Take a moment to recall a few times over the past month in which you felt some tension with friends, family, or coworkers about who was right, who was being too bossy or controlling, who was getting a better deal, or similar issues. These can involve anything—moments of casual discussion, deciding where to go out to eat, or determining who left a mess in the kitchen. Jot down a couple of these.

_____

_____

_____

Now imagine how much easier it would be to get along if you no longer cared about being right or whose needs were being met more often. This is not to say we should sign on for unbalanced, abusive relationships—but rather that everything goes very differently when both parties are less concerned with "me."

I Had a Little Shadow ...

One of the problems in developing an identity is that it involves excluding the aspects of "me" that don't fit. As I mentioned in Chapter 6, if I think of myself as an intelligent, compassionate, generous man (on good days), I'm going to have difficulty whenever I notice my stupid, unfeeling, selfish side (the rest of the time). In fact, when these other sides of my personality emerge in an interaction, I'll probably get upset—and feel angry with *you* for bringing these out. The famous psychiatrist C. G. Jung described these parts of our personality that we don't acknowledge because they don't fit our conscious identity as our *shadow*. We all have one, made up of everything we don't like about ourselves. You can find yours with a little reflection right now:

FINDING MY SHADOW

First make a list of some of your favorable qualities or virtues—the things that you like about yourself and that you feel good about when others notice.

1. _____

2. _____

3. _____

4. _____

5. _____

6. _____

Now look at each item on the list above and describe its opposite below on the corresponding numbered line:

1. _____

2. _____

3. _____

4. _____

5. _____

6. _____

Picture a person who embodies these negative qualities. This is a rough portrait of your shadow.

By illuminating how we construct our identity, mindfulness practice helps us recognize and accept our shadow moment by moment. Every desirable and undesirable feeling, thought, and image eventually arises in meditation, and we practice noticing and accepting them all. We see our anger, greed, lust, and fear along with our love, generosity, care, and courage. Seeing all of these contents, we gradually stop identifying with one particular set and rejecting the other. We eventually see that we have a great deal in common with everyone else—including those we are tempted to judge harshly. We see for ourselves why people in glass houses shouldn't throw stones.

> Mindfulness practice helps us understand why people in glass houses shouldn't throw stones.

It has been said that *mindfulness practice is not a path to perfection but a path to wholeness.* We don't wipe out the aspects of our personality that don't fit our desired identity, but rather make friends with these elements. This is humbling but also freeing. An ancient Zen teacher once put it this way: "The boundary of what we can accept in ourselves is the boundary of our freedom." By simply practicing awareness of present experience with acceptance, we can see ourselves and others more clearly, not distorted by the desire to see ourselves in a certain light.

Working with our experience in this way helps us celebrate our ordinariness while tearing down some of the barriers that separate us. There was a comedy troupe some years ago that created a record titled *I Think We're All Bozos on This Bus.* One routine went something like this: "Are you a Bozo?" "I'm a Bozo too." "My mother was a Bozoette in college." Despite all of our attempts to distinguish ourselves from one another, we share so many human foibles. We naturally start to relate to others with compassion when we see they're just like us. We also come to appreciate that we're unique—just like everyone else.

Embracing emotion

Mental health professionals use the phrase *affect tolerance* to describe the ability to fully feel emotions without running away from them. This is another essential skill for getting along. If I cannot recognize and tolerate my own feelings, I'm going to either project them onto you (for example, imagine that you're angry with me when in reality I'm angry with you) or blame you for "making" me feel a certain way. Mindfulness practice cultivates affect tolerance and thereby gives us much greater freedom in relationships. A classic Japanese story captures this well:

A cruel, sadistic general rode into town one day with his army. His men immediately set about stealing whatever they could and wreaking havoc. They raped women, killed children, burned down houses, and destroyed crops. When the general caught wind that there was a revered Zen master in town, he set out to vanquish him too.

The general galloped his horse up the hill on the edge of town and rode right into the main hall of the Zen temple. There, meditating on a cushion, was a little old man. The general brought his horse up next to him and held his bloody sword over the man's head. The man looked up. "Don't you realize I could run you through with this sword without blinking an eye?" asked the general. "Don't you realize I could be run through with that sword without blinking an eye?" asked the Zen master. At this point it is said that the general became disoriented, bowed, and left town.

Now, I'm not suggesting that this will always work as a military intervention. Nonetheless, it illustrates a powerful aspect of mindfulness practice. By spending time with both pleasant and unpleasant experiences and not escaping into entertainment or distraction, we become better at tolerating discomfort. Furthermore, by seeing ourselves as part of the larger world, and seeing how our sense of a separate self is constructed moment by moment, we become much less preoccupied with self-preservation—whether literal, as in this story, or symbolic, as in most interpersonal conflicts. This gives us enormous flexibility in how we respond to others. If the Zen master can be run through with a sword, we might be able to hear our partner's complaint about the dishes in the sink without launching a full-scale counterattack.

It's Not Personal

Another way that mindfulness practice helps us tolerate our feelings is by helping us see their impersonal nature. When we observe feelings arising during meditation practice, we focus on how they're experienced in the body. We see the tension associated with anger or fear; the feeling in our throat, chest, and eyes that comes with sadness; the lightness that comes with joy. Attending to emotions in this way, the "I" becomes extra. We experience not "my" but "the" anger, love, fear, joy, sadness, or lust arising in the body. As we come to believe less in our usual narrative thoughts ("I hate you because you were so mean to me"), it gets much easier to tolerate a full range of feelings. In fact, even negative emotions can become interesting—we watch them come and go, reach crescendos and fade. They become like other bodily events, such as an itch or an ache. This new perspective adds to our flexibility in responding to them.

A classic metaphor compares emotions to salt in water. If we dissolve a tablespoon of salt in a glass of water, it's difficult to drink. If, on the other hand, we dissolve the same tablespoon of salt in a clear pond, drinking it isn't a problem at all (or at least wasn't before so many ponds were polluted). Mindfulness makes the mind like a clear pond—able to integrate all sorts of contents without becoming overwhelmed by them. Because the mind has become expansive, we no longer feel compelled to get rid of unpleasant feelings or hold on to pleasant ones. We can practice *being with* all the emotions that arise in relationships. We can then be much more flexible in responding to interpersonal situations, no longer so afraid of having our feelings hurt.

> Mindfulness helps us embrace intense feelings and thereby makes us less afraid of being hurt.

Listening to one another

Another enormous benefit of learning to tolerate our feelings, especially when combined with an increased capacity to pay attention, is being able to listen to others. Often this isn't easy. Other people's concerns touch on ours and bring up painful reactions. When our friends tell us about their parent who is sick or their child who is struggling, we're reminded of our own loved ones' vulnerabilities. Just being with another person's anger, fear, or sadness can be difficult, because feelings tend to be contagious. And yet being with another in this way can be both helpful to the other person and enriching to the relationship. (In fact the word compassion comes from the Latin, *com pati*—to "suffer with.") I learned this lesson from a patient early in my clinical training.

I was a young psychology intern at a municipal teaching hospital. While the facility had excellent personnel and was associated with a prominent medical school, the physical plant was terrible. The old nurses' residence had been converted into clinical offices. It was once a stately building with high ceilings and enormous windows, but had long ago fallen into disrepair. Because it was due for renovation soon, the cash-strapped hospital had stopped virtually all maintenance. Once, after an angry patient tore a toilet out of the men's room, it sat in the hallway for weeks.

My particular office was a nice-size room on the third floor. There was an old wooden desk and two institutional chairs. The paint on the walls was peeling, and there were no curtains on the window. The office was lit by a single incandescent bulb, and at night the window was a gaping black rectangle.

It was in this setting that I saw a very depressed young man. He was convinced that he had no possibility of happiness, no chance of finding friends or love. Week after week he would tell me of his hopeless situation. I made feeble attempts to help—suggesting other ways to handle interactions, offering the possibility that things could turn out better than he expected. We looked at his past and why he might feel the way he did. We discussed the possibility of his taking medication. He found none of these suggestions useful.

Often I would leave one of these sessions quite depressed myself, thinking, "I'm a bright guy. I could've gone into so many fields. I'm clearly not cut out for *this*." Sometimes after a particularly depressing session my patient would come back the next week looking a little brighter. Sometimes he'd even suggest that our last meeting had been a little helpful. I would think, "To *you*, maybe—it just made me depressed."

After a while I began to understand what was happening. If I could actually hear him and feel the same stuckness he felt, it would somehow help. He finally felt a little understood, a little less alone. My challenge was being able to really *be with* him—to feel and tolerate his deep sadness and sense of no path forward. It took me a while to change tack, but I eventually got better at just being present. Instead of frantically trying to help, I learned to listen to his experience and note how his sorrow, loneliness, and grief resonated in my own mind and body. The shift probably looked subtle on the outside—but people are extraordinarily sensitive to these things. It helped him connect to his own feelings and even over time to begin to connect to other people.

While all of our interpersonal interactions aren't as intense or difficult as those psychotherapy sessions, similar principles apply. When we can actually be with someone and empathize with his or her experience, even when it's very painful, the relationship deepens. How often do we hear of romantic relationships, marriages, or friendships breaking apart because one or both parties feel that the other one doesn't really pay attention? "You never really listen to me." "You don't try to understand." "You're always lost in _____ [your computer; your work; the football game; that soap opera; phone calls with _____]." And while this skill is important for all relationships, as we'll see soon, it's absolutely essential to effective parenting.

Life with and without a space suit

Just as our attempts to avoid discomfort can trap us into anxiety, depression, and stress-related medical conditions, they can also isolate us from others. In our struggles to avoid feeling hurt, we don protective layers that leave us isolated. We discussed in Chapter 1 our shared reluctance to tell others of our difficulties—nobody wants to be thought of as a loser in this land of plenty. If we are unhappy, we assume it's because we have made mistakes—chosen the wrong career, spouse, or consumer product. After all, the people in commercials all seem to be doing so well.

By trying to appear happy and not exposing our vulnerabilities to others, we wind up alone and, paradoxically, more vulnerable. The Beatles got it right years ago when they sang, "It's the fool who plays it cool by making his world a little colder." Unfortunately, to varying degrees, we are all that fool.

Mindfulness helps us see that life is difficult for everybody—that we are indeed in the same boat. As the Dalai Lama put it, "Through compassion you find all human beings are just like you." If we think about what makes us feel close in love relationships or friendships, it is usually openly communicating our shared vulnerability.

Ironically, many people are drawn to meditation with the hope of becoming *invulnerable*—no longer feeling needy, insecure, or dependent on others. But it doesn't work out that way. Instead, mindfulness practice teaches us how to be vulnerable. There is a myth of a lost paradise called Shambhala that predated the arrival of Buddhism in Tibet (like most myths, it can be understood to relate to a mythical kingdom or a psychological realm). A special breed of warriors lived there. They were not warriors in the conventional sense—defeating external enemies in battle—but psychological warriors. It is said that they had the courage to live life *like a cow without its skin*. They trained themselves to be exquisitely vulnerable to feelings—sensitive to everything. This is the opposite of living life in a space suit, protected by defenses. Being this sensitive, this vulnerable, allows us to really connect with one another. Peeling off our protective layers allows us to touch and be touched.

Most of us fear this level of vulnerability, associating it with weakness. After all, we live in a culture in which a politician can ruin his or her career by admitting to having been in psychotherapy. But this reveals a confused understanding of what strength is psychologically and interpersonally. There is a traditional Japanese adage that captures the confusion:

Which is stronger, a mighty oak tree or a reed of bamboo? Many assume the oak; but the true answer is a reed of bamboo. When a monsoon comes, the mighty oak easily loses a branch or splits in two. In even a gentle breeze, the reed of bamboo bends. It may nearly fold over in a strong wind. But as soon as the storm passes, the bamboo stands upright again.

> Mindfulness helps us become more resilient at the same time as it makes us more vulnerable and sensitive.

Mindfulness practice helps us develop an emotional life like the reed of bamboo or the Shambhala warrior. We become vulnerable and sensitive but recover easily when difficulty passes. By practicing awareness of present experience with acceptance, we notice a full range of feeling responses and are vulnerable to them all. But because we feel them fully, they leave fewer traces when they pass—so we are freshly open to the next moment. Being present in this way enables us to connect deeply to others. We can be with our friend's joys and sorrows because we can welcome our own. My patient's experience illustrates nicely why we put on space suits and how mindfulness practice can help us take them off:

Larry hated being so sensitive. As a little kid, he would worry about doing well in school, felt homesick when he went away to summer camp, and was often self-conscious. Other kids made fun of him for crying, and his parents both told him he should toughen up.

In high school he started to come into his own—he grew tall and became good at sports. He started to feel more confident and was able to hide his insecurities.

By college Larry had become something of a player. He was quite good looking now and picked up women easily. He often drank with his buddies and occasionally did other drugs. He liked being cool and having a lot of friends.

As an adult, Larry's sensitive side began to give him trouble again. He married a loving woman and landed a respectable professional job but started to feel inadequate at work. He hated feeling weak. He developed insomnia and stomach distress—both stress-related. He also noticed that he was drinking more.

To deal with his stress, Larry took up mindfulness practice. While it helped him relax, it also highlighted just how sensitive he really was. He noticed that almost all interactions with other guys made him feel vulnerable—wondering what they thought of him and debating how assertive he should be. He often felt angry after encounters—even those that on the surface went well. Larry also realized that he was sentimental about little things—random acts of kindness, a child crying, someone taking care of an animal. Watching these feelings come and go was confusing. He wished he could be tougher but also saw that needing to be tough was like being in a prison. Eventually he felt how deeply he just wanted to be accepted for who he was—to not have to be so cool anymore.

So Larry started taking more risks. He told his wife about some of his feelings, and luckily she was understanding and appreciative. He even started being more honest with a few of the guys at work and developed real friendships there. His insomnia and indigestion diminished as his connections to others deepened.

Mindfulness in relationship

Connecting with others not only allows us to get along but also enriches our lives. Researchers find that when we feel close to friends and loved ones we experience greater energy and vitality, a greater capacity to act, increased clarity, an enhanced sense of value or dignity, and both the desire and capacity for more connection. Interpersonal connection feels "right" and is self-reinforcing. When my colleague and I understand and support one another, creative ideas flow and work becomes a pleasure; when my wife and I feel close and loving, we're eager to engage the world and face whatever life brings.

We have seen how our individual mindfulness practice can change our relationship to our own emotions in ways that allow us to connect to one another. There are also mindfulness techniques that we can practice with others to deepen relationships.

You will need a partner for this exercise. While it can feel rather intense and intimate, the exercise can work with loved ones and with people you know less well. Both you and your partner should have at least a little experience with meditation practice before trying this. Allow 20–30 minutes.

—————————— *Breathing Together** ——————————

Begin by sitting facing one another, spines relatively erect. Close your eyes, and do 10–15 minutes of concentration practice. Bring your attention to the sensations of your breath in your belly. Notice how your belly rises with each inhalation and falls with each exhalation. Whenever you find your attention wandering, gently return it to the sensations of the breath. You may notice some feelings of anxiety or apprehension doing this while facing another person. Just allow those feelings to come and go, returning your attention to the breath.

Once you've developed a little bit of concentration, gently open your eyes. Allow your gazes to rest on one another's bellies. Watch the breath of your partner as you also continue to notice the rising and falling sensations in your own body. Perhaps your breathing will start to synchronize; perhaps it won't. Either way, just try to remain aware of your own breathing and that of your partner for the next five minutes.

The following phase can feel rather intense, so feel free to adjust your gaze as you see fit. Try raising your gaze to silently look into the eyes of your partner. Don't try to communicate anything in particular—just take in the experience of being with him or her. Allow yourself to notice your breath in the background while you focus most of your attention on looking into your partner's eyes. If this starts to feel too uncomfortable, feel free to lower your gaze to your partner's belly again. You can shift back and forth between the belly and the eyes to adjust the intensity of this experience.

---

*Available in audio at *www.mindfulness-solution.com*.

Once you've gazed into your partner's eyes for several minutes, begin to imagine what he or she was like as a young child. Imagine him or her having a mother and father and growing up with other children. Imagine how he or she went through the same stages you did—going off to school, becoming a teenager, perhaps eventually leaving home. Be aware that your partner has had thousands of moments of joy and sorrow, fear and anger, longing and fulfillment—just like you.

Now begin to imagine how your partner will look as he or she gets older. Be aware that, just like you, your partner will be dealing with the next stages of the life cycle. He or she will probably have to wrestle with infirmity and old age. Imagine how this will be for him or her—both the pleasant and unpleasant aspects.

Finally, be aware that, just like you, someday your partner will die. The molecules in his or her body will recycle back into the earth or atmosphere and be transformed into something else.

Once you've imagined your partner at all stages of the life cycle, bring your attention back to how he or she looks in the present. Then drop your gaze down to your partner's belly and breathe together again for a few minutes.

Finally, finish the exercise with several minutes of meditation with your eyes closed. Notice the different feelings that accompany each phase of the exercise.

Paying Attention in Relationship

The *Breathing Together* exercise can be both interesting and a bit overwhelming. It illuminates how most of the time we're less attentive and more defended against really connecting with the other person. It can also help bridge gaps that we feel between ourselves and others by highlighting our commonality. And it can spur us to be compassionate and follow the ancient injunction, usually attributed to Plato: "Be kind, for everyone you meet is fighting a hard battle."

Of course, most contact with other people won't be quite like the *Breathing Together* exercise (if you insist on it, you probably won't have too many friends). Nonetheless, there are ways to practice mindfulness in relationship less formally.

My friend and colleague Janet Surrey has been studying ways to use mindfulness practice during both psychotherapy and everyday interactions. She points out that whenever we're talking with another person we can bring our attention to three objects of awareness. First there are the body sensations, thoughts, and feelings happening in us. We're familiar with these from meditation practice—we simply notice them while interacting with the other person. Second, there are the body sensations, thoughts, and feelings that we sense in the other. We intuit these through the words, body language, and facial expression of our partner. Third—and this one may seem strange at first—we can bring our attention to our *felt sense of connection and disconnection* with the other person.

There is a classic scene that has unfolded countless times in marital counseling (please forgive the gender stereotypes): The wife says to her husband, "Honey, I hate it that every time I get upset, you disappear." He looks confused and says, "But sweetheart, I'm sitting right next to you." She starts to get frustrated and says, "I don't mean you *literally* disappear; I mean you disappear *emotionally*." "But I'm listening to all of your feelings," he says, bewildered.

The conversation often breaks down at this point, with neither party understanding the other. What the wife is describing is her felt sense of connection or disconnection with her husband. This is a subtle experience—not easy to measure or define clearly. Yet it's an important aspect of all relationships.

By attending to our felt sense of connection and disconnection, along with our inner emotions and those of our partner, we can feel more richly related to other people. There is an informal mindfulness practice that you can try whenever in conversation:

Three Objects of Awareness

Just as you would pay attention to your feet moving through space and touching the ground when doing walking meditation, bring your attention to these three objects of awareness when talking with another person:

1. Your body sensations, thoughts, and feelings
2. Your partner's words, body language, and facial expressions
3. Your felt sense of connection and disconnection with your partner

When your mind wanders from these three objects, gently bring it back.

You can try this informal practice when with friends, loved ones, coworkers, or anyone else with whom you have more than passing contact.

Beginner's Mind

Have you ever said or done something and been surprised by the other person's reaction? We go about our business, thinking that we're being decent, reasonable people—and suddenly find ourselves in trouble. This is disturbing enough in public situations: A student thinks she's just answering a question and can't understand why her teacher is suddenly annoyed; a supervisor doesn't see how he could have possibly offended his subordinate. But when it happens in intimate relationships, it can make both parties thoroughly miserable.

Russ could hardly believe what had happened. It was Friday night, and he was happy to be going home. He had been working hard all week, and he and Nancy had scarcely had time to talk. He was looking forward to finally relaxing and spending some time with her.

When he got there, Nancy looked great. She had on a new outfit and had done her hair differently. They hugged and kissed, and he started telling her how stressful his day had been and how glad he was to see her. After they had talked for a little while, Nancy asked, "So where are we going tonight?" Russ replied, "I don't know. What would you like to do?" She didn't answer right away. Russ started to sense that something was wrong. "I guess it doesn't really matter," she replied after a few seconds.

The evening started to go downhill from there. Nancy suddenly seemed cold. Russ asked her if she was upset about something. He couldn't imagine what might be the problem. It took quite a few minutes, but eventually she told him that she thought he had said he was going to take her out and she was angry that he hadn't made a plan. Russ hated the feeling that he had somehow failed her again and started to react defensively, saying that all they had discussed was "spending time together" Friday night. Nancy said something about this kind of thing happening "a lot" since Russ had been so tied up in his work. He said something about her always thinking he wasn't doing enough. It didn't take long before they were both hurt and angry, thoroughly convinced that the other was being unfair.

How might mindfulness practice have helped? Mindfulness meditation cultivates what the Zen master Shunryu Suzuki called *beginner's mind*—the ability to let go of prior conceptions and see things with fresh eyes. He famously said, *"In the beginner's mind there are many possibilities, but in the expert's there are few."* Mindfulness practice does this by helping us not take our thoughts too seriously but seeing how they change with our moods, and by helping us notice what is actually happening in the moment.

In intimate relationships, it can be especially difficult to see things with a beginner's mind. We become so accustomed to our assumptions about the other person, and so influenced by our emotions, that we don't see our partner very clearly.

Had both Russ and Nancy been able to approach their situation more mindfully, they might have each responded differently. Approaching the situation with open curiosity and a willingness to fully feel feelings could have made a big difference.

When Nancy looked upset, Russ might have practiced *Three Objects of Awareness*, and tried just to listen to her while watching his own emotional reactions—instead of responding defensively. He would have considered the possibility that she was annoyed because she was hurt and that she was hurt because she loved him and missed him. He would have been able to feel and stay with the pain of her disappointment, rather than immediately seeing it as a reflection of his shortcomings. And he would have been able to imagine what it had been like to be Nancy over the past weeks when he'd been so wrapped up in his work.

When it became clear that Russ hadn't made plans, by practicing mindfulness Nancy might have more clearly noticed the hurt beneath her anger. She would have been able to experience and tolerate her longings for connection and feelings of being neglected more easily. Rather than assuming he didn't make plans because he didn't care about her, she might have heard that Russ really wanted to be with her too and might have told him how she had missed him.

If they each had been able to see the other with fresh, clear eyes and open to both their own and the other's pain, they might have responded to one another with empathy and understanding. This would have enabled them to reconnect emotionally, compromise on plans for the evening, and have a nice night together.

Parenting

Anyone who has ever cared for children—even briefly—knows that it's an emotional adventure. A diligent meditation student once complained that her mind was full of desire. She had read of spiritual seekers who renounced worldly pleasures and thought that she perhaps should be trying this herself. She asked Jack Kornfield, a well-known psychologist and meditation teacher, "How can I get beyond my constant desiring? What practices should I pursue to become a renunciate?" Jack asked her what she did each day. She replied, "Not much. I'm a stay-at-home mom—I take care of my three kids—and try to find time to meditate." He said, "You've already got more than enough opportunities to practice renunciation."

By caring for another we're challenged to let go of our focus on fulfilling our own desires. Many times this is a relief. We get a sense of meaning or purpose in caring for others that's missing when we're focused on trying to make ourselves happy. But doing it isn't easy. Children need a lot of care and attention and have a way of highlighting all of our unresolved emotional issues and vulnerabilities. Parenting is a difficult job for which most of us have little formal training. Luckily, mindfulness practice can help us do it more skillfully.

Being Present

Over the past several decades, psychologists have learned a lot about how parent–child interactions shape development. Babies are born with exquisitely sensitive communication capabilities—but they don't arrive with a translator. Parents face the challenge of understanding their children's preverbal language from day one. Anyone who has ever cared for a crying infant has been through the checklist: (1) diaper wet? (2) too cold? (3) too hot? (4) hungry? (5) sleepy? Sometimes none of these is the problem and the baby just needs to be held.

Once the basics are covered, this last need is critical. Children rely on their caregivers for emotional regulation. We discussed in Chapter 2 the balance between the intensity of unpleasant experiences and our felt capacity to bear them. When this capacity is strong, we can deal well with considerable misfortune. When this capacity is weakened, little things easily overwhelm us. The younger the child, the less he or she can deal with unpleasant experiences alone. Instead, children are designed to "borrow" our capacity to bear discomfort.

We've all seen how a young child in terrible distress can settle quickly when held by Mom or Dad. This holding is actually a very complex process. Researchers have recorded interactions between a parent and a baby by videotaping both of their faces. Slowing down the tapes, they can observe microcommunications. The baby begins to smile, the parent responds; the parent's eyes shift, the baby responds. These microcommunications happen as quickly as *ten times per second*. It's through this process that the baby feels the parent's presence, and it turns out that if the parent can bear the emotion of the moment, the baby often can too. Of course this isn't important just for babies. When children get older, our capacity to "hold" them when they're distressed is equally important.

Seen more broadly, the human capacity to bear difficult experience is contagious. This becomes particularly clear during times of crisis. One graphic example described by Thich Nhat Hanh involved people fleeing Vietnam at the end of the war:

Conditions on the crowded refugee boats were terrible. The passengers had experienced horrible trauma; many were separated from their families and afraid for their lives. Most had lost all of their possessions. The boats themselves were overloaded and vulnerable both to attacks by pirates and to sinking. Even if they made it to their destination, it wasn't clear whether the refugees would be accepted or sent back out to sea.

In this atmosphere it was very easy for panic to break out. Sometimes there would be a nun, monk, or other person with a strong mindfulness meditation practice on board. Passengers near that person would tend to be more settled. It was as though there were concentric rings of acceptance surrounding him or her. The closer people were to the meditator, the stronger the influence. The opposite effect could be seen elsewhere. If a passenger was hysterical or hostile, others around that person tended to be agitated as well.

Mindfulness practice helps us provide holding for our children in two ways. First, by helping us pay attention, it helps us read their communications more accurately. While we may not be fully conscious of subtle signals being transmitted back and forth ten times a second, we can be more aware of our child's emotional state and our own reactions to it. Second, mindfulness practice increases our capacity to bear discomfort. Since it's

> Through mindfulness practice we learn to read our children's communications more accurately and to comfort them more effectively.

particularly difficult for most of us to see our children in distress, the greater our capacity to bear this, the better our chances are of being able to help them deal with difficult emotions. For Stacey, this was a life saver.

As a young mother, Stacey had a lot of trouble whenever her daughter cried. She herself had been raised by alcoholic parents who weren't available emotionally. Her daughter's cries reminded her of her own early tears—but she was at a loss for how to respond.

To deal with the stresses of being a mother, Stacey took up yoga and learned mindfulness meditation. When doing formal sitting practice, Stacey began to have memories of feeling abandoned by her parents. She became aware of deep feelings of fear and sadness. She realized that she had never really felt seen or loved.

Recalling how alone she had felt as a child, Stacey committed herself to being more present to her daughter. Instead of responding out of fear or shutting down, she practiced really looking at and listening to her daughter when she was upset. Gradually Stacey was able to see how her daughter responded to her own state of mind—if Stacey could trust that she herself would be okay, her daughter would settle when she held her. Caring for her daughter this way felt like healing her own wounds.

While many of us have had better parenting than Stacey, we can all use mindfulness practices to become more aware of our own emotional responses and to attend more skillfully to our children. Several of the practices and exercises discussed in Chapter 6, especially *Noting Emotions in the Body*, *Surveying Emotions in the Body*, and *Observing Emotions throughout the Day*, can be particularly useful when we notice realms of emotion that make us either recoil or overreact. The *Three Objects of Awareness* practice can also help us be more present and observant with our children.

Entering a Child's World

One challenge to communicating with children involves cultural differences. Even if you're raising your biological child in the same community in which you grew up, a child's world is very different from an adult's. Children's culture involves a different sense of time and reality.

The younger the child, the more the boy or girl lives in the present moment. When my children were little, I asked Karlen Lyons-Ruth, a well-known developmental psychologist, what she thought about the "terrible twos." Why are toddlers so tough to manage at this age? She explained that kids' emotions aren't really so different at age two than at age one. What changes is their capacity to think about the past and future. When a one-year-old girl wants a cookie and I say, "No," she gets upset. But if I say, "Look at Teddy—I think he wants to play," she quickly gets involved in the present and turns her attention to the bear. By age two, when I introduce Teddy, she smiles, looks at the bear, and then demands the cookie again. This capacity to think about things from the past and imagine a future gets stronger each year until children are, like their parents, mostly living in their thoughts about the past and future.

To connect well with young children, we need to be able to return to the present ourselves. Mindfulness practice helps. If we can learn to be present following our breath, we can certainly be engaged looking at our baby or even reading *Goodnight Moon* or playing Chutes and Ladders yet another time. Our ability to be present for whatever is happening in the moment, even if it doesn't hold a lot of entertainment value, is very useful with young children.

Children also live in a different reality. The younger the child, the less the girl or boy lives in a world of logical concepts and the more she or he lives in a kaleidoscopic world of images. What adults call fantasy and reality blend seamlessly. Here, too, mindfulness practice can help us be with young kids. The more we practice mindfulness, the less seriously we take our own concepts and the more open we are to the fluid experience of moment-to-moment awareness. We notice how our own fantasies interweave with experiences that we think of as "reality." As we become more comfortable with this aspect of the mind and more aware of how its contents shift and change, we become more attuned to children's magical worlds.

We can see this vividly when we play with kids. It's interesting to think about how work and play differ. Work tends to be goal oriented, focused on doing rather than being, and favors result over process—the bottom line is getting the job done. Play, on the other hand, is goalless, focuses on being rather than doing, and favors process over result—the only goal or result is a good time. As adults, we can get so caught up in work that it's difficult to play. Doing chores, paying bills, responding to e-mail, and running errands—we get in the habit of just trying to finish things so we can get to the good stuff.

Mindfulness practices help us recover the ability to play. By cultivating awareness and acceptance, they teach us to be with experience in the moment rather than only pursuing goals. If we follow a regular practice pattern including both formal meditation and informal practice throughout the day, mindfulness training can help us remember how to play with our children.

> Mindfulness helps us connect with our children by tuning in to our own fantasy world and by helping us remember how to play.

Love and limits

When my twin daughters were young, I was horrified to notice how often I said, "No." I recall a visit to their pediatrician when they were toddlers. He gave them both an exam, inquired about their sleep and eating habits, and reassured us that they appeared to be physically healthy. He then asked if we had any other concerns. I said, "My only concern is that they are both acutely suicidal." They would try to wander into the street, touch the hot stove, climb the stairs, and otherwise endanger their lives. In response, I protectively said, "No ... No ... No" all day long.

Talk about puppy training. As parents of young children, we spend hour after hour trying to either protect them from physical harm or socialize them to be able to get along with others ("What's the magic word?" "Hitting isn't allowed!" "You have to take turns."). This requires a constant stream of criticism—since a lot of what comes naturally to young children is often either dangerous or socially unacceptable.

It's remarkable that any kids grow up to like themselves. What balances our constant disapproval is love and the ability to separate the deed from the person. If we can maintain a deep sense of love and acceptance while working to correct our kids' behavior, the chances of their hating themselves are drastically reduced. It also helps to be really present when we read stories, play checkers, toss a ball, and cuddle.

Regular mindfulness practice, including particularly the *Loving-Kindness Meditation* described in Chapter 4 and the *Breathing Together* practice described earlier in this chapter, helps us do this. The more we practice accepting ourselves and seeing ourselves as part of the larger universe, the more we can really accept our kids, even if they aren't behaving optimally. And the more we practice being present generally, the easier it is to be present when playing with our kids or sharing in their experiences of wonder and discovery. During tough times, we can turn to loving-kindness practice as a life preserver to keep ourselves afloat and avoid getting caught in a storm of critical thoughts toward our child.

Again, It's Not Personal

Perhaps the biggest obstacle we face in accepting our children involves taking their behavior personally. What parents haven't felt that their child's good behavior reflects positively on them, while feeling ashamed of their kid's bad behavior? To some degree, even though we know we shouldn't, we all view our kids as extensions of ourselves. Now not only are we concerned with our own rank in the primate troop, but we're worried about theirs. Whose child is a better athlete? Whose is a better student? Whose is kinder or more mature? Whose is more attractive? Every dimension we've ever worried about in our own life becomes an arena for worrying about our child's success or failure.

This usually leads to trouble. It makes us push our kids to achieve goals that may not be in their best interest. It makes us feel anxious or overwhelmed at precisely the times that our kids most need us to be present for them. It is the engine behind many of our parenting mistakes.

If you are a parent, or have cared for children, think of the moments during which you were most upset by a child's behavior. Take a moment to recall one incident before reading on. What were you feeling inside at the time? Did you feel ashamed or humiliated? The realization that we can't get a child to behave, or the thought that we've raised our child poorly, puts most of us over the edge. In these moments, when we take our kids' behavior as a reflection of our own competence, we become least effective. An experience I had after moving to a new community brought this home:

Our new town had a lot of conservation land and attracted an out-doorsy crowd. Each year around 20 families would participate in a multi-day community hike in the White Mountains. The trails were challenging, involving considerable change in altitude, sometimes in hot, buggy weather.

A couple of hours into our first hike my kids were beginning to feel tired. One of the veteran mothers said, "You're hiking with your kids. It may go better if you hike separately." I thought that this was an odd comment, until a couple of hours later, when things took a turn for the worse.

My wife and I started to argue—first with our kids and then with each other. The veteran mom offered to hike with our kids for a while and let us hike with another group. We took her up on her offer, and everything got a lot better. My kids finished the hike tired but happy.

What made the difference? We can care for children best when we don't take what they do personally (kids of course also behave better with adults who are not their parents). I had no problem dealing with other children's complaints—they didn't reflect on me. Similarly, other parents were better able to support and redirect my kids when they had trouble.

By loosening the preoccupation with "me," helping us see how identity is constructed, and increasing our capacity to bear emotions, regular mindfulness practice helps us to not take parenting as personally—to respond to our own children with the compassion and objectivity we might have with someone else's. The same way that it helps us to be less concerned with our own successes and failures, it allows us to take our kids' successes and failures less seriously. And this makes it much easier to enjoy loving them.

Setting Limits

Most of us have little difficulty knowing what skillful parenting might look like. We just have trouble putting it into action. It's easy to understand that clear limits with consistent consequences help children behave well. Reward good behavior; ignore or thoughtfully punish bad behavior. Don't yell, criticize, or shame the child, but follow through with your plan. It's pretty simple.

The problem is, most of us have trouble responding appropriately in the heat of the moment. Much of the time we respond to our feelings automatically. This is so much a part of our everyday experience that our language around it is confused. If I say, "I got angry," what do I really mean? Do I mean that I felt anger arising in my mind and body? Do I mean that I expressed my anger to another person? We are so unaccustomed to having a gap between feeling and behavior that we don't have an easy way in English to distinguish these two responses.

Mindfulness practice creates the necessary gap—what in meditation traditions is called *recognizing the spark before the flame*. It helps us notice a feeling arising and notice the impulse to act

> When we say "I got angry," our language demonstrates that we hardly recognize a gap between having a feeling and acting on that feeling.

that follows. Mindfulness practice allows us to feel the urge to act on that impulse and to decide whether doing so would be skillful right now. It offers the possibility of taking a breath and grounding ourselves in what we're experiencing at the moment, *before* taking action.

Behavior Modification for Parents

Children regularly enroll their parents in behavior modification programs. A boy wants his mother to buy him a toy. His mother says, "No," and the boy starts to whine. He complains that she never gets him anything he wants but always gets his sister stuff. As they walk around the store, he carries on more and more. Finally, exasperated, his mom buys the toy. Voilà! The boy is happy and cooperative again. Mom receives reinforcement for buying the toy and will be more likely to give in again the next time.

Children train us to yell with similar techniques. "It's time to clean up your toys." Fifteen minutes later, nothing has happened. "Really, sweetheart, you have to clean up before dinner." Ten minutes more, no progress. "I'VE TOLD YOU TWICE. IT'S TIME TO CLEAN UP!" Now the child starts putting things away—and Dad receives positive reinforcement for yelling.

Mindfulness practice can help us avoid this sort of behavioral training. In the first instance, it can help us tolerate the feeling of disappointing our child. In the second, it allows us to open a gap between feeling, impulse, and action—so we have the opportunity to change course.

While establishing a regular mindfulness practice will generally help us respond more appropriately to these sorts of challenges, in the heat of the moment the *Three-Minute Breathing Space* described in Chapter 6 can be a particularly handy life preserver. Taking a brief break from the drama to notice our thoughts, feelings, and body sensations, take refuge in the fact that the breath is still there, and relax into the feeling experience of the moment can help us tolerate what is happening and discern the best response.

Absolution

My friend and colleague Trudy Goodman calls our mistakes raising children *parenting crimes*. We all have our own rap sheet of indictments and convictions. These are the incidents in which we yelled at our kids, humiliated them, made them feel rejected or inadequate, failed to set effective limits, burdened them with adult worries—the list goes on and on.

They include all the moments in which we're grateful for child protective services. Like the day in the Home Depot that I managed to restrain myself from strangling one of my young daughters by thinking, "It would be very embarrassing as a clinical psychologist to be reported for child abuse."

Convicting ourselves of parenting crimes is rarely helpful. It propels us to overcompensate for our mistakes (giving in to demands after having been too harsh or becoming too harsh after giving in). These convictions also make us more insecure and less able to deal with the next challenge.

Mindfulness practice generally, and *Loving-Kindness Meditation* in particular, can help here too. When we learn to take the whole drama less personally and see how our own responses come out of our personal history and conditioning, we don't convict ourselves so harshly. We start to see our foibles as parents as part of human vulnerability and foibles generally—not just our particular shortcomings. We see all the self-critical thoughts as just more judgments, rather than as solid realities. And we notice that, try as we might, there's no way we can be perfect parents or protect our children from difficulty. They will face the same challenges of loss and change as other human beings. They will face joy and sorrow, pleasure and pain, no matter what we do.

Putting it all together: practicing relational mindfulness

Most of the ways that mindfulness practice improves our relationships are gradual and cumulative. Sometimes when I lecture on this topic I'm glad my wife isn't in the audience. She might stand up and object like people are invited to do at weddings and say, "I don't think this stuff works. After all of his mindfulness practice, he's really not very good at intimacy. *He's still a guy.*" She may be right, but her objection leaves out an important possibility alluded to in the Preface. We don't have a control group. Who knows what I would have been like *without* years of mindfulness training?

For most of us, getting along with others will never be effortless, with or without mindfulness practice. Nonetheless, engaging regularly in formal and informal mindfulness practices, and remembering to use life preservers when we find ourselves caught in storms of feeling that might otherwise drive us to behave rashly, can help.

As part of establishing a general mindfulness practice of the sort described in Chapters 3 and 4, *Loving-Kindness Meditation* is particularly important for generating acceptance—not only toward yourself but also toward others. You can try directing positive intentions toward both people you like and those you don't. The guiding principle is not to force false sentiments but rather to accept whatever arises. As discussed in Chapter 4, this may involve acknowledging all sorts of negative or paradoxical responses.

If you have a partner who is interested in mindfulness practice, the *Breathing Together* exercise described in this chapter can be very powerful. Periodically doing this together can help reinforce a feeling of connection with one another.

During the rough and tumble of daily interactions, the *Three Objects of Awareness* practice can help you be more fully present. It can be very enriching to take ordinary conversations as opportunities for informal mindfulness practice—since even our simplest exchanges reveal a lot of emotion and meaning when we attend to them fully. If you're having difficulty knowing what you actually feel in a relationship, practices and exercises discussed in Chapter 6, such as *Noting Emotions in the Body,* *Surveying Emotions in the Body,* and *Observing Emotions throughout the Day,* can help you become more aware of these. If you're getting stuck in repetitive, obsessive thoughts about a relationship, *Thought Labeling* (Chapter 6) can help you see the pattern more clearly, while *Thoughts Are Just Thoughts* (Chapter 5) can help you let them go.

And then there are the inevitable moments in which we might "lose it" in one way or another. These are interactions in which anger or fear takes over and we find ourselves in danger of saying or doing things we may later regret. In these moments, the *Three-Minute Breathing Space* (Chapter 6) can be a valuable life preserver. It may require excusing yourself briefly from the interaction but has the potential to save you and the other person a great deal of grief.

Sometimes we've had time to think about our response to another person and realize what the best course of action is but are having trouble resisting the urge to do something foolish. This might happen during moments of jealousy with a partner, anger at a disobedient child, or frustration with a friend. Here *Urge Surfing* (Chapters 7 and 9) can be another life preserver. You can watch the urge to make a phone call, send an e-mail, or drive to the person's house arise, reach a crescendo, and pass—without acting on it. Similarly, there are times that we get so preoccupied with a relationship drama that we need to clear our heads by attending to something that's neither personal nor interpersonal. Here *Nature Meditation* (Chapter 5) can be useful either as a formal or informal practice.

Because there are even more varieties of relationship issues than there are of anxiety, depression, or stress-related problems, no single prescription will fit everyone. Here's one way that mindfulness practices fit together to enhance a person's relational life. Your own experience will likely be somewhat different:

Stuart was a hardworking mid-level manager and father of three who tried to do well at work while still being there for his wife, kids, and ailing parents. Though he loved his family, he was often stressed out and missed his younger days when he had time to himself.

To try to relax, Stuart took up mindfulness practice. He got into the routine of meditating several times a week before work and doing informal practice during both his commute and weekend chores. As he began to feel calmer and more present, Stuart noticed that his relationships also started going better. He picked up books and articles about meditation and found himself changing his priorities.

On his job, the big difference was that Stuart took things less personally. He became aware of what a huge role ego played when things went wrong—everyone always blaming each other and getting defensive. He started to see how his own efforts to impress others caused him needless worry, so he focused more on doing a good job and less on being recognized. Stuart now took everything less personally—he didn't get so pumped up when things went well or think so poorly of himself when they didn't. The more he focused on helping the business succeed instead of protecting his self-image, the smoother work relationships became.

At home, mindfulness practice made Stuart see how distracted he had been. His wife had often complained of feeling neglected, which hurt him because he had tried so hard to please everybody. In an effort to both deepen his practice and respond to his wife's needs, he began treating their conversations as times to practice *Three Objects of Awareness*. He noticed that when his attention wandered or he felt pressed to attend to his to-do list, she'd get upset. He realized that by bringing his attention back to what was happening between them in the moment, he would feel closer to her, and they got along better.

Being mindful during his interactions with his kids, Stuart realized that he was often impatient with them. When one didn't understand something or needed his help, he sometimes acted annoyed—which invariably upset his kid and led to either an argument or a meltdown. After seeing this pattern repeat over and over, he started trying to take a *Three-Minute Breathing Space* when he got tense. He wasn't always successful, but at least sometimes he could notice the feelings underneath his impatience—whether anxiety, pain about his child's difficulty, or anger connected to one of his own childhood memories. On good days, seeing these and taking the time to breathe and tune in to his feelings allowed him to respond more skillfully to his kids.

Stuart's relationship to his ailing parents also benefited from his mindfulness practice. While they had tried to be good to him, they themselves had been raised in chaotic families, so this didn't come naturally. Stuart still had a lot of leftover disappointment and anger about his own upbringing, which was triggered whenever his parents were bossy or controlling. By attending more carefully to his feelings when with them and using the *Three-Minute Breathing Space* when he was about to lose it, Stuart got better at helping his parents without being driven crazy.

With all of this going on, Stuart needed a way to clear his head and take a break from his intensely interpersonal life. *Nature Meditation* provided a welcome respite—he was grateful for occasional opportunities to just pay attention to the natural world.

Mindfulness practices for living the full catastrophe: relationships

Once you've established a foundation of regular formal and informal practice as described in Chapters 3 and 4, you can use the following to enhance your relationships.

Formal Meditation Practices

- *Breathing Together* (page 232) to feel connected to your partner and sense the common ground between you
- *Loving-Kindness Meditation* (page 84) to cultivate compassion toward others and absolve yourself from parenting crimes and other infractions
- *Noting Emotions in the Body* (page 145) to increase awareness of your feelings in response to others
- *Thought Labeling* (page 154) to identify and let go of obsessive thoughts about a relationship
- *Thoughts Are Just Thoughts* (page 125) to allow obsessive thoughts about a relationship to arise and pass

Informal Practices

- *Three Objects of Awareness* (page 234) to attend to your felt sense of connection and disconnection with other people

Also, all of the following can help bring attention to the here and now throughout the day and thereby help you be more present in your relationships:

- *Walking Meditation* (page 67)
- *Nature Meditation* (page 128)
- *Eating Meditation* (page 263)
- *Driving, Showering, Tooth Brushing, Shaving (etc.) Meditation* (page 90)

Life Preservers

- *Three-Minute Breathing Space* (page 157) when you're about to act impulsively out of anger, fear, or other passion
- *Urge Surfing* (pages 191 and 273) when you're feeling compelled to do something foolish in a relationship despite having thought of the consequences
- *Nature Meditation* (formal or informal; page 128) to clear your head when you need a break from interpersonal life

Developing a plan

You may find it useful to jot down an action plan for using mindfulness practices in relationships. You can photocopy the form on the following pages and make different plans for different relationships.

When your relationship needs more help

It's remarkably easy to get stuck in destructive patterns with others. While mindfulness practice can help interrupt these, sometimes the perspective of a neutral third party is needed.

If despite your best efforts things aren't improving and a relationship problem is taking a toll on someone's health, happiness, or functioning at school or work, consulting with a mental health professional may

PRACTICE PLAN

Begin by reflecting on relationships you find challenging.

Relationship I Want to Work On: _____

_____

Situations I Want to Address: _____

_____

My Experience during These Situations:

Physical (what happens in my body): _____

_____

Cognitive (thoughts): _____

_____

Behavioral (things I do or avoid): _____

_____

Times I Most Need a Life Preserver: _____

_____

_____

Now, based on what you've read about and experienced with the different practices, jot down an initial practice plan (you can vary this as your needs change).

Formal Practice	*When*	*How Often*
_____	_____	_____
_____	_____	_____
_____	_____	_____

(cont.)

Informal Practice	When	How Often
_____	_____	_____
_____	_____	_____
_____	_____	_____

Life Preserver	Likely Situation
_____	_____
_____	_____
_____	_____

make sense. Many psychotherapists work not only with individuals but also with couples and families. If your conflict is with someone at work or school, you might consult a therapist individually—since it's often not practical to take your teacher, boss, or coworker into therapy. When the problem is in a couple, between siblings, or between a parent and child, family therapy is usually optimal. If your partner or other family member doesn't want to participate, you can always consult a therapist yourself as a first step to explore options for proceeding.

A small but growing number of psychotherapists use mindfulness-based approaches to couples and family therapy. While other approaches can also be very useful, you may find that working with a therapist who is trained this way will support your mindfulness practice as you work on interpersonal issues. You can find suggestions for finding a couple's or family therapist, along with other resources for working with relationships at the back of the book.

Relationship difficulties of one kind or another are inevitable. Usually it's our behavior that gets us into trouble—we know intellectually what would be best but have trouble following through. This happens in a lot of other areas too. In the next chapter we'll tackle our tendency to fall into bad habits—and see how mindfulness practices can help us make better choices in everything from eating and exercising to TV and sex.

CHAPTER 9

Breaking bad habits

Learning to make good choices

*E*ver have trouble doing the right thing? Feel bad about things you've done? So far we've discussed how mindfulness practice can help us work with inner experiences and connect more deeply with others. While we've touched on how mindfulness can give us flexibility in our behavior—by facing fears or responding more skillfully to others when they annoy or disappoint us—we've emphasized mindfulness as a way to work with inner thoughts and feelings.

But our actions can cause trouble in so many ways. We make hundreds of choices each day that affect our welfare and that of those around us: choosing whether to have one more drink or piece of cake; choosing whether to get sleep or to stay up; choosing whether to do our work or goof off; choosing whether to tell the truth, help out a friend, or turn on the TV. It turns out that a lot of our suffering comes from the consequences of bad habits. Some of these consequences are external (getting into trouble with others or ruining our health) while others are internal (feeling down on ourselves for being "bad"). Some choices have both kinds of consequences, like when a couple of drinks too many makes us say things we shouldn't, causes a hangover that hinders our job performance the next day, and leaves us feeling embarrassed and ashamed.

How can we make decisions more wisely? The first step is to actually realize that we're making choices. Some of our habits are so ingrained that we're hardly aware of deciding to drift to the refrigerator, make up an excuse, or spend more than we had planned. Living mindlessly can leave us wondering how in the world we gained three pounds "overnight," why we're getting the cold shoulder from our friends, or what thief has access to our credit card. With mindfulness practice, we can better notice what we're doing when we do it.

And once we make a choice, how do we develop the strength to follow through with it? How do we close the refrigerator door, admit the truth, and put away the charge card? While this can be harder still, mindfulness practice can help here too.

There's no limit to the number of troublesome habits we can fall into. Take a moment to see how often you indulge in each of these greatest hits:

A BAD HABITS INVENTORY

0—Never   1—Rarely   2—Sometimes   3—Often   4—Very often

Using this scale of 1 to 5, rate how often each of the following happens:

- Eat more than you need (____) _____
- Eat unhealthy food (____) _____
- Drink too much alcohol (____) _____
- Drink at inappropriate times (____) _____
- Use too much of another intoxicant (____) _____
- Use another intoxicant at inappropriate times (____) _____
- Smoke cigarettes (____) _____
- Go to sleep too late (____) _____
- Spend too much time surfing the Internet (____) _____
- Spend too much time watching TV (____) _____
- Bite nails, scratch or pick at skin, pull out hairs, or other nervous habit (____) _____
- Multitask when driving (dialing cell phone, combing hair, etc.) (____) _____
- Work too much (____) _____

(cont.)

- Put off doing work (____) _____
- Put off doing chores (____) _____
- Exercise too much (____) _____
- Put off exercising (____) _____
- Buy things you don't really need (____) _____
- Gamble excessively (____) _____
- Flirt excessively (____) _____
- Engage in inappropriate sexual relations (____) _____
- Tell little white lies (____) _____
- Tell more substantial lies (____) _____
- Exaggerate a story to entertain or impress (____) _____
- Exaggerate a business or tax expense (____) _____
- Act grumpy or unkind to people who don't deserve it (____) _____
- Engage in a troublesome habit not listed above (____) _____
- Engage in another troublesome habit not listed above ☺ (____) _____

_____

Now take a moment to go back to the items you rated higher than zero. Jot down on the line next to each one its external and/or internal consequences.

What did you notice? Except for the occasional saint, most of us fall prey to some of these. Might your life be better if you had a little more control over these behaviors?

Guilt, shame, and other delights

Most of us hate how we feel inside when we fail to live up to our own standards. Inner guilt and shame gnaw at us and drive us to more misbehavior. We're also not big fans of speeding tickets, prison time, divorce, unemployment, or other external costs of bad habits. Luckily, by practicing mindfulness regularly, we can limit all of these consequences.

Chapter 5 discussed how cultures use different approaches to help their members get along with one another. While they almost all have rules against stealing, lying, killing, and adultery, some teach that it's a sin even to think about doing such a thing, while others allow for the thought or impulse but prohibit the deed. We've also seen how trying to banish unwanted thoughts and impulses can tie us in knots and contribute to depression, anxiety, and a host of stress-related medical conditions.

When we practice *awareness of present experience with acceptance*, we notice that a remarkable variety of noble and not-so-noble impulses regularly enter the mind. We also become aware of a lot of ambivalence—mixed feelings toward other people, our jobs, our bodies, and the myriad choices we make each day. We find that we make many decisions with an angel on one shoulder and a devil on the other. "Should I or shouldn't I?"

How might you choose? A very basic way is by considering the risk of punishment. We reduce our speed on the highway or wait at the "No Right Turn on Red" sign based on a quick calculation: the police may be watching. Most of us feed the parking meter at least in part because we don't like to pay fines.

Of course sometimes our behavior is governed instead by our conscience. Freud called this the *superego*—literally the "over I." Almost all of us have a sense of someone or something inside that watches over our actions and judges them as morally good or bad. This first develops in childhood when we internalize adults' relentless reminders about right and wrong behavior. We feel guilty when we violate these internal rules in secret and feel ashamed when we get caught. Since both guilt and shame are unpleasant, we learn to restrain ourselves in order to avoid them.

There are other, more nuanced bases for making choices that go beyond avoiding punishment, guilt, or shame. When we pay close attention to our experience, we notice that harmful behavior *creates waves of disturbance in the mind*. It's difficult to have a peaceful meditation session after a long day of lying and stealing or raping and pillaging. So through mindfulness, we make healthier, wiser decisions (and minimize the pain of doing the opposite) because we're more sensitive to the subtle effects of those decisions.

We start noticing that certain mental states tend to follow certain actions, which naturally leads us to more ethical and skillful behavior. For example, if I watch my mind after being mean to my wife, I'm likely to notice several disturbing consequences. On the most basic level, I'll worry that she'll be angry and may act cold or even try to hurt me back. At the next level, I'll feel guilty or ashamed that I've been a bad person, not living up to my inner image of a good husband. Even more subtly, I'll become aware of the suffering that I've caused her and will notice that she's a human being like me who feels the same sort of pain that I feel when mistreated. I'll also feel disconnected from her and more alone in the world. All of these experiences are unpleasant—if I can remain mindful, they'll discourage me from behaving badly next time. Of course if I remain mindless, I might be mean over and over—until I'm shocked to find myself being served divorce papers.

On the other hand, if I'm kind or generous with my wife, I'll notice a very different set of consequences in the mind. I'll have less fear of retribution, fewer self-critical thoughts, and probably have pleasant empathic feelings when I see her happiness. I'll also feel more connected to her and less alone. If I'm mindful of these pleasant experiences, I'm more likely to act thoughtfully again next time (and less likely to be served the papers).

In this way, mindfulness practice helps us see that it's actually in our own self-interest to behave fairly and compassionately. The only way we actually "get away with" unethical behavior is by not really noticing its consequences in our own minds. By illuminating the subtle effects of our actions, mindfulness practice helps us make wiser choices.

Practicing mindful ethics

The challenge is developing enough continuity of mindfulness to stay aware of these cause-and-effect relationships. Establishing a regular practice as described in Chapters 3 and 4 is a good way to start. Beyond this, when dealing with other people, regularly practicing the *Three Objects of Awareness* described in Chapter 8 will help clarify your inner experience as well as how others react to you. It will highlight the anxiety that arises as soon as you bend the truth and the pain the other person experiences when you're mean.

You can cultivate awareness of the subtle effects of other actions by doing informal practice throughout the day. If you're mindful when filling out your tax return, you'll notice the slight fear or guilt that arises when you consider overstating a business expense. If you're mindful when shirking a bit of work, you'll notice the anxiety and guilt that ensues. These passing, sometimes subtle feelings become natural correctives, gently encouraging us to do the right thing.

Practicing mindfulness in this way also helps us see the benefits of fixing mistakes. When we respond to our misgivings about what we've done by setting things straight, we notice the relief that comes from no longer carrying the burden. This becomes reinforcing, motivating us to set things right again the next time. Over time, making these adjustments can alleviate a lot of fear, shame, and guilt.

> By highlighting the pain that follows from our unskillful behavior, mindfulness naturally motivates us to do the right thing.

The Failure of the Pleasure Principle

Behaving wisely and ethically actually becomes easier over time. With a continuity of mindfulness we see over and over that unskillful behavior almost always comes from seeking gratification. Trying to hold on to pleasure and avoid pain can not only lock us into depression, anxiety, chronic pain, and a pattern of failed relationships (as discussed in Chapters 5–8) but can also cause subtle suffering in small moment after small moment.

Our impulses to be deceptive or hurtful to others all involve grasping at pleasure and trying to avoid pain. We might lie about having plans so we can stay home and read a good book rather than go out with someone we find trying, get our coworker to do the boring part of a project to sleaze out of work, or exaggerate our accomplishments to bask in the glow of admiration. We imagine that we'll be happier if we hide the truth, avoid the unpleasant tasks, or puff ourselves up. But the disturbing effects of failing to live up to our ideals have a way of coming back to haunt us.

And it's not just about feeling guilt and shame—our ethical lapses also leave us looking over our shoulder. "Will he find out that I stayed home that night?" "Will she realize she did most of the scut work?" "Do they think I'm full of hot air?" Our lapses make us paranoid—we expect others to treat us the way we treat them. So when we go through life cheating in little ways, we're left living in a world where we expect to be cheated.

Seeing clearly that this grasping causes suffering and that pleasure and pain will come and go no matter what we do, it becomes easier to be fair and generous with others. Instead of fretting over what we'll have to give up, we realize that acting greedily is a no-win situation. Just as we learn to walk away from a carnival game once we see that it's rigged and we have no chance of winning, we let go of overly self-serving behavior once we understand that it doesn't really make us feel better for very long.

At an even more subtle level, as discussed in Chapter 8, mindfulness practice can help us make just and ethical choices by shifting our view of who we think we are. As we begin to see ourselves as part of the wider world, as cells in a larger organism, our tendency to grab too much for ourselves starts to relax. Much as our right hand is happy to put a glove on our left hand, we become less concerned with "me" and more concerned with "us." We don't have to remind ourselves of the golden rule, because the separation between "me" and "you" becomes less significant.

Most of us experience this softening of boundaries at least occasionally in our families. Many couples share finances, so that there's no distinction between "my money" and "your money." Or when we spend on our young child, it doesn't feel like "my" money going to "you." On good days, when a close relative needs our help, we give it freely, without feeling like we're sacrificing something—it's all in the family.

Mindfulness practice has the potential to broaden this sense of family to include everyone. Of course it's the rare person who is aware of his or her interrelatedness all the time. But when we glimpse through mindfulness practice that it's possible to experience ourselves and others this way, we know it's also possible to retain some awareness of our interconnections even when fretting that things aren't turning out as we'd like. This awareness usually leads to wise behavior, making episodes of guilt and shame less likely.

> Being in touch with our interconnectedness naturally leads us to wiser choices.

Some people are already pretty ethical but can use mindfulness to make refinements leading to greater peace and ease. Others have a long way to go—and may need mindfulness practice to help climb out of an abyss:

If you met Mary today, you'd see a streetwise but honest woman. If you had known her 15 years ago, you would have been a fool to trust her.

Mary grew up in an upper-middle-class suburban neighborhood. Her father was a hard-drinking businessman who cut corners and made risky deals. Her mother, while loving, was afraid to cross her father. Mary wasn't much of a student, and by the time she was in high school she and her father were at war. When other kids in her class were preparing for college, she couldn't take it anymore and left home.

Living on her own was tough. She lied about her age and got a job at a strip club. She sold pot, bootleg cigarettes, and knockoffs of expensive watches. She dated a lot of guys, all of whom turned out to be jerks.

Through it all she somehow avoided getting involved in hard-core prostitution or violence. She even managed to learn about investing and put away some money.

At 24 Mary had a daughter. Her boyfriend soon left, and Mary was at a crossroads. She's not entirely sure what tipped the balance, but having another person depending on her made a difference. She felt that her own parents had done an atrocious job and desperately wanted to do better by her own child. So she set about trying to straighten out her life.

Mary was in touch with a friend from high school who had become a nurse. The friend was teaching mindfulness meditation at the hospital and encouraged Mary to come to a class. Mary knew she was stressed out, so she took her friend up on the offer.

Sitting with her thoughts and feelings wasn't easy. Mary was used to scheming, setting up deals, making connections, and evading the law. She had a lot of difficulty staying with her breath for more than brief periods, but did better with walking and eating meditation, as well as informal practice. Being mindful at the club was practically impossible— she felt overwhelmed by the pain of the other dancers' broken lives and interactions with the customers who treated her like a piece of meat. She noticed how sad, angry, and frightened she felt. Like everyone else there, she relied on alcohol or drugs for anesthesia.

At first, mindfulness practice showed Mary that she was even more stressed than she had realized. It made her notice that each time she got high she felt relief from her anxiety, anger, and sadness, but they soon returned when the drugs wore off—along with lousy physical feelings. She saw the cycle of emotional pain, getting high to escape it, being in more pain when she came down, and wanting to get high again. She also saw that she trusted very few friends and was wary of most people. And she started thinking about her family—feeling the hurt and anger, along with a wish to somehow make things better so her daughter could have grandparents.

Mindfulness practice revealed to Mary that she was never going to be at peace unless she disentangled herself from this life. This prompted her to start psychotherapy, which over time made it even clearer that she needed to make some changes.

With considerable trepidation, Mary began training to be a medical assistant. What a contrast with her life at the club. At the doctor's office everything had to be done right and it all had to be documented. Busy with a baby and a job, she found it really hard to keep up any formal mindfulness practice. But when her self-doubts and anxiety about succeeding at her new job became overwhelming, she went back to classes. Difficult as it was, she also kept up her informal practice whenever possible.

As Mary continued her therapy and tried to live more mindfully, she realized how deeply ingrained her habits had become. She found herself covering little mistakes, lying when she was late, and pretending to know things that she didn't. Her practice helped her see how every one of these moves added to her anxiety, guilt, and shame even if they didn't have any external consequences (she hadn't been caught—yet). Gradually, she experimented with telling the truth more. People usually responded well, and it was a relief not to have to worry about being found out.

Over the next few years Mary did a lot of psychological work and gradually became happier in the process. It was not an easy road. Being a single mother was hard enough—doing it with her troubled background made it harder. Bit by bit she felt the anger, sadness, and longing for closeness she had blocked out while living with her parents and working at the club. Being more aware of all her feelings, she was better able to connect with her daughter, whom she grew to love deeply. Learning to tolerate her own childhood emotions helped her reconcile somewhat with her parents, who turned out to be better with their granddaughter than they had been with Mary.

Learning to find and live by inner values meant a lot. Mary now felt like she was a decent person and a good mother. She made a few friends she could trust at the office and among other moms. While it was exhausting to be a single working mother, she was actually less stressed now living with integrity than before her daughter was born. It was a relief to no longer worry about getting busted by the police or caught lying about a deal and to no longer fear weird customers or her own walled-off feelings. She even was able to give up drugs once her life straightened out—which as we'll soon see, many people can't do so easily.

Addicere

Often we understand intellectually which choices will lead to the greatest well-being for all involved but still have trouble acting accordingly. The English word *addiction* comes from the Latin *addicere*, which means "to be awarded to another as a slave." It's remarkable how often we're enslaved by our immediate desires. We have trouble making wise choices around eating, exercise, sleep, drinking, drugs, smoking, gambling, shopping, surfing the Internet, telling the truth, work, love relationships, and sex—to name just a few. Even those of us who don't think of ourselves as "addicts" usually have difficulty making sensible choices in some arenas. Almost any behavior can become an addiction—and for some of us many do at one time or another. Often the problem involves overindulgence, though we can also get into trouble by becoming too ascetic in our effort to *avoid* overindulgence.

Eating

If you tried the *Raisin Meditation* in Chapter 3, you may have noticed that this raisin was not like other raisins. We eat mindlessly most of the time. Besides causing us to miss out on one of life's great pleasures, mindless eating sets us up for all sorts of health problems. Nearly two-thirds of Americans are overweight, and one-third fit the criteria for obesity. One to four percent of young women suffer with anorexia, bulimia, or binge eating. While other animals eat when they're hungry and stop when they're full, many of us have clearly developed a weird relationship with food.

What's involved in mindless eating? It depends on whether we're chowing down or trying to diet. When we're chowing down, we're usually thinking about other things and not really tasting our food. In these moments, we respond to the sight of food with the impulse to devour it— whether or not we're actually hungry. We miss more subtle sensations of fullness and anticipate the next bite before we finish chewing the current one. Usually we gather more on our fork or spoon long before we finish swallowing what is already in our mouth. We may eat to self-soothe— distracting ourselves from unpleasant thoughts or feelings with the pleasant sensations of eating. Not tasting, we don't really appreciate the food and almost certainly miss seeing the effort that went into growing and preparing it. Eating this way may be temporarily comforting, but it isn't very rich or meaningful, and it often leads to health problems.

Mindless eating takes on other dimensions once we start to struggle with calories. When we diet, we become preoccupied with food. Each meal becomes a battle between desire and willpower. We become black-and-white thinkers—succeeding or failing at every meal. We congratulate ourselves on our restraint in one moment, only to find ourselves suddenly overindulging in the next. This brings on what are called *abstinence violation effects*—the self-hatred and impulse to give up that we feel when we fall off the wagon. On top of this come all sorts of self-critical thoughts about being fat, ugly, weak-willed, self-destructive, undisciplined, or unhealthy. Self-reproach about losing control, combined with negative judgments about our appearance and character, makes us miserable. How do we respond? Naturally—by visiting the refrigerator again to soothe ourselves.

Mindfulness practice offers an alternative. Many people experience this quite powerfully when they attend a silent meditation retreat. During intensive retreats the entire day is spent in silence, observing the mind and body. Usually a good deal of concentration develops, and we notice inner and outer events that are otherwise outside awareness.

Since most of the day is spent alternating between sitting and walking meditation, mealtimes are a big treat. They are an opportunity to do something different and gratifying. Add to this the fact that retreat center food is usually quite good and you can imagine how meditators salivate at the sound of the meal bell.

At the first meal, newcomers in particular usually fill their plates high with goodies. The offerings are tasty and healthy, so why not? Meals are structured as meditation sessions and are eaten slowly and silently. Instead of focusing on the breath or footsteps, participants focus on the experience of eating.

It doesn't take long before most people realize that they've taken too much. After 30 minutes their plate is still half full, but they're already stuffed. The mind resolves to be more restrained next time.

By the next meal, however, hunger and anticipation have both returned, as has the temptation to fill one's plate. Most people serve themselves less food the second time but still overshoot the mark. Usually it takes several meals to learn how much food is actually enough.

While I'm not particularly over- or underweight, I find that the only times I'm not at all eating disordered are during such silent retreats. I actually taste and appreciate my food and—after some trial and error—learn to eat only what my body needs. During the rest of my life, I'm less fully conscious when eating and invariably use food to self-soothe or distract myself from unpleasant thoughts or feelings.

> Mindfulness can interrupt cycles of deprivation, followed by bingeing, followed by overeating to soothe the guilt or shame of having binged.

Most of us won't spend our lives on retreat or eat every meal as a silent meditation, but we can still learn to eat more mindfully. Instructions for formal eating meditation were presented in Chapter 3. Whether or not you have struggles with food, I encourage you to see what a rich and rewarding experience it can be to practice mindfulness while slowly eating a meal in silence. Practicing this from time to time infuses all of our eating experiences with more mindful attention.

It is also possible to use ordinary meals as opportunities for informal mindfulness practice. You might try this the next time you eat alone.

Informal Eating Meditation

Turn off the TV and put away the newspaper. Take a few minutes to settle into your chair. Notice your breath and how the body feels. Observe where there is tension and whether hunger is present or absent. Notice whether you're experiencing any cravings and whether any emotions are present. Try to observe the thoughts that arise without judging them. See if you can discern your motivation for eating at this moment—is it hunger, boredom, a craving, or a need to eat now because of your schedule? Try not to pass judgment on the motivation, but be aware of it.

Now allow yourself to eat. Depending on your circumstances, this needn't be a slow concentration exercise, but try to notice when you taste your food and when you don't. Try also to keep track of feelings of hunger and satiety—the sense that your belly is empty or full or the sense that you've had enough of a given taste. Notice what happens to your emotions and thoughts as you eat and how you make the decision to stop or have more.

When we bring mindful attention to the process of eating, we tend to notice experiences that otherwise pass undetected. We see the relationships between thoughts, feelings, and eating. We might see ourselves eating more rapidly when something upsets us and slowing down when we are more at peace. We become better able to recognize and tolerate emotions rather than automatically turning to food to dampen them. We can also use eating as an opportunity to appreciate our connection to the world outside ourselves, as in the story about eating a tangerine presented in Chapter 8. We can appreciate all of the efforts that went into producing, transporting, and preparing the food, as well as the remarkable natural processes by which the energy of the sun has been transformed into what appears on our plate.

Once you've tried a few silent meditation meals and have experimented with *Informal Eating Meditation*, you can also try to eat mindfully when with other people—you'll just need to split your attention between the food and the conversation.

Another useful practice is to experiment with eating problematic foods mindfully. It can help you enjoy them on occasion without going overboard:

———— *Troublesome Foods Meditation* ————

This usually works best added to the end of a period of regular breath or walking meditation. First do the *Raisin Meditation* described in Chapter 3 (if you don't like raisins, you can choose another small piece of dried fruit or similar healthy morsel). Then try the same slow, deliberate eating meditation with a food such as chocolate, fudge, potato chips, ice cream, or other seductive (and not so healthy) food.

Many of us routinely snarf these foods down without really savoring the experience. Eating such treats mindfully can change our relationship with them—allowing us to indulge in moderation.

Another area where people frequently lose control is in settings with unlimited food. Parties, buffets, and banquets are all dangerous—they encourage bingeing. One approach for mastering these situations is to periodically visit them as a deliberate mindfulness practice:

———— *Buffet Meditation* ————

Go to a party or buffet with the intention of practicing mindful eating. See if you can notice when hunger plays a role versus when your "eyes are bigger than your stomach." Pay particular attention to sensations of fullness. Eat slowly enough so that your digestive system has time to signal your brain when you've had enough. Once you feel full, practice saying "No thank you" to people who offer you more. Notice all the thoughts and feelings that arise while eating in this setting.

The more you can deliberately practice *Buffet Meditation*, the easier it will be to eat mindfully at such occasions in the future.

Forgiveness Meditation

For people trying to regulate their eating, self-criticism around lapses in discipline plays a big role (recall the abstinence violation effects mentioned earlier). Mindfulness-oriented approaches to eating problems therefore emphasize awareness over discipline. When we notice what we're doing from moment to moment, we become more likely to make wise choices. This approach helps us avoid the familiar seesaw pattern— ascetic and self-depriving one day, only to suddenly throw off our self-imposed shackles and pig out the next, and then eat poorly on the third day to sooth the resulting self-hatred. If you find yourself getting stuck in these sorts of patterns, certain mindfulness practices can help.

One particularly useful approach is to highlight the negative thoughts that come up after a binge and use mindfulness practice to put them into perspective. Some mindfulness-based eating programs integrate cognitive-behavioral therapy (CBT) techniques involving imagery to do this. The following exercise makes a good life preserver after a binge if you are in danger of throwing in the towel and pigging out again. Approach this playfully so that you don't wind up taking the thoughts too seriously:

Thought Parade

Imagine that you're watching a parade, and each of the marchers is holding up a sign. Each sign contains one of your self-critical thoughts:

- "I am an elephant."
- "My stomach is hideous."

- "I have no willpower."
- "I am a pig."
- "Everyone else can eat sensibly, but I'm a big baby and can't stop myself."
- "I'm disgusting."

Allow each of the marchers to walk by, carrying their sign with them. Just watch the parade and observe your feelings.

Another approach to these negative thoughts that can also serve as a life preserver involves the loving-kindness practices discussed in Chapter 4. After starting with a period of breath meditation to develop some concentration, you might silently repeat "May I be happy," "May I be peaceful," "May I be free of suffering," "May I accept myself exactly as I am," or "May I forgive myself for pigging out." As discussed earlier, some people find it easiest to start these practices with the image of a benefactor—directing loving, compassionate energy first toward someone who embodies compassion and later turning it toward yourself. The idea isn't necessarily to counter your self-critical thoughts but rather to illuminate them. If your mind argues back, "But I really am disgusting" or "I really deserve to be shot," simply observe that thought arising and passing and return your attention to the loving-kindness phrases.

Putting It All Together: Mindful Eating

You can weave these different techniques together to suit your particular relationship with food. They all rest on the foundation of a regular mindfulness practice of the type described in Chapters 3 and 4. To the extent that your lifestyle allows, try to periodically make one of your formal practice periods *Eating Meditation*. Being mindful when eating a small meal will require at least a half hour—it's important not to rush. This will both enable you to savor your food and enable your digestive system to signal that you're full (food needs to digest a bit for some of these signals to be generated). If you have a friend or partner who is interested, you can eat mindfully with him or her, maintaining silence during the meal.

The next component involves eating more normally paced meals mindfully—*Informal Eating Meditation*. This, too, is best done either alone or silently with others. A key element is noticing the thoughts and feelings that arise around food, including the impulses to soothe or distract yourself. Once you've practiced this a number of times, you can try eating mindfully at a meal with conversation—though your attention will be more divided.

If you have certain foods that are your downfall—junk food like chocolate, potato chips, and French fries or comfort foods like toast with butter and jam, pizza, and salted nuts—try the *Troublesome Foods Meditation*. Eating these from time to time as a formal meditation practice will cue you to slow down and be attentive when you eat them at other times. Similarly, if you tend to overindulge at buffets or parties, trying the *Buffet Meditation* will help inoculate you against losing control in these settings.

Most people who struggle with overeating fall prey to abstinence violation effects and are tempted to give up after overindulging. This is where the *Thought Parade* and *Loving-Kindness Meditation* can come in handy as life preservers. Experiment with them both to see which works best for you—identifying the thoughts and poking fun at them with the *Thought Parade* or gently soothing yourself with *Loving-Kindness Meditation*.

Learning to be mindful around food will play out differently for different people. Here's how it worked for one of my patients:

John spent his whole life struggling with his weight. His family liked food and spent a lot of time at meals. Nobody was particularly disciplined. Other kids were able to eat anything they wanted, but every calorie stuck to his body. John was teased as a kid—though he got a reprieve when he could use his weight to his advantage playing football in high school.

By the time he was in his 30s weight became a big concern again. He wasn't morbidly obese, but he was heavy enough for his weight to get in the way of his social life. John's doctor suggested a mindfulness-based approach and sent him to see me.

It was clear early on that John was obsessed with his weight. He had painful memories of being teased. He knew that he ate to soothe himself, recalled his parents offering food when he was upset, and realized that he never knew how much was enough.

I introduced John to mindfulness practice. We did the *Raisin Meditation* together, and he was amazed—he saw that he rarely actually tasted his food. We then ate a silent meal together. This was also eye opening—John realized he was always thinking about the next bite and had little awareness of his body. In fact, John came to feel that he had divorced himself from his body because he felt so bad about being fat. In the process he had lost touch with both taste sensations and feelings of fullness. The more John could be mindful at meals, the less he ate. He didn't need to struggle—he just needed to pay attention. It took some time, but he was eventually able to reach a more comfortable weight.

Mindfulness practice can go a long way toward resolving eating difficulties. If such problems have taken over your life, however, you may also benefit from the structure of outside help. A mental health professional who specializes in eating disorders can help you identify the thoughts and feelings behind your behavior and find healthier ways to work with them. Some of these clinicians now use mindfulness-based approaches, so you should ask about this. A particularly well-researched program that uses an approach similar to the one described here is *Mindfulness-Based Eating Awareness Training* (MB-EAT) developed by Jeanne Kristeller and colleagues at Indiana State University.

Intoxicants

According to government figures, approximately 8% of Americans over age 12 reported using illegal drugs in the month before they were asked and 25% smoked cigarettes. Fifty percent of us drank during the past year, while 22% have had over five drinks in a single evening. Intoxicants clearly play a big role in many of our lives. (Here's yet another area where the other animals generally don't share our problem—though in this case they occasionally do when given the means. Most animals won't abuse substances too badly unless experimenters make their life miserable by depriving them of food, raising them in isolation, or otherwise being mean to them. They're not too different from us in this regard.)

While some use of intoxicants is harmless and may even offer health benefits,* we all know that they can create serious difficulties for both the user and those around him or her. What draws us to alcohol and other drugs? We discussed in Chapter 2 the part played by *experiential avoidance*. Pretty much all intoxicant use is designed to deaden one experience and enliven another.

Take normal social drinking as an example. When asked why we drink, most of us say that alcohol makes us feel more "relaxed" or allows us to have more fun at gatherings (yeah, I know, some people say they like

---

*While the mechanism isn't clear, it appears that regularly drinking moderate amounts of alcohol (two drinks per day for men under age 65, one drink per day for men over 65 and all women) may help to prevent cardiovascular disease and other problems.

the taste). I was taught early in my training that the superego (conscience) is the part of the mind that is soluble in alcohol. And it can indeed be a relief to live without this for a while. Investigate a little deeper, and we discover that without alcohol we feel some social anxiety—a little self-consciousness here, some competitive feelings there—which alcohol anesthetizes.

When I was in training, a psychiatrist at Harvard Medical School named Edward Khantzian suggested that we could determine something about a person's psychological difficulties based on his or her drug of choice. Intoxicants are a form of self-medication, and people learn to choose the medicines that most effectively address their problems. Perhaps drinkers medicate anxiety, while cocaine or amphetamine users medicate feelings of inadequacy. While there may be other reasons for particular drug choices (like our social class or ethnic background), the fact remains that we use intoxicants to alter unwanted states of mind.

Mindfulness practice can help to illuminate how and why we take drugs. As with eating, it's possible to turn our attention to the moment-to-moment experience of using a mind-altering substance. Of course, this works only at the beginning—unlike food, over a certain dose alcohol and other drugs can make it difficult to really pay attention to our experience.

Here's an interesting exercise to try whether or not you feel that you have a problem with substances (assuming you're not abstinent). I'll describe the exercise using alcohol since it's the most commonly used recreational drug, though this can be done with most mind-altering substances. You may need 45 minutes for this one—and don't plan to drive afterward:

——————————— *Mindful Intoxication* ———————————

Start with a few minutes of sitting meditation practice. Settle into your seat, notice your breathing, and try to follow the breath for complete cycles. Give yourself 10–20 minutes of breath meditation before imbibing. Notice thoughts or feelings that arise—both pleasant ones, such as anticipation of what you are about to do, and unpleasant ones, which you'd rather escape.

Once your mind has settled a bit and you can attend to your experience, have a drink. Take just enough to bring about some

changes in your awareness but not so much as to seriously interfere with your ability to pay attention. Then go back to following
your breath. Notice what you experience in your body; notice the
thoughts and feelings that arise in the mind. Let yourself be aware
of the aspects of alcohol that are pleasant and those that are unpleasant. If urges to drink more come up, watch them arise, reach crescendos, and perhaps diminish.

After a few minutes of being with intoxicated experience,
drink some more and observe what happens. Continue alternating
between drinking a little more and meditating on the effects until
you reach a point that seems like enough to you.

What did you discover being mindful of your drinking in this way?
How did you determine your stopping point? Perhaps the exercise will
lead you to want to change your habits;
perhaps not. See if you can carry some of
this awareness into normal circumstances
in which you drink alcohol.

> Mindfulness practices can
> help interrupt patterns of
> excessive drinking or drug
> use by giving us insight into
> why we use intoxicants and
> helping us remain conscious
> of their effects once we start.

Getting Motivated

There is an approach to habit change
used by addiction professionals called
motivational interviewing. It focuses on
the theme of an old joke: "How many psychologists does it take to change
a light bulb? Only one—but first the light bulb has to want to change."
Motivational interviewing begins by exploring what a person likes about
his or her habit. If you struggle at all with the use of alcohol or other substances, you might find this exercise helpful. Begin by jotting down your
answers to the questions on the facing page (they can also be adapted to
work with unhealthy eating or other behaviors).

Using mindfulness practice to observe substance use can support
this sort of inquiry. Simply paying attention to the thoughts, feelings, and
sensations in our awareness before and after ingesting naturally illuminates the pros and cons of the behavior. This can be an important step
toward evolving a wise relationship with alcohol or other intoxicants.

In college, Joey was a beer pong champion. He could aim and throw

A MOTIVATIONAL INTERVIEW

- What feels good about drinking (smoking cigarettes, using another drug)?

_____

- What benefits does it offer?

_____

- What might you lose if you were to give it up?

_____

After getting a sense of its benefits, explore its drawbacks:

- Does drinking (smoking cigarettes, using another drug) cause you any difficulties?

_____

- Do you imagine it might some day?

_____

- Does it create any risks?

_____

And finally:

- On balance, does it enrich your life or detract from it?

_____

- Have you tried to stop or cut back? If so, what happened?

_____

with precision even when drunk. He and his fraternity brothers played almost every weekend—though sometimes he'd abstain if he had a big paper or test coming up.

He had good luck when girls came over and often managed to hook up with one of them. It was a lot of fun, even though he didn't always remember the details the next morning. His relationships didn't last very long, but he figured there was no need to settle down yet. He was not the most introspective young man on campus.

Now that he had been out of school for several years, fewer friends wanted to party. He was living with his older brother, who started bugging him about laying off the beer. His brother said their father was an alcoholic—it's true that Mom used to hassle him about drinking too much—but Joey didn't think it was an issue. Besides, he didn't really know how else to have a good time. His job was boring, so naturally he looked forward to drinking on the weekends.

Joey probably wouldn't have done anything about his drinking if not for meeting Megan. She was new at work and very hot. He was thrilled when they started dating. Megan was into meditation and convinced Joey to come with her to some classes (he would have taken up needlepoint if she'd asked). The practice was difficult at first because he wasn't used to looking inward or being without entertainment, but then he liked it when he noticed that he felt a little "high" after meditation—sensory experiences were more intense. He especially enjoyed making love with Megan after they meditated together.

Everything was going well except Megan was bothered by how drunk Joey would get when they went out. He tried to cut back, but each time after a drink or two he found himself having several more. His brother, who was still nagging him about his drinking, convinced him to speak to an addictions counselor friend.

Joey had a motivational interview. On the pro side, alcohol was "fun," made him relax, gave him something to do, and had helped him feel cool and hook up with women. Ever since he entered college it had been part of his identity. If he gave it up, he was afraid he'd feel bored and awkward at parties and might not be so cool. On the con side, he didn't like feeling hung over the next day. He felt this more clearly since he had started meditating. He also didn't like putting on weight—and peering into the future, he didn't want to wind up looking like Homer Simpson. His circle of drinking buddies was also shrinking. Most important, Megan didn't like it—and he really liked Megan.

The other thing that caught his attention was how hard it was to stop after a couple of beers. Since meditating with Megan he was more curious about his thoughts and feelings and he didn't really understand why it happened. By paying more attention—more or less practicing *Mindful Intoxication*—he noticed fear appeared after a couple of drinks. He'd worry that the feeling of excitement and freedom he got from his first beers wouldn't last—that he'd crash—and this drove him to have more.

And once he was a little drunk, his thinking went out the window. So he'd drink until he was pretty far gone.

Mindfulness-Based Relapse Prevention

We saw in Chapter 6 how mindfulness-based cognitive therapy (MBCT) can help prevent relapses of serious depression. In a similar way, mindfulness-based relapse prevention (MBRP), developed by Alan Marlatt and his colleagues at the University of Washington, has been shown to help prevent relapses of substance abuse. In this program, participants who have been sober for at least a month are taught to use mindfulness practice to remain alert and aware of the choice points where they might start using again.

Participants use mindfulness practice to explore feelings of craving in detail, noticing the thoughts, feelings, and situations that serve as triggers. They then get into the habit of practicing mindfulness in high-risk situations that might lead to using. Participants are also taught to notice that thoughts are indeed just thoughts—they come, go, and change regularly—and therefore needn't define reality. By using mindfulness practice to stay with difficult feelings, the program helps people see that these are indeed tolerable and it's not necessary to turn to alcohol or drugs to make them go away.

Discovering this for oneself is at the heart of most mindfulness-based recovery programs. One way to do this is to see that our urges to respond to cravings are like waves—which we can learn to surf. This is similar to urge surfing impulses to escape physical pain, which was discussed in Chapter 7. The practice is a life preserver that you can try the next time you feel an unwise urge to use an

> Through mindfulness practice we can learn to ride out our cravings without acting on them.

intoxicant. (It works equally well for urges to eat unwisely or to engage in any other problematic behavior):

——————— Urge Surfing for Cravings* ———————

Close your eyes and feel the urge to use a substance arising in your body. Your breath will be your surfboard, allowing you to ride the wave without being wiped out. Visualize the craving as a wave in the ocean. Notice how it begins as a small wavelet that builds and

---

*Available in audio at *www.mindfulness-solution.com*.

builds until it crests. Use your breath to ride the wave—don't worry; as long as you stay with the breath you won't be overwhelmed. Allow each wave to rise up as high as it wants. Ride each one until it peters out near the shore.

We can understand waves of craving as conditioned responses. You may recall the experiment in which the Russian scientist Ivan Pavlov conditioned dogs to salivate at the sound of a bell by repeatedly pairing that bell with food. After a while just ringing the bell would make the dogs salivate. Similarly, if we have used substances to escape difficult emotions in the past, we develop a conditioned response of craving them whenever painful emotions or difficult situations arise. Here, instead of acting on those urges—which would deepen the conditioned connection between negative emotions and substance use—we surf the urges. Doing this eventually loosens the association between difficult experiences and substance use, making it easier to surf the urge next time.

Joey's urges to keep drinking after the first couple of beers felt like conditioned responses. Once he was a little drunk, it was hard to resist the temptation to drink more. When Megan started pulling back, however, he decided to really try. He set a two-beer limit for himself and started using mindfulness practice to deal with his urges to keep going. He saw the tension increase in his body when the fear of the good feeling wearing off came and experimented with riding this out. While not always successful, sometimes it worked. He could surf the urges and stick to his limit. He even experimented with not drinking at all some nights. It actually wasn't so bad—he could still enjoy himself, and he felt better the next day. With continued mindfulness practice, Joey developed a more balanced relationship toward alcohol—and a better one with Megan too. He still overdid it at times, but he now definitely had more control.

Putting It All Together: Being Mindful of Intoxication

Intoxication use runs the gamut from unproblematic to life destroying. Mindfulness practice can help us see where our own use fits on this continuum and if need be to do something about it. As with all of the other issues we've discussed, establishing a regular pattern of formal and informal practices is a good way to start.

If, like Joey, you're not trying to be abstinent, an interesting next step is to try *Mindful Intoxication*. This can help you see both the desirable and undesirable effects of intoxicant use on your particular mind and body. It may also help you moderate your use the same way mindful eating helps us eat in a more balanced way.

Another way to assess your relationship to intoxicants is through *A Motivational Interview*. You can complete this for whatever substances you use—your answers may well be different for each. This can help you see the positive and negative roles intoxicants play in your life, which will provide clues as to where you might want to be more mindful.

Should you come to the conclusion that you're using intoxicants to self-medicate difficult experiences and it would be wiser to cut down or stop, *Urge Surfing* can be a helpful life preserver. You'll need to have already established a general mindfulness practice for this to be most effective. When cravings arise, bring your attention to them while using your breath to surf the urge until it reaches a crest and dissipates.

If you're trying to cut back or stop using and you notice yourself giving up as soon as you have a setback, the life preservers we discussed for slips related to eating can work for intoxicants as well. You can modify the *Thought Parade* to suit your circumstance, using signs saying "I'm a weakling," "I'm a hopeless drunk [drug addict, etc.]," "I'm a bum"—whatever thoughts your mind generates after you fall off the wagon. You can also use *Loving-Kindness Meditation* (Chapter 4) to counteract self-critical spells, again modifying the phrases if necessary: "May I be happy," "May I be peaceful," "May I be free of suffering," "May I accept myself exactly as I am," or "May I forgive myself for using again."

If the use of substances has become a major problem in your life, mindfulness practices can help, but other supports are usually needed too:

The Intersection

Carla was a bright, successful, hardworking businesswoman in her late 30s. She was disciplined in many areas but had smoked pot, drunk, and occasionally used other drugs since high school.

When she was little, Carla always felt she was too sensitive. She would cry easily when things went awry and felt anxious about what other kids thought of her. While she made friends as she got a little older, she never felt like part of the in crowd. She was hurt when she wasn't invited to a party and crushed when she wasn't chosen to be a cheerleader.

Pot and alcohol became good solutions. They connected her to other users and helped her feel cool. They also took the edge off her social anxiety and allowed her to weather daily ups and downs without so much pain. She didn't feel so sensitive when she got high—she felt she could handle things better.

Only recently, when she started taking opiate painkillers to deal with a back problem, did she see her reliance on drugs as a problem. She became physically dependent and struggled with withdrawal symptoms.

It was under these difficult conditions that she first tried mindfulness practice. I initially taught her *Separating the Two Arrows* (Chapter 7) as a way to deal with her back pain. Desperate for relief, she practiced this along with other formal and informal techniques. She was eventually able to kick the opiates and in the process became more aware of her emotional states. The ordeal made her see how reliant she was on substances to manage her feelings.

Carla also began to see how this was getting in the way of her emotional development. She still felt very young and insecure around other people. The drugs had not only insulated her from pain for all these years but also had robbed her of normal opportunities to learn how to interact and how to tolerate negative feelings.

Carla then had a powerful recurring dream. She was walking a maze. Time and again she came back to the same intersection. To the left was a steep, rocky, difficult path going upward. To the right was a clear, smooth, easy path that sloped gradually downward. Naturally, time and again she went to the right, only to discover that this path led back to the beginning of the maze. Each time she awoke from the dream, she realized that the steep path was actually the way out. (I'm not making this up—this was exactly the dream she reported.)

Carla realized that she had been taking the easy path—relying on intoxicants to anesthetize feelings—for her entire adult life. With encouragement she continued her mindfulness practice now with the express purpose of learning how to tolerate unpleasant emotions. She began to realize that she could indeed bear many thoughts and feelings that in the past were triggers to get high.

It was nonetheless slow going. She needed motivational interviewing in therapy to see what the drugs provided as well as their costs. She needed to practice *Urge Surfing* every day. She repeatedly needed to use *Loving-Kindness Meditation* to forgive herself for falling off the wagon. She needed support from a community in Alcoholics Anonymous. And she needed to continue a pattern of regular formal and informal mindfulness practice. With these supports, Carla learned to *be with* many difficult states of mind and in the process get control over her habits.

Mindfulness practice can help each of us see how our personal maze is constructed. By noticing the moment-to-moment consequences of our actions, we eventually come to see which paths lead to freedom and which ones keep us trapped. Even if you don't have the same degree of difficulty with substances as Carla, these practices can help you work creatively with adversity, rather than respond to it compulsively.

As was the case for Carla, substance issues can require outside help. If you suspect that you have a problem and the techniques discussed here aren't enough to resolve it, a combination of professional help and community support may be in order. You might try to find a mental health professional who works with substance abuse problems and is also familiar with mindfulness practice. If they are familiar with MBRP, all the better. Twelve-step programs such as Alcoholics Anonymous or Narcotics Anonymous have also helped millions, and their approach dovetails well with mindfulness-oriented approaches. Information about where to find twelve-step programs, along with additional guides for using mindfulness practices to work with substance abuse problems, can be found in the Resources at the back of this book.

Work, gambling, shopping, and sex

Ethical decisions, food, and intoxicants are not the only realms in which bad habits can lead to suffering. Work, gambling, shopping, and sex are also ripe for trouble. Each of these lends itself nicely to compulsive behaviors driven by our desire to avoid unpleasant experience—and these compulsive behaviors usually lead us to grief.

Many people either work or avoid work compulsively. In the former it's often fear of failure, or fear of being with one's own mind absent the structure of work, that drives us. We're left chronically stressed, unable to relax and relate to others. People who avoid work compulsively may also fear failure or fear difficult or uncomfortable elements of a job. Shirking work can lead to repeatedly disappointing those who rely on us.

By practicing mindfulness, we get to see in both situations the unwanted feelings that our behavior wards off—we see how overworking and slacking off are actually both forms of experiential avoidance. By turning our attention to these feelings rather than avoiding them, we can become far more balanced in our relationship to work.

Gambling also causes a lot of trouble. Whether at the casino, at the track, or on Wall Street, the fantasy of striking it rich can be very seductive. Psychologists have long observed that variable-ratio intermittent reinforcement creates extremely strong habits. Slot machines are a perfect example—they pay out after a certain number of bets, but that number keeps changing. And we keep pulling the handle. Other forms of gambling are addictive in the same way. As with other potentially troublesome habits, when we're engaged in gambling we tend to be distracted from our concerns. Since winning feels so good, we get hooked on the fantasy that a big win would keep us happy. In the process, however, we might go broke or neglect our other responsibilities.

Shopping is a bit like gambling, but with more reliable results. As mentioned in Chapter 2, we do it a lot. When shopping becomes a problem, it usually involves predictable phases—each with a corresponding inner experience:

1. Imagine acquiring something new—desire arises (*Think about buying a car*)
2. Search out and examine the possibilities—excitement builds (*Check out cars on the road, read about them online, visit showrooms*)
3. Buy something—feel gratified (*Drive the shiny new car off the lot*)
4. Get used to having it—gratification fades (*Stop noticing so often that you're in a new car*)
5. Imagine acquiring something new—desire arises again (*Think about buying something else*)

With mindfulness practice we see how short-lived the gratification from shopping usually is. We might also notice other feelings, such as guilt, shame, or anxiety about spending too much money, cluttering our house with too much stuff, or using up more resources than we really need. Being mindful of these phases, including the after-effects of buying things, can go a long way toward helping us develop balanced shopping habits.

Sex, when it becomes a problem, is a bit like shopping. We go through the same five phases—just use your imagination to change the wording of the list a little. When sex becomes an addiction, it disrupts relationships and leaves behind a string of injured partners. Here, too, being more mindful of our experience can help us find balance.

Putting It All Together: Mindful Work, Gambling, Shopping, and Sex

With some minor adjustments, the mindfulness practices we discussed for ethical decisions, food, and intoxicants will work here too. In each instance, developing a regular pattern of formal and informal practice is the best way to begin. Next you can try modifying the *Informal Eating Meditation* and *Mindful Intoxication* exercises to suit your particular habit. This will shed light on what triggers it, what feelings the habit helps alleviate, and what its consequences are. A *Motivational Interview* will further illuminate these dynamics. Should you decide to try to make changes, *Urge Surfing* can be used as a life preserver when you're tempted to give in to cravings, while variations on *The Thought Parade* and *Loving-Kindness Meditation* can help you work with abstinence violation effects when you slip.

Since we humans can use almost anything to escape unpleasant thoughts or feelings, the opportunities for addictive habits are limitless—as are the opportunities to use mindfulness practice to free ourselves from them. In some arenas, such as drinking or gambling, we might decide that abstinence is our best strategy. With others, such as food, shopping, or work, this isn't really an option (though some people may choose to abstain from fudge, megamalls, or corporate law jobs). As we take more moments of our lives as occasions for mindfulness practice, we see what lies behind our cravings and compulsive behaviors. Gaps then open up between impulse and action that allow us to choose our course a little more wisely.

If compulsive behavior around work, gambling, shopping, sex, or a related area is interfering with your life or becoming part of a vicious cycle, consulting with a mental health professional is a good idea. While most well-trained clinicians will be able to help, some therapists specialize in particular problems such as gambling or sexual addiction. Suggestions for finding an appropriate therapist can be found at the back of the book.

Mindfulness practices for bad habits

All of the following rest on a foundation of regular formal and informal practice as described in Chapters 3 and 4. They can be adapted to most troublesome habits in the ways just described.

Formal Meditation Practices

- *Raisin Meditation* (page 75) to lay a foundation for other eating meditations
- *Eating Meditation* (page 79) to practice eating mindfully
- *Troublesome Foods Meditation* (page 264) to cultivate mindfulness in the presence of dangerous treats
- *Buffet Meditation* (page 264) to deal with parties and other unlimited food situations
- *Thought Parade* (page 265) to gain perspective on self-critical thoughts after falling off the wagon
- *Loving-Kindness Meditation* (page 84) to soothe self-critical chatter after bingeing
- *Mindful Intoxication* (page 269) to increase awareness of the effects of intoxicants and thoughts and feelings about using them
- *Urge Surfing* (page 273) to learn to tolerate cravings

Informal Practices

- *Three Objects of Awareness* (page 234) to observe your reactions to encounters with others and how others react to you—making wise choices clearer

All of the following can help bring attention to sensory experience throughout the day and illuminate impulses to engage in bad habits:

- *Walking Meditation* (page 67)
- *Nature Meditation* (page 128)
- *Eating Meditation* (page 263)
- *Driving, Showering, Tooth Brushing, Shaving (etc.) Meditation* (page 90)

Life Preservers

- *Thought Parade* (page 265) or *Loving-Kindness Meditation* (page 84) when about to binge further after slipping
- *Mindful Intoxication* (page 269) when finding yourself continuing to use a substance after already being somewhat intoxicated

- *Urge Surfing* (page 273) for moments when cravings are driving you toward unwise choices
- *Nature Meditation* (formal or informal; page 128) to anchor your attention in the world outside your cravings

Developing a plan

You may find it useful to jot down an action plan for working with your troublesome habits. The following chart can help you organize your thoughts. You might photocopy this to use with different habits.

PRACTICE PLAN

Begin by reflecting on how the habit is affecting your life.

Problematic habit: _____

Situations in Which You Do The Behavior: _____

_____

Triggers:

Physical (sensations that precede the behavior): _____

_____

Cognitive (thoughts that precede the behavior): _____

_____

Behavioral (things you do that lead into the behavior): _____

_____

Consequences: _____

_____

(cont.)

Times I Most Need a Life Preserver: _____

_____

_____

Now, based on what you've read about and experienced with the different practices, jot down an initial practice plan (you can vary this as your needs change).

Formal Practice	When	How Often
_____	_____	_____
_____	_____	_____
_____	_____	_____

Informal Practice	When	How Often
_____	_____	_____
_____	_____	_____
_____	_____	_____

Life Preserver	Likely Situation
_____	_____
_____	_____
_____	_____

Bad habits of one kind or another are inevitable and almost guaranteed to contribute to our suffering. One of the few areas where distress is equally likely is the focus of the next chapter—dealing with aging, illness, and death. If this topic doesn't seem relevant to you at the moment, just wait a little while.

CHAPTER 10

Growing up isn't easy

Changing your relationship
with aging, illness, and death

One purpose of mindfulness practice is to enjoy
our old age.

— SHUNRYU SUZUKI

Notice any changes in your body or mind over time? When we're young, these are great: "See how big and strong I am?" "I'm almost all grown up!" As we move through adulthood, however, sooner or later most of us lose our enthusiasm for maturation: "I'm putting on weight and don't have much energy these days." "My mind is a sieve—I can't remember a thing." "When did that spot [wrinkle, lump, etc.] appear?" When we're children, old people seem alien, like Martians. Look at their weird bodies—bald heads, gray hair, wrinkly skin, and odd bumps. You can even see the veins in their hands! It's hard to imagine that this might be our fate—if we're lucky to live long enough.

What we fear

We've discussed how many of our psychological problems stem from resisting change and loss. This is particularly apparent when we contemplate aging. Take a moment now to reflect on your feelings about age-related changes. Jot down on the following chart a few of the welcome and unwelcome changes that you've noticed over time in your appearance, physical abilities, mental abilities, and life situation (relationships, work, housing, etc.).

283

FEELINGS ABOUT AGING

Welcome Changes   Unwelcome Changes

Appearance

_____   _____

_____   _____

_____   _____

_____   _____

Physical Abilities

_____   _____

_____   _____

_____   _____

_____   _____

Mental Abilities

_____   _____

_____   _____

_____   _____

_____   _____

Life Situation
(relationships, work, housing, etc.)

_____   _____

_____   _____

_____   _____

_____   _____

What did you find? Do you have more concerns in one category than another? Is it easier, perhaps, to name unwelcome changes than welcome ones? As we grow older, a remarkable amount of suffering results from our difficulties accepting the inevitable. And on top of resisting changes that have already occurred, we fear those we imagine are coming.

In an interesting study, nearly 40,000 adults from around the world were asked to name the age-related changes that they worry about most. It turns out that different cultures fret about different things: Germans worry most about losing their memory or mental alertness; Dutch about gaining weight; Thais about failing eyesight; Brazilians about losing sexual drive and teeth; Belgians about incontinence; Indians about losing their hair or having it turn gray; and Americans about loss of energy, difficulty caring for themselves, memory loss, and weight gain. (For reasons that nobody can figure out, Egyptians report very few concerns about aging.)

Take a moment to return to your chart. Which changes do you worry will increase as you go forward? Are there changes you fear that have yet to begin?

In the cross-cultural study, people seem to worry most about the particular attributes they rely on to define their sense of self or to maintain their rank in their primate troop (family, friends, and coworkers). A good friend of mine got particularly caught up in this:

Carlos was unusually talented intellectually. He had always been at the top of his class and managed to earn doctoral degrees in two different fields. Anyone could tell after talking to him for even a few minutes that he was brilliant.

As he entered his 50s, Carlos started to worry about losing his intellectual sharpness. He was embarrassed that he couldn't recall names and dates the way he once did. He didn't particularly care that he had put on weight, lost hair, and had a graying beard—all that mattered was his mental acuity. Despite still being one of the brightest men I knew, he started making plans to retire early so that no one would see him functioning below his peak.

While we each worry about different changes, few of us accept aging without concern or protest.

Self-Improvement

Fearing the inevitable, many of us try to ward off changes with self-improvement projects. We imagine how good we'll feel someday when we reach our goals:

"After this diet, I'll be so thin—I'll look great."

"I'll feel so much better once I start working out."

"When I finally meet the right man [woman], I'll be happy."

"If only I could afford Botox—I'd really be happier without these wrinkles."

"Someday I'll get a really high-paying job and not have to worry about money anymore."

"If I keep meditating, I'll become completely peaceful and calm and everyone will love me."

While working toward self-improvement goals can certainly help us live healthier, more productive lives, it also focuses our attention on an imaginary future, taking us away from appreciating what is actually happening in the present. It keeps us looking for answers to our problems in places where we may never find them. And as we age, this approach becomes less and less tenable—it becomes harder to imagine that our future will be rosier than today.

What Doesn't Work

The research results are in: most of what we think will make us feel better won't. In fact, it turns out that humans are very poor *affective forecasters:* we don't make accurate predictions about what will make us happy or unhappy. In general, we err in the direction of assuming that external life events will have enduring effects on our mood, only to discover that they don't. We have *happiness set points*—built-in tendencies to return to our habitual level of well-being. While positive and negative events certainly influence our mood, we have a remarkable tendency to return to our accustomed level.

For example, despite our fantasies to the contrary, once our basic needs are met wealth doesn't make us happier. The same is true of education or high IQ. Couples with children are not happier than those without. Even living in a sunny climate doesn't work. While sunny days may cheer us up after a week of rain, they stop having their effect

> We tend to overestimate the power of external circumstances—from being married to living in a sunny climate—to make us happy.

if the sun shines every day (we habituate to sunshine the same way we habituate to everything else).

Not only are we bad at predicting future feelings, but we also have faulty recollections of the past. As we age, most of us long for some aspect of the good old days. We envy those with younger bodies who have their whole life ahead of them. We don't realize that on average younger people aren't actually happier. Monitoring the moods of people ages 19–94, researchers found that older people experienced positive emotions longer and had negative emotions subside more quickly than younger people. In one study, scientists found that on average people ages 20–24 were sad 3.4 days a month, while those ages 65–74 were sad only 2.3 days a month.

As long as our basic needs are met, much of our well-being or misery has more to do with how we *interpret* our situation than with the situation itself. I remember talking about money to a mentor many years ago. I explained that my parents had lived through the Great Depression, so I naturally picked up from them a tendency to worry about not having enough. He had come of age in the 1930s but said that he took away a completely different message: "We lost practically everything, and yet life went on. I learned that you can have almost nothing and still be okay."

What we learn through mindfulness practice is that it is our attachment to how we see ourselves and our circumstances, rather than age-related changes themselves, that causes much of our difficulty with growing older. Once again, it is our wish to avoid unpleasant experience that's at the root of our unhappiness.

> It's our attachment to a particular self-image that makes us unhappy as we age.

Mind over matter

An alternative to seeking eternal youth was suggested by the famous baseball pitcher Satchel Paige: "*Age isn't a problem. It's a question of mind over matter. If you don't mind, it doesn't matter.*" Mindfulness practice helps us not mind so much. It does this by awakening us to four important insights: (1) everything changes—and clinging to changing phenomena makes us unhappy, (2) all we actually ever "have" is the present moment, (3) our thoughts are not reality, and (4) we are part of an interdependent web of life.

You may recall the Buddha legend from earlier chapters. After growing up sheltered in the palace he went on several unauthorized chariot rides and saw for the first time old age, illness, and death. These experiences were so disturbing that they inspired him to leave the palace to seek psychological awakening—to find a way to live in light of these realities. In a way, most of us play out the same story. As young people we don't fully grasp the reality of old age, illness, and death; but as we get older, they become clearer. Just as mindfulness practice helped the Buddha awaken, it can help us embrace the inevitable changes in our life and live more richly and fully with them.

Facing Reality

Earlier chapters described how our impulse to avoid uncomfortable experiences—including anxiety, sadness, anger, and physical pain—locks us into those experiences. The same applies to dealing with aging, illness, and even death. What we learn from mindfulness practice is that it is both possible and rewarding to face these realities. In ancient texts, students are encouraged to meditate on the following points:

Five Subjects for Frequent Reflection

- "I am sure to become old. I cannot avoid aging."
- "I am sure to become sick. I cannot avoid sickness."
- "I am sure to die. I cannot avoid death."
- "All things dear and beloved to me are subject to change and separation."
- "I am the owner of my actions; I will become the heir of my actions." (Anguttara Nikaya 5.57)

At first glance, this meditation seems like a bad idea. Won't it just make us depressed to think about these things? As long as we imagine that we can stay eternally young, avoid illness, live forever, hold on to our loved ones and possessions, and escape the consequences of our actions, these reflections are indeed upsetting. But the reality is, trying to hold on to these delusions doesn't *really* make us happy. In fact, it leaves us feeling constantly threatened, as every day we hear of someone else who has fallen ill, suffered another loss, or died. The energy we put into trying not to notice reality is draining. In fact, our efforts at denial are at the root of a lot of our suffering.

Everything changes

One way that mindfulness practice helps us embrace the inevitability of age-related change is by revealing that our fantasies of eternal youth are—surprise—just fantasies. When we attend to the moment-to-moment unfolding of experience, we see that everything is indeed always changing. No two breaths are alike; no two meditation sessions are the same. Moods come and go, thoughts come and go, pleasures and pains come and go. Even the stories we tell ourselves about the future come and go. With age, we get to see how these stories change over time.

Take, for example, buying a new house. We begin full of fantasies of the future—what we will do in each room, how we will use the yard, where we will put our things. Perhaps we imagine raising our children there, spending time with our spouse, or entertaining friends. Perhaps we are proud to own the property. A new house is so solid, so permanent. We expect to live there practically forever.

But things don't turn out quite the way we imagine. Each day living in the house is different. Relationships change and (if we're lucky) our children grow up. Someday the house becomes too small or too big, no longer suiting our needs. We may be shocked to realize that we just borrowed the house for a while and will be passing it on to others. Mindfulness practice helps us understand the inevitability of these changes from the beginning. Embracing this reality can make it much easier to enjoy the ride, feel less encumbered, and take pleasure in the fleeting moments that constitute our lives.

When we allow ourselves to notice the inevitability of change, we relate to our changing bodies and mental faculties differently. When I was young, I remember being warned that I would have to live with misfortunes like breaking a grown-up tooth "for the rest of my life." That was a very daunting prospect. With age we begin to grasp that "the rest of my life" isn't forever and the human body is like a car—expected to wear out. Distressing as it is to realize this, it is also a key to living life well.

> It is wiser to contemplate the law of
> impermanence than to try to repeal it.
> —LARRY ROSENBERG

Becoming more comfortable with aging can also keep us from wasting our energies on projects that promise eternal youth. Extramarital affairs, exotic sports cars, hair transplants, and face-lifts become less tempting when we realize they won't stop time. Relationships also have a better chance of flourishing if we can embrace the aging of our parents, children, partners, and friends.

Midlife isn't a crisis when we accept the inevitability of change.

One way to warm to changes in our body and mind is by attending to them through regular mindfulness practice of the sort described in Chapters 3 and 4. Repeatedly bringing attention to present experience can go a long way toward helping us embrace the inevitability of change and cling less to images of the good old days.

Still, there are times when despite regular practice we rail against the changes. This often happens when we discover we're no longer so competent at a skill, feel rejected for being too old, fall in, or notice we no longer fit in with a younger set. To prepare for these times a tailored formal meditation practice can be particularly useful. While initially disturbing, the following exercise can help you embrace, rather than avoid, the aging process. You can return to it as a life preserver whenever aging is causing you grief. It requires about 20 minutes to complete the first time:

—————— *Befriending the Changes** ——————

Begin by settling into your seat and finding your breath. Spend five or ten minutes just observing the in-breath and out-breath, gently returning your attention to these sensations whenever your mind drifts into thought.

Once you've developed a bit of concentration, allow yourself to imagine how you felt when you were a child. Imagine yourself sitting in your current posture with your childhood body. What might you have been wearing? How did you feel in your body? Be the child you once were for a few minutes.

Next imagine yourself, still as a child, but now naked, looking in a mirror. Start at your feet and gradually "look" at your legs, midsection, chest, neck, and head. Take in both how you appeared on

---

*Available in audio at *www.mindfulness-solution.com.*

the outside and how you felt from the inside. After inhabiting your child body for several minutes, allow your attention to return to the present and follow the breath.

⚘

Next imagine yourself sitting as a young adult (if you are currently a young adult, try imagining how you were a few years ago). Imagine how you felt sitting as you are now but in your younger body. Be the young adult you once were for a few minutes.

⚘

Now again imagine yourself naked, looking in a mirror, only as a young adult (or as you were a few years ago). Start at your feet and gradually "look" at your legs, midsection, chest, neck, and head. Take in both how you appeared on the outside and how you felt from the inside. After "looking" at yourself in the mirror for a few minutes, return again to your breath for a little while.

⚘

Continue this exercise by envisioning yourself at your current age, first from the inside, sitting, and then looking at yourself naked in the mirror. Then move into the future. Imagine how you will look and feel at future milestones such as middle age, retirement, or old age. In each circumstance, take some time to imagine how you would feel sitting in your current posture and how you would look naked in the mirror. Notice in particular which aspects of the different ages you readily accept and which ones you resist.

If you discover that one age is particularly difficult, you might try directing loving-kindness toward the image of yourself at that age. For example, if it's difficult to be with the image of being quite old, hold that image in mind and suggest to the person you see, "May you be happy, may you be peaceful, may you be free from suffering" or similar intentions.

What did you discover? Was it hard? Most people find it initially disturbing to look at their life cycle this clearly. Nonetheless, the more we can embrace reality, the more gracefully we can pass through the stages of our lives.

Michael was the favorite son of a successful businessman father and an adoring stay-at-home mom. Even as a young boy he was good at sports and well liked. He was voted most likely to succeed in high school and won an athletic scholarship to a selective college, where he became captain of the track team, dated popular girls, and earned high grades. He went on to a prestigious law school, passed the bar on his first try, and landed a plum job in a big firm. Soon he fell in love, married a beautiful paralegal, and started a family. In a few years he made partner and moved into a lovely suburban home.

While there were of course some highs and lows, Michael remained upbeat and confident through his 30s. He seemed to live a charmed life.

While Michael didn't like to think of himself as vain, he cared about his looks. As he got into his 40s, his hair began thinning and he put on weight. His wife, while still attractive, was no longer a knockout. Although he was earning big bucks, he didn't find the law that interesting. For the first time in his life, Michael started to feel unsettled. He had compelling fantasies about younger women and became nostalgic for his college and law school days. He did the math: it was 22 years since he had graduated from college; in another 22 years he'd be 66. How did this happen? Had he passed his peak?

Michael began to wonder about what really mattered. All his life he had been building toward the next great thing, and now that he was married and financially secure he didn't know what that might be. He realized that earning more money wasn't going to matter much, and even though he thought a lot about other women, he didn't want to destroy his family by having an affair.

Encouraged by one of the guys at the office, he went to a lecture at a local meditation center. The teacher spoke about how sooner or later our ambitions let us down and the inevitability of aging, illness, and death dawns on us. The teacher's words rang true. So, with his friend's encouragement, Michael began practicing mindfulness. He soon got into the habit of meditating for 20 minutes most mornings, doing informal practice when he could, and attending weekly talks at the meditation center.

One talk was about embracing impermanence. The teacher had the group do an exercise similar to the *Befriending the Changes* practice. Michael did well recalling earlier stages of his life—feeling lively and cute when little, sexy and virile as a young man. But as he looked at himself currently and imagined himself in years to come, he experienced disgust. Clearly he had to do something about his attitude.

It was all very disorienting. His whole life had been about the future and things getting bigger and better. Now Michael realized that he needed to notice what was happening at this moment and deal with the fact that it's all impermanent. Luckily, his mindfulness practice started to work. Over the next months he began to worry less about being over the hill and became more interested in making his life now worth living.

Michael stopped going to the fancy hair salon and tried the local barber instead—risking a less stylish haircut. When he needed a new car, he bought a Honda instead of a Porsche. He stopped trying to impress everyone at work and get the most lucrative cases and started listening to his coworkers more. He showed more appreciation toward his family and friends. He spent less time managing his investments on the Internet and more time talking with his wife and playing board games with his kids. He paid attention to the ordinary, everyday moments. He began to live as though this wasn't a dress rehearsal.

Working with illness

Like aging, illness is unavoidable. While some of us are fortunate to be relatively healthy and others are afflicted with serious disease, *no body* escapes sickness entirely. We discussed in Chapter 7 a number of illnesses that are caused or maintained by psychological factors—either by our general emotional state or by our reactions to our symptoms. While many illnesses have such a psychological component, others do not. We saw how mindfulness practice can help us work our way out of stress-related illnesses. Fortunately, it can help us deal skillfully with the other types as well.

Is It Serious?

When we begin to pay attention to bodily sensations, we notice that they are endlessly varied and ever present. Whenever a new symptom shows up we wonder, "Is it serious? Should I see a doctor? Can I treat it myself?" If we're young and have been pretty healthy, we're likely to assume that most symptoms are *probably nothing*. We expect that our body will recover naturally from minor infections and injuries, so we make few adjustments in our routines to take care of each new development. This can be an effective strategy—after all, the body does usually heal itself successfully. Of course, this strategy can also lead us to overlook important warning signs. The mole that turns out to be melanoma or the "weird cough" that turns out to be bacterial pneumonia could both have been treated more effectively had we caught them sooner.

If we are older or have had or been around more severe illnesses, we tend to assume that new symptoms *may be serious.* Here our imagination knows no bounds. Every lump is a malignancy; every new sensation is a debilitating neurological disease. Germs lurk everywhere, and no amount of Lysol and Purell can keep us safe. Reading *Prevention* magazine and going to the health food store reminds us of how much can go wrong with this fragile body. For many people this leads to endless medical visits, as they seek reassurance by ruling out one or another disorder. As we saw in Chapter 7, fear itself can cause many ailments.

You can try a brief exercise to see their mechanism in action. Leave your eyes open so you can read the directions as you go along. It will take only a few minutes.

INDUCING AN ILLNESS—PART I

Begin to focus on your breath and settle into where you are sitting or lying right now. Feel the sensations throughout your body, starting at your feet and progressing up your legs, through your belly, back, chest, and neck. Notice how your arms feel holding this book and (if you are sitting), how your head balances on your neck.

Now bring your attention to the sensations inside your head. Right now, as you read this, see if you can notice a little bit of pressure somewhere—the kind that were it to grow might turn into a headache. Focus your attention on that pressure and see if you can notice it beginning to form an actual headache. Take a minute to really concentrate on the pressure to allow it to grow. Notice exactly where you feel the pressure and how easily it could transform into pain. (Close your eyes now to pinpoint the sensations.)

Did you feel a bit of pressure in your head? If you knew someone who suffered from a brain tumor, or if you had had trouble with headaches in the past, you would naturally be sensitized to this sort of sensation. When we anxiously scan for it, the pressure is not hard to find. If we then react to it with fear or concern, the pressure can easily build into a bona fide headache.

Now try another little experiment.

INDUCING AN ILLNESS—PART II

Imagine you've just learned that you have been exposed to lice. Someone with a bad infestation spread them to the furniture on which you are currently sitting or lying. Take a moment to check out the sensations all over your body. Might there be a little itching somewhere? Maybe on your scalp? Is there perhaps itching in more than one place? Take a few moments to feel these sensations. Could they actually be lice? (Close your eyes for a few moments to feel the little beasts.)

And finally one more:

INDUCING AN ILLNESS—PART III

Right now, bring your attention to the sensations in your left foot. Notice them carefully. Do you feel a little tingling or numbness? Might the sensations in your left foot be different from those in your right foot? Take a few moments to really pay attention to them. (Close your eyes briefly to feel the sensations.) Could this be the first sign of neuropathy?

Because our bodies create millions of sensations each minute, we have limitless opportunities to become concerned about illness. Combine this capacity with living in the information age, where we get to hear about maladies afflicting people everywhere, and we have a setup for illness anxiety. In illness anxiety our concern about a symptom amplifies our experience of that symptom. As discussed in Chapter 7, it can also tighten muscles in the back, neck, or jaw; disrupt sleep–wake cycles and sexual responses; and cause the digestive system and other organ systems to malfunction.

How Mindfulness Practice Helps

What are we to do? We can get into trouble by ignoring symptoms, and we can get into trouble by attending to them. Though it cannot fully resolve our dilemma, mindfulness practice can help us work with it more skillfully.

By being attentive to the sensations in our bodies we are more likely to notice new ones that might require attention. While ultimately we are going to have to use our thinking, gather information, and perhaps consult a health care professional, having data about what sensations arise in the body under different circumstances can help us respond more appropriately to them.

Mindfulness can also be very useful in working with our anxiety about symptoms once we understand them. It can help us learn to tolerate discomfort and see the distinction between uncomfortable sensations and our distress about those sensations (the "two arrows" discussed in Chapter 7). It can also help us notice anxiety about symptoms as they arise and thereby see how anxiety might be contributing to our problem. When acceptance is the key to interrupting a fear–symptom–fear cycle, mindfulness practice can help us cultivate that acceptance. This can be especially powerful when a symptom is amplified by illness anxiety:

Laurie was very concerned about the tingling and burning in her feet. Her father was diabetic and had serious problems with circulation, so she knew this could be a serious matter. Her primary-care doctor sent her to a well-known neurologist, who did a thorough evaluation and told her she had mild peripheral neuropathy.

Shaken by the diagnosis, Laurie's attention went straight to her feet each morning. Was this going to be a good or bad day? She had taken to wearing padded sandals—even in the winter—to limit her discomfort. Some days even the trip from the bed to the bathroom was difficult.

When her doctor suggested she see me, a psychologist, Laurie was put off. "Are you suggesting this is all in my head?" she protested. He tried to explain that he understood her pain was real but thought I might help her live with it better.

She arrived at my office quite desperate. Since she had already been evaluated by a skilled neurologist and told there was no need to adjust her activities, we focused on her reactions to her symptoms. After gathering some history and learning of her worries related to her father's condition, I taught her the *Separating the Two Arrows* practice from Chapter 7. She quickly became aware of how much fear and sadness surrounded her symptoms. When she practiced simply attending to the sensations themselves, she realized they were actually not that painful. But she was extremely disturbed by the fact that her feet "weren't normal." When her feet felt worse, she panicked, thinking her disease was progressing.

I invited Laurie to try formal sitting practice several times a week along with informal mindfulness practice throughout the day. I asked her to notice whenever her mind *wasn't* focused on her feet. She saw that she attended to her feet more when she was anxious and was more anxious whenever she felt odd sensations in her feet. It was a vicious cycle. I suggested she practice saying "yes" to these sensations, no matter how odd. While initially she protested that they were too uncomfortable to tolerate, eventually she was able to do it. To her surprise, she started having times when her feet didn't bother her so much and she could turn her attention to other things.

> Mindfulness can help us see the distinction between discomfort and our distress over feeling discomfort.

After a couple of months she concluded that the sensations weren't getting progressively worse but were coming and going. Especially when she could relax her aversion to them, they weren't so bad.

Using Illness to Support Mindfulness Practice

Not only can mindfulness practice help us work with illness, but illness can provide an opportunity to practice mindfulness. It can afford a retreat from the busyness of life and awaken us to realities that support our practice. Even the discomfort of illness can provide support.

A Mini-Retreat

Staying home from work or school because of illness gives us an extra chance to cultivate mindfulness. It can be hard to find time to meditate during a busy week, and sick leave provides an opportunity. Of course if you're very feverish or tired, you may find it difficult to focus your mind. But if you're reasonably awake, being in bed can be a great opportunity to develop both concentration and mindfulness. The *Breath Awareness Meditation, Body Scan Meditation,* and *Eating Meditation* described in Chapter 3 can all be done while sick in bed, as can the *Loving-Kindness*

Meditation and other practices described in Chapter 4. Since illness puts goal-oriented activity on hold, it lets us focus on *being* rather than *doing*. It can even provide insight into the nature of reality.

Pain also provides an opportunity for practice. Have you ever seen a picture of a yogi lying on a bed of nails? Pain sensations can anchor the mind, bringing our attention to the present. They can also give us an opportunity to work with our habitual impulse to pull away from discomfort—to practice approaching difficult experience rather than avoiding it.

On top of this, illness challenges our fantasies of control. Since it comes upon us by surprise, it reminds us that "humans plan while God laughs." Psychologist and meditation teacher Jack Kornfield tells the story of a revered teacher at a forest monastery in Thailand who was known for pointing this out to his students repeatedly. A student would tell him, "I won't be at the monastery tomorrow. I am going to Bangkok to take care of some financial business." The teacher would reply, "*Maybe.*" The same teacher would say that you could sum up all the insights gained from meditation practice with one phrase: "*Not always so.*"

Silver Linings

For many of my patients, learning to work with a problem like Laurie's or recovering from a stress-related medical problem like those described in Chapter 7 has silver linings. I have had more than one person say (once they were better), "I'd never wish this back pain [or other problem] on anyone, but I'm glad it happened to me." Working their way through the difficulty taught them how to let go, experience the moment, face fear, and connect with a full range of emotions. It also taught them to notice and embrace the fact that everything changes—like it or not. They discovered the truth behind the saying "*I finally got a grip when I learned to let go.*"

Of course, while we can learn from any illness, they all can't be resolved through mindfulness practice. Sooner or later, one comes along that we can't overcome. It's important not to become too attached to health or to blame ourselves when such an illness strikes. Some people assume after learning about the role that the mind and behavior can play in illness that every malady is somehow "my fault." I like to remind my patients what happened to all the great ancient meditation masters. No matter how wise, skillful, or compassionate they were, their bodies all fell apart in the end.

Death

If you don't want to die, don't be born.
—LARRY ROSENBERG

Astronomers estimate that the sun is 4.57 billion years old—about halfway through its life cycle. In another 5 billion years, the sun will expand to encompass what is now the earth's orbit. Scientists are divided about what this will mean for us. One group says that in about 200 million years the earth will become too hot for humans and that in 500 million years the oceans will evaporate. Another group disagrees. They say that as the sun gets bigger, its gravitational pull will weaken, the earth will move farther away, and everything will freeze. Either way, you know our prognosis.

How can we live in light of this? People respond in different ways. The most common approach is denial. As the Zen master mentioned in Chapter 1 pointed out, we have a remarkable ability to live as though death is not real. Modern culture conspires to support this denial. We put young people on pedestals and hide the elderly in nursing homes. We sanitize the dead in funeral parlors, trying to make them look attractive and alive. We do everything possible to keep death out of our awareness.

Is anything wrong with this? After all, death is pretty unpleasant— who wants to think about it all the time? Like so many things we do to try to feel better, our efforts here also make matters worse. As the meditation teacher Larry Rosenberg puts it, "Death is not waiting for us at the end of the road. It is walking with us the whole time." Our attempts to block this reality out of awareness actually add to our daily stress and rob us of the opportunity to live our lives fully.

They do this in many ways. First, there is anxiety. Try as we might to block out thoughts of death, we still occasionally notice it. This is particularly problematic if we watch the local news, where "if it bleeds it leads." So while we generally avoid acknowledging our mortality, we do hear about other people's deaths from time to time. If we try to hang on to delusions of immortality, each bit of news frightens us.

Next there are our foolish pursuits. You've seen the bumper sticker "Whoever dies with the most toys wins." Whether it's wealth, prestige, power, popularity, or sex, chasing things that ultimately fade causes endless disappointment. We're much less likely to take these pursuits seriously if we recognize the reality of death.

And then there's our difficulty really connecting with others. When people are facing either their own demise or the loss of a loved one, they need friends and family. To whatever degree we're in denial about death, we can't really be with them because we can't fully face what they're going through. Other people sense our distance and feel more isolated themselves.

Denying death also keeps us from living in the present by locking us into fantasies of the future—a mythical time in which we'll get security, relaxation, free time, recognition, a fit physique, or some other dream. It keeps us from enjoying and appreciating today.

A Death Theme Park

Some twenty years ago I visited a Thai Buddhist monastery that could best be described as a "death theme park." There were real human skeletons in glass cases and pictures of corpses on the walls. People in local towns donated the bodies of their loved ones to the monastery so the monks could perform "spiritual autopsies." The monks would dissect the bodies—not to gain medical knowledge but to see for themselves that we really are just made of flesh and blood, and that death is real. Despite all this emphasis on death, the monks and nuns were not a depressed lot. They used these practices to remind themselves that life really is short—so that they might wake up and fully experience this moment right now.

A well-known Zen story exhorts us to do the same: While walking across a field, a man encountered a tiger and was promptly chased off a cliff. He managed to stop his fall by clutching a hanging vine. Far below, another tiger had come, hoping to eat him. Above, the first tiger waited hungrily. Two mice, one white and one black, began nibbling through the vine. Just then, the man spied a luscious strawberry. Holding the vine with one hand, he plucked the strawberry with the other. How sweet it tasted!

Occasionally, a similar attitude has taken root in the West. From 1861 through 1865 as many American soldiers died in the Civil War as in the American Revolution, the War of 1812, the Mexican War, the Spanish-American War, World War I, World War II, and the Korean War combined. Historian Drew Faust points out that this made death very real to everyone and contributed to a new attitude. In mid-1800s America, it was thought to be essential to think about death every day—not to be morbid, but to take *today* seriously.

Can continuous awareness of death really enrich our lives? Can it help us live each day more fully? Yes, but we need to use this awareness deliberately to support our awakening. One way is by trying to keep life's inevitable losses in perspective:

A Zen master was sitting in his temple chambers while a novice monk dusted and swept. The centerpiece of the room was a beautiful ancient vase that had been at the monastery for hundreds of years. In a moment of inattention, the young monk accidentally knocked the vase off of the shelf. It fell to the floor and shattered. The monk was beside himself. He apologized profusely to the master and frantically tried to gather up the ceramic shards. He expected the master to be angry, but the old man didn't look upset. Once the monk began to calm down a little, he asked the master, "Aren't you angry?" "No," the master replied. "Why not?" asked the monk. "It was a precious, ancient vase, and I destroyed it with my carelessness." The master paused for a moment and then said, *"To me, the vase was already broken."*

By being aware that everything (including us) falls apart in the end, we can live more lightly—and be less shocked and distressed by change and loss. It can also help us take ourselves less seriously, which can be a tremendous relief. Another story, from closer to home, captures this:

A young man who was feeling adrift heard of a wise rabbi living in Brooklyn and decided to seek his counsel. He traveled to New York and made his way to a small apartment in a poor part of town where he was to have his meeting. The rabbi was welcoming and spent several hours with him.

The man asked questions about biblical teachings and Jewish history and sought advice about what to do with his life. While he very much appreciated the rabbi's insights, the young man kept wondering about the rabbi's life. There was almost nothing in the apartment except a desk, a couple of chairs, a mattress, and a few books. Gathering up his courage, he asked the rabbi if this was where he lived. The rabbi answered, "Yes, for many years." Puzzled, the young man asked, "Where are all of your things?" "You're looking at them," the rabbi replied. Then he pointed to the young man's backpack and asked, "Is this all you have with you?" "Yes," said the young man, "but I am only passing through."

> Awareness that everything falls apart in the end can relieve us of the stress of trying to keep things together—including ourselves—that will inevitably crumble.

"*So am I*," responded the rabbi.

Dropping the Hot Coal

Of course most of us don't relate to loss, and especially our own death, like the Zen master or rabbi. There is a famous *New Yorker* cartoon where a man is looking at the obituary page in a newspaper. The obits are labeled "Two Years Younger Than You," "Twelve Years Older Than You," "Three Years Your Junior," "Your Age on the Dot." When we read obituaries, we are reminded of death and often look for reasons why the other person died and we won't: "He was probably a smoker." "She looks like she didn't exercise." "He was really old." "She lived in a bad neighborhood." We have to expend a lot of psychological energy to avoid noticing the inevitability of our own death. Yet think of all the concerns that would fall away if only we could embrace it.

Most of our worries become trivial in light of our death. My friend and colleague, Paul Fulton, once told me about his strategy to deal with public speaking anxiety. He would write across the top of his notes, "SOON DEAD." What difference would it make if people liked his talk? All the concerns about "me"—how I look, what others think, what I own, whether I'm good or bad—stop mattering in light of the great leveler. It is sometimes said that our preoccupation with our survival and well-being is like holding tightly to a hot coal—it's a relief to drop it.

One way to practice dropping the coal is by constructing our own death theme park. In doing this, we may come to notice that we are not actually afraid of dying but are frightened of our fantasies about it. As with other psychological difficulties, it is the negative thoughts about our experience and our resistance to it, rather than our experience itself, that are most disturbing.

There are several ways to practice becoming aware of death. We can take time to visit a cemetery, read the tombstones, and let the reality of our coming and going sink in. We can read the obituaries regularly. And we can actually allow ourselves to imagine our own death.

One particularly effective way to do this, if you are open to the adventure, is by writing your own obituary (see the facing page).

People have all sorts of reactions to this exercise. Many choose not to do it. (It can be emotionally intense, and perhaps now isn't the best time to embark on the project.) Other people find that it brings up all sorts of feelings, often centered on sadness about leaving behind loved ones or not fulfilling dreams. Many times the exercise makes us aware of how much others matter to us and how unimportant our other preoccupations are. Whatever arises for you, try to take it in with awareness and acceptance.

WRITING MY OBITUARY

Set aside an hour or so—enough time to complete the project. You'll need a quiet place, a newspaper, and either paper and pen or a computer. Begin by meditating for a few minutes. Bring your attention to the present by focusing on your breath and noticing the sensations in your body at the moment. Next read a few of the obituaries. Notice what they include: where people were born, how their lives unfolded, whom they touched. Notice too how your mind reacts to the stories.

Now imagine an age at which you might die. Write your obituary as it might actually read if someone who knows you well wrote it. Let it be honest—there is no need to ever show this to anyone. Include the aspects of your life that you feel good about as well as those you wish were different. Mention the people, places, and events that have mattered and the people you will be leaving behind.

As you write the obituary, notice all the different thoughts and feelings that arise. Observe the ones that are difficult to bear and how the mind responds to these. Notice too any positive feelings that arise. Try to stay open to the whole experience.

Traditional Death Meditations

Many religions have developed meditations on death. They are usually designed to reduce self-preoccupation. Some of the most graphic come from Buddhist traditions, where the emphasis on embracing change and impermanence as a way to become free of suffering figures prominently. These are not for the faint of heart, as they vividly challenge our resistance to acknowledging our own impermanence. In one such meditation, students are encouraged first to contemplate the aspects of the body that we don't usually consider attractive (viewer discretion advised):

—— *Unpleasant Parts of the Body Contemplation* ——

[Reflect] ... on this very body from the soles of the feet on up, from the crown of the head on down, surrounded by skin and full of various kinds of unclean things: "In this body there are head hairs, body hairs, nails, teeth, skin, flesh, tendons, bones, bone marrow, kidneys, heart, liver, pleura, spleen, lungs, large intestines, small intestines, gorge, feces, bile, phlegm, pus, blood, sweat, fat, tears, skin-oil, saliva, mucus, fluid in the joints, urine."

Once we have a sense of the body as it actually is rather than as we like to imagine it, we are encouraged to systematically imagine the fate of our body left at a burial ground to decompose. We are asked to imagine the various stages:

Cemetery Contemplation

- A corpse cast away in a charnel ground, picked at by crows, vultures, and hawks, by dogs, hyenas, and various other creatures
- A skeleton smeared with flesh and blood, connected with tendons
- A fleshless skeleton smeared with blood, connected with tendons
- A skeleton without flesh or blood, connected with tendons
- Bones detached from their tendons, scattered in all directions—here a hand bone, there a foot bone, here a shin bone, there a thigh bone, here a hip bone, there a back bone, here a rib, there a chest bone, here a shoulder bone, there a neck bone, here a jaw bone, there a tooth, here a skull
- The bones whitened, somewhat like the color of shells, piled up, more than a year old
- The bones decomposed into a powder
  (Adapted from the *Kayagata-sati Sutta*)

The student is further encouraged to realize that this is the "nature of my body, such is its future, such its unavoidable fate."

It isn't easy. Like the *Befriending the Changes* and *Writing My Obituary* practices, these are designed to bring us face to face with reality so as to make it easier to accept. Like those other exercises, they're best attempted on a day when you're feeling reasonably stable and up for a challenge.

Connecting

In some philosophical traditions, the fact of our death is seen as a problem. Existentialists discuss how it underscores our fundamental separateness—after all, even if surrounded by loved ones, we die alone. From another perspective, however, death is part of what ties us together.

We are all hurt and lonely at one time or another. We can feel alienated from our family, friends, or romantic partner—mistrustful of their intentions, *different* from other people. If we're sad, frustrated, angry, or anxious, we can feel we're suffering because there is something wrong with us. We sink into what psychologist and meditation teacher Tara Brach calls a *trance of unworthiness*. Our friends are enjoying their work, going to the movies, and having fun at parties. We feel damaged or inadequate because we feel disconnected. During these moments of isolation, seeing our common fate can be a great relief.

Of all the changes and losses we face, death is not only the one we deny most; it is also the most universal. There is an ancient story that captures how seeing this reality can break us out of our loneliness:

The Mustard Seed

A poor woman in ancient India was said to be "psychotic with grief" because her only son had just died. She carried his lifeless body around the village, wailing, asking everyone she saw for help. People wanted to do something but didn't know how to ease her pain. Eventually someone suggested she visit with a wise teacher who was camped near the village.

The woman carried her son's body to the camp, where she found the Buddha and his followers. She showed the Buddha her son's body and begged him to tell her how to bring the boy back to life. The Buddha listened carefully and then said, "I think I can help." "Please, please, I'll do anything," she replied. He told her that all she needed to do was to return to the village, get a mustard seed from a neighbor, and bring it back to him. In India at the time mustard seeds were as common as salt or pepper would be in a Western home, so the woman was heartened and set off right away. As she was leaving, the Buddha said, "Just one more thing. Make sure the household from which you get the seed hasn't known death."

The woman set off hopefully and knocked on the door of the first house she came to. She told her story. The man was very sympathetic and immediately offered her a mustard seed. As she was leaving, she remembered to inquire, "If you don't mind my asking: has this home been touched by death also?" The man became sad and told the story of his cousin, who had been tragically killed the year before. The woman thanked her neighbor and set off to the next house.

At the next house she was greeted warmly again and given another mustard seed, but at the end heard a story about a mother who had died in childbirth. She thanked this neighbor too and moved on. The pattern repeated at house after house, until she had visited every home in the village. She received many mustard seeds but also heard many sad stories.

The woman returned to see the Buddha and said, "Thank you—I think I'm beginning to understand." She went on to become one of his students and eventually became a great teacher in her own right.

Recognizing our mortality and our shared vulnerability to the mortality of our loved ones can powerfully connect us to one another. It moves us out of isolation and into life-affirming connection. It also helps us see how our preoccupation with differences—gender, culture, age, and rank in the primate troop—is trivial compared to what we have in common.

And we don't share mortality just with other humans but with all living organisms. By recognizing the reality of birth and death, we connect to the wider world and experience ourselves as part of the web of life. This is a very good thing, given our challenging individual prognoses.

We all have opportunities to feel this connection every day, though usually we devote so much energy to thinking about what will make us feel better or worse that we forget to notice it. Just turning our attention to these opportunities can help us feel more connected. You can do this intentionally with a brief meditation. This exercise also works nicely as a life preserver when you are feeling oppressed by a sense of isolation or alienation. You'll need about 10 minutes:

———————— *Getting beyond "Me"* ————————

Begin by finding your seat and settling into the breath and the experience of being where you are. Spend a few minutes just practicing being present.

Once you've settled a bit, recall moments in your life when you felt connected to something larger than yourself. These might be moments of connection with nature; friends, a lover, family, or community; music or art; spiritual teachers or practices; religious figures or images. Perhaps they were moments of intense sensual involvement, such as when riding a roller coaster, swimming in a lake, making love, or skiing down a mountain; or subtle wonder, such as beholding a flower. Allow yourself to recall as many of these moments as you can, remembering how they each felt.

Now take a moment to jot down a few of the moments that came to mind and the feeling that accompanied each one:

Connected Moment	Feeling
_____	_____
_____	_____
_____	_____
_____	_____
_____	_____

It is only by connecting to the wider world that we can be at peace with mortality. Luckily, mindfulness practice helps us make this connection. You'll probably notice if you review your list that your moments of connection each involve being present for an experience—we don't usually feel connected in the moments that we are planning for the future or reviewing the past. In fact, you may have noticed that it is your thoughts and judgments that keep you from experiencing your interconnection with other people and the rest of life. Luckily, mindfulness practice helps us take these thoughts more lightly—so that they're less likely to get in the way of connecting.

Putting it all together: embracing impermanence

While all of these ideas may make sense intellectually, most of us still instinctively recoil from aging, illness, and especially death. These are

Connecting to the wider world helps us make peace with our mortality.

not easy realities to accept, despite the fact that resisting or denying them traps us into needless suffering.

In the Buddhist traditions in which many mindfulness practices evolved, embracing impermanence—particularly the inevitable decay of the body—gets a lot of attention. Coming to grips with this reality is both one of our biggest psychological challenges and one of our most potentially liberating undertakings. Difficult as it is, facing the inevitability of aging, illness, and death can free us from suffering while empowering us to do the same for others who are struggling.

Establishing a regular pattern of formal and informal practices as described in Chapters 3 and 4 will help bring your attention to the changing nature of all things and lay a good foundation for this effort. This is true whether or not illness and death are occupying your mind at the moment.

Unwanted events can also propel us forward in this work. If you or a loved one is seriously ill, or if someone close to you has recently died, thoughts and feelings about impermanence will already be with you. The best way to work with these will depend on your circumstances at the moment.

In dealing with this difficult realm, it is important to choose between *stabilizing* practices (cultivating a sense of safety) and *moving toward the sharp points* (facing what you would rather avoid). If you're feeling overwhelmed by emotional pain or having to manage a lot of caretaking duties, it's probably best to begin by cultivating stability. Externally focused practices such as *Walking Meditation* (Chapter 3), *Eating Meditation* (Chapter 3), or *Nature Meditation* (Chapter 5)—done either as formal practices or informally during the day—can help you take refuge in the present moment and be less caught in distressing thoughts. Inner-focused formal practices such as *Loving-Kindness Meditation* (Chapter 4) and the *Mountain Meditation* (Chapter 5) can help you to feel more accepting of what is happening. These can all also be used as life preservers when you feel overwhelmed by feelings, while the *Three-Minute Breathing Space* (Chapter 6) can be especially useful if you need to come back to the present in the midst of an immediate crisis.

When you're feeling less overwhelmed, moving toward the sharp points may be in order. Doing this can help you come to grips with the inevitability of impermanence whether or not illness or death is upon you at the moment. Practices and exercises described earlier in this chapter, such as *Five Subjects for Frequent Reflection, Befriending the Changes, Writing My Obituary, Unpleasant Parts of the Body Contemplation,* and

Cemetery Contemplation, can serve to bring you face to face with the impermanence of the body. They can all be integrated into your regular practice routine or applied at moments when you find yourself particularly resistant to the reality of aging and death.

If you are ill, consider using any time off you may have from work and other responsibilities to do more mindfulness practice. You can use the *Breath Awareness Meditation, Body Scan Meditation,* and *Eating Meditation* described in Chapter 3 to create your own mini-retreat. If you suspect that illness anxiety is contributing to your condition, try the *Separating the Two Arrows* practice and other approaches described in Chapter 7 to accept, rather than fight, the symptoms.

As in all of the applications of mindfulness practices we've discussed throughout this book, there is an art to sensing what is most needed when. If the more challenging practices are overwhelming, they can be mixed with the stabilizing ones. And whether you're trying to overcome your resistance to seeing the impermanence of the body or trying to get through a day filled with dealing with illness or death, the prescription in "The Mustard Seed"—seeing the universality of loss—will help. You can also use the *Getting beyond "Me"* practice either as a regular meditation or as a life preserver when feeling overwhelmed. It can help remind you of your connection with the wider world—a world that will outlive your body and those of your loved ones.

While resistance to change of one sort or another is part of all psychological suffering, the challenges of aging, illness, and death are sometimes at the heart of our struggles:

Harry was a bright, worldly man in his late 60s who was determined to live past 100. He was recently retired and took excellent care of himself—eating the right foods, exercising regularly, and practicing yoga. He was financially secure, played golf regularly, and enjoyed taking in museums, concerts, and other cultural events. While generally in excellent health, Harry came to see me on the advice of his doctor because of recurrent neck pain. It didn't interfere much with his functioning, but he hated having something wrong with his body. Tests showed disk degeneration typical for his age but nothing more.

As I got to know him, it quickly became apparent that Harry liked to have his ducks in a row. He was a very competent guy who researched everything thoroughly and made careful decisions. He read *Consumer Reports* from cover to cover. He seemed to imagine that if he did everything right nothing would go wrong.

I was particularly intrigued when he told me that he wanted to live past 100. At first I thought he was kidding, but he wasn't. As we discussed his plans, he told me of all the things he needed to accomplish and how much time they would take.

I asked him his thoughts about death. Not surprisingly, he didn't like to think about it. He needed to improve his golf game, learn Spanish, and write a novel before he died in order to feel successful—his accomplishments to date were not enough.

Since he already practiced yoga, Harry took readily to my suggestion to try mindfulness meditation. A naturally disciplined man, he soon made formal and informal practice part of his daily routine. Once he had a feel for cultivating mindfulness, I gave him a copy of the *Five Subjects for Frequent Reflection* to keep on his desk. He found this unsettling, though intriguing. Then I had him try the *Befriending the Changes* and *Writing My Obituary* practices. Neither of these was easy. He felt resistance to both and in the process realized how much energy he'd been putting into trying to control things and ward off the inevitable. It became clear to us both that his neck pain stemmed in part from the tension this created.

Harry realized that he would need to start letting go—of everything. In his quest to pass 100 he was making life in the present more fearful and less joyful. So he stopped trying so hard to block out news of illness and death and became more accepting of his and his wife's wrinkles and sags. He tried making a few purchases without thorough research. He even traveled to Europe without planning every day in advance. As he worked on this shift and kept up his regular mindfulness practice, the tension in his neck subsided and his already fulfilling life became even better. He may not make it to 100. But however many years he has left, he's likely to enjoy them more.

Mindfulness practices for working with aging, illness, and death

The following rest on a foundation of regular formal and informal practice as described in Chapters 3 and 4. They can all be used to work with aging, illness, and death in the ways just described.

Formal Meditation Practices and Exploratory Exercises

- *Five Subjects for Frequent Reflection* (page 288) to remind yourself regularly of the reality of change and loss
- *Befriending the Changes* (page 290) to cultivate acceptance for the cycle of life

- *Writing My Obituary*, *Unpleasant Parts of the Body Contemplation*, and *Cemetery Contemplation* (pages 303 and 304) to embrace the reality of your own impermanence
- *Mountain Meditation* (page 129) to cultivate stability and acceptance in the face of difficult changes
- *Inducing an Illness* (Parts I–III; pages 294 and 295) to observe how anxiety and hypervigilance can create illness
- *Separating the Two Arrows* (page 186) to practice accepting, rather than fighting, symptoms
- *Breath Awareness Meditation*, *Body Scan Meditation*, and *Eating Meditation* (page 54, 72, and 79) to conduct a mini-retreat when ill
- *Loving-Kindness Meditation* (page 84) to cultivate acceptance when feeling especially resistant to or frightened by illness, aging, or death
- *Getting beyond "Me"* (page 306) to remind you of your connection to the wider world that extends beyond your life

Informal Practices

The following can bring attention to sensory experience throughout the day. They can help you take refuge in the present moment while illuminating the changing nature of all things:

- *Walking Meditation* (page 67)
- *Nature Meditation* (page 128)
- *Eating Meditation* (page 263)
- *Driving, Showering, Tooth Brushing, Shaving (etc.) Meditation* (page 90)

Life Preservers

- *Nature Meditation* (page 128), *Walking Meditation* (page 67), and *Eating Meditation* (pages 79 and 263), formal or informal, to anchor your attention in the present when fear of illness, aging, or death becomes overwhelming
- *Loving-Kindness Meditation* (page 84) when fear or resistance to illness or death creates great distress
- *Mountain Meditation* (page 129) to increase stability and acceptance in the presence of unwanted change

- *Getting beyond "Me"* (page 306) to identify with the wider world when concerns about your personal prognosis become difficult
- *Three-Minute Breathing Space* (page 157) to cope with a crisis when dealing with illness or death

Developing a plan

You may find it useful to jot down an action plan for working with aging, illness, and death. The following chart can help you organize your thoughts:

PRACTICE PLAN

Begin by reflecting on how aging, illness, and death currently impact your life.

Situations you find challenging:

Physical (symptoms or changes that disturb you): _____

_____

Cognitive (thoughts about impermanence): _____

_____

Behavioral (things you do to deal with aging, illness, and death)_____

_____

Times I Most Need a Life Preserver: _____

_____

_____

Now, based on what you've read about and experienced with the different practices, jot down an initial practice plan (you can vary this as your needs change):

(cont.)

Formal Practice	When	How Often
_____	_____	_____
_____	_____	_____
_____	_____	_____

Informal Practice	When	How Often
_____	_____	_____
_____	_____	_____
_____	_____	_____

Life Preserver	Likely Situation
_____	_____
_____	_____
_____	_____

When you could use more help

As with all of the other life challenges we've been discussing, our reactions to aging, illness, and death can be overwhelming. If you are involved in a particular religious tradition, seeking guidance from a clergy member can be a valuable source of support at these times. Hospice professionals are another possible resource for both individual and group counseling. While virtually all psychotherapists are accustomed to working with concerns about aging, illness, and death, some also specialize in working with chronic disease or end-of-life issues. Tips for finding professional help, along with other resources for working with these challenges, can be found at the back of the book.

We've seen how mindfulness practices can help us work skillfully with worry and fear, sadness and depression, and all sorts of stress-related medical problems. We've seen how they can help us with the wild and wacky issues we have trying to get along with each other, how they can help us break destructive habits and make wise choices, and even how they can help us work with our ultimate challenges—aging, illness, and death itself. So many of our troubles stem from our highly adaptive tendencies to seek pleasure, avoid pain, think, and plan. Because mindfulness practices help us embrace our experience in the present moment, they can help with most everything that ails us.

While mindfulness practices are remarkable in their ability to resolve both day-to-day and more serious difficulties, they actually have a potential that reaches even further. The practices were developed as part of an ancient path to happiness that goes beyond resolving particular difficulties, promising full psychological awakening and liberation from suffering.

Until recently, modern scientific research had little to say about human happiness and positive states of mind—being dedicated instead to studying psychological distress. It's heartening to see that researchers are now beginning to back up the centuries-old reports of monks, nuns, and other dedicated spiritual seekers. While I've been something of a slow student on this path, others, who either started the journey with more awareness or have practiced more diligently, tell us that freedom and awakening is indeed possible *in this lifetime.* So before you put this book down, please read a little further to get a glimpse of where else these practices can lead.

CHAPTER 11

What's next?

The promise of mindfulness

here is a peculiar line in the American Declaration of Independence. It counts among our inalienable rights "life, liberty *and the pursuit of happiness.*" What does it say about us that we need to *pursue* happiness—as though it were some sort of fugitive?

We've seen how accidents in our evolutionary heritage can make happiness remarkably elusive. This is especially true when we seek it in the wrong places. As the philosopher Joseph Campbell pointed out, many of us climb the ladder of success only to find that it has been leaning up against the wrong wall.

And it's no wonder. We're hardwired to pursue pleasure and avoid pain, enhance our rank in the primate troop, and protect our loved ones—but we live in a world where pain, failure, illness, death, and other disappointments are inevitable. We're also hardwired to think incessantly of ways to ward off these difficulties using a brain honed to anticipate and recall disasters—a brain exquisitely designed to bathe us in distressing thoughts.

Mindfulness practices were first developed thousands of years ago in response to this predicament. We've seen how they're an effective antidote to the experiential avoidance that gets us stuck in anxiety, depression, stress-related disorders, and all sorts of counterproductive habits. We've even seen how they can help us get along better with one another and grow older more gracefully. As your life unfolds, difficulties of all sorts will no doubt continue to arise, and you can use the practices we've been discussing to deal more effectively with them.

But mindfulness practices were originally developed to go even further. As my friend and colleague Charles Styron points out, they are actually part of a very ambitious happiness project. With roots in Buddhist psychology, they were designed not only to help us deal with day-to-day distress but as part of a path toward the lofty goal of enlightenment—complete liberation from psychological suffering.

Until relatively recently, modern Western psychology hasn't paid a lot of attention to positive states of mind—much less enlightenment. Sigmund Freud said famously that the goal of his psychoanalytic treatment was to turn "hysterical misery into ordinary human unhappiness." As Martin Seligman, the contemporary psychologist who spearheaded the study of positive mental states, put it, our field has focused most of its attention on how to move people from "minus five to zero." While this has certainly been a noble pursuit, most of us hope for more.

Luckily, scientists have made some strides in this area over the past decade or so. We now know something not only about what makes us miserable but also about what can make us happy. Many of these discoveries parallel what people have observed over the centuries by practicing mindfulness.

The Hedonic Treadmill

As we see so clearly in addictive behavior, trying to amass pleasurable experiences as a path to well-being doesn't work for long. All pleasant experiences pass, and we can make ourselves very unhappy by constantly chasing new ones. Furthermore, this pursuit often harms either us (too many brownies, too much alcohol) or others (sexual misbehavior, theft, violence).

We also discussed earlier the failure of success. Winning competitions is a losing strategy, because we habituate and recalibrate. No matter how successful we are in pursuing wealth, status, knowledge, power, or other temptations, the mind soon becomes accustomed to what we have and seeks more.

Scientists call the mechanism by which seeking pleasure becomes unsatisfying the *hedonic treadmill*. It is as though we were running on a treadmill—no matter how fast we move, we wind up in the same place emotionally. Whether it is my patient who sold his oil-trading business for $30 million cash but still felt unsuccessful, the lottery winner who now feels adrift, the movie star who is depressed despite being adored by thousands of fans, or the gourmet who is bored by yet another fancy meal, neither winning nor experiencing new sensual pleasures brings lasting happiness or psychological freedom. As one multimillionaire put it when asked how much money is enough, "just a little bit more." Mindfulness practice reveals what scientific psychology is discovering: constant wanting and grasping makes us unhappy, while the opposite—appreciating what *is*—makes us happier.

Of course hearing this doesn't immediately stop us from imagining that the next acquisition or accomplishment really will bring fulfillment. Winning, getting what we think we want, and sensual pleasures all feel great in the short run. Almost everyone enjoys being promoted, starting a new romantic relationship, or getting a new car. Because we enjoy the experience of moving from not having to having and from discomfort to comfort, we easily become hooked on getting more. We feel good temporarily, but since it doesn't last, we soon want something else.

No matter how successful we are in getting what we think we want, before long we're captured by new desires.

Are we therefore doomed to cycles of wanting, briefly being gratified, and then wanting more? Researchers say no. There are alternatives, but we need to know where to look for them. Luckily, mindfulness practice can help us find these alternate paths to well-being.

Appreciating What Is

Conventional wisdom cajoles us to "stop and smell the roses" and "count our blessings." Both turn out to be good ideas. One powerful antidote to becoming trapped in constantly pursuing new pleasure is to appreciate what we already have.

By mindfully savoring experience, we move our attention away from our stories about life toward actually living our moment-to-moment experience. Eating meditation is a nice example. We're satisfied with much less food when we actually take the time to taste what we consume. A simple walk, commuting to work, and buying groceries all also become rich and interesting when we're paying attention. Traveling in a foreign country, we appreciate the little things—the simple daily life of local people is fascinating because we take the time to observe it carefully. Mindfulness practice allows us to appreciate our *own* daily life by experiencing it afresh each moment.

While most mindfulness practices are nonverbal, we can use a simple verbal exercise to help us appreciate *what is*. This exercise has actually been shown to enhance happiness significantly:

THREE GOOD THINGS

Each evening for a week, write down three things that went well that day and what caused them to go well.

That's all there is to it. Remarkably, in large-scale surveys of people who tried this, most found that it significantly decreased depressive symptoms and increased positive moods for the next six months.

A particularly fruitful arena in which to practice appreciating what is involves other people. Scientific research suggests that moving beyond preoccupation with "me" is very important to our well-being. Ironically, while getting more for "me" is very gratifying in the short run, in the long run it leaves us flat. Another simple but more intense exercise offers us the opportunity to simultaneously appreciate what is and get outside of ourselves. While this is not a mindfulness practice per se, it moves us in a similar direction:

EXPRESSING GRATITUDE

Begin by thinking of someone in your life who made an important positive difference, who is still alive, and whom you never properly thanked. It can be anyone—a parent or other relative, a friend, a teacher, a coworker. Next set aside some time and write a 1–2 page testimonial to that person. Make it clear and concrete, telling the story of what the person did, how it made a difference to you, and where you are in life now as a result. Once you've completed your testimonial, call the person up and say that you'd like to come for a visit. If he or she asks why, suggest that you would rather not say—it's a surprise. Finally, visit the person and read your testimonial slowly, with expression and eye contact.

This exercise is not always easy. Even imagining doing it can bring up powerful feelings. Nonetheless, it proves to be effective for enhancing well-being. I suspect that it works so well because it simultaneously helps us appreciate reality as it is and deeply connect with another person.

Service

In Chapter 1 we discussed our existential predicament: sooner or later we lose everything and everyone that matters to us; we're hardwired to try to enhance our self-esteem but can never win at this game; and our individual prognosis is terrible. It's therefore not surprising that research finds seeking more for "me" ultimately makes us unhappy. Pleasure hunting is subject to the hedonic treadmill and soon loses its luster.

Appreciating what we have and connecting to other people are more reliable alternatives. In fact, using our talents to make a contribution to something bigger than "me" ultimately turns out to be more satisfying than pleasure seeking. We discussed in Chapter 8 how mindfulness practice helps us see how our sense of self is constructed moment by moment and how by noticing our interdependence we can connect more readily to others. We also explored in Chapter 9 how this can help us act ethically. Experiencing our interconnectedness also can make us happier.

While "I" won't last very long, the larger universe will. If I can begin to see myself as part of this vast web of matter and energy, participating in the circle of life, I will suffer much less as everything continues to change. As mentioned earlier, I will also naturally feel an impulse to care for this wider world, much as my right hand wouldn't hesitate to bandage my left.

We all sense the interconnected nature of things at times, though we call it by different names. Some people see it as God, or perhaps as his creation. Other people use terms like *nature, ecosystem,* and *web of life* to describe it.

Whatever our language, when we grasp the world as one fantastically complex organism, we feel a natural impulse to be helpful. Some of us are more moved by a wish to be useful to other people, while others are most drawn toward helping other animals or the environment as a whole. Of course it isn't always easy to see this clearly and act accordingly. Albert Einstein described our challenge beautifully:

> A human being is a part of the whole, called by us "Universe," a part limited in time and space. He experiences himself, his thoughts and feelings as something separated from the rest—a kind of optical delusion of his consciousness. This delusion is a kind of prison for us, restricting us to our personal desires and to affection for a few persons nearest to us. Our task must be to free ourselves from this prison by widening our circle of compassion to embrace all living creatures and the whole of nature in its beauty. Nobody is able to achieve this completely, but the striving for such

achievement is in itself a part of the liberation and a foundation for inner security. (In a letter of 1950 written in reply to a rabbi who was trying in vain to comfort his 19-year-old daughter about the death of her sister, a "sinless, beautiful 16-year-old child.")

An important finding from research on happiness is that freeing ourselves from the prison of our "optical delusion" and devoting our energies to some aspect of this wider world is vital to our well-being. Among other things, it provides the uniquely human experience of *meaning*. Other creatures seem to have all sorts of desires and needs, and may even be altruistic in their behavior, but probably only human minds experience events as meaningful or meaningless. When we're focused solely on our own pleasure, life tends to lack meaning. As Seligman put it, we feel as though we're "fidgeting until we die." On the other hand, when we can experience ourselves as part of the larger world and dedicate our efforts to being useful, our lives feel meaningful. By allowing us to see our interconnectedness, mindfulness practice helps bring meaning to our lives.

Generosity

Acting generously—a natural outcome of being less preoccupied with oneself—also seems to help. A group of scientists at the University of British Columbia devised a simple experiment that elegantly demonstrated how giving to others can increase happiness. They gave college students envelopes containing either a $5 bill or a $20 bill that they had to spend by the end of the day. They told half the group to spend the money on themselves and instructed the other half to spend it on a gift for someone else or a charitable donation. The students were all asked to rate their level of happiness at the end of the day. Regardless of the amount, those who spent the money on others reported feeling significantly happier than those that spent the money on themselves.

Meanwhile, other scientists are beginning to demonstrate that meditation practice can directly increase our compassion for others, altering our spending habits. Dr. Richard Davidson and his colleagues at the University of Wisconsin trained subjects in *Loving-Kindness Meditation* (Chapter 4). He then exposed them to images of people suffering, such as a child with an eye tumor, while scanning their brains. Compared to a control group of nonmeditators, the meditators had more activation in the insula, a part of the brain associated with empathy, in response to the pictures. Those with the most activation reported the highest levels of well-being and were more generous when offered an opportunity to donate part of their honorarium to charity.

Flow

Researchers have also identified another important path to happiness that is not subject to the hedonic treadmill. Not surprisingly, this one too involves relaxing the focus on "me" and appreciating what is. We all have moments in which we are fully involved in what we're doing. Athletes describe this as being in the *zone*; artists describe it as finding their muse or creative energy. The Hungarian psychologist Mihály Csíkszentmihályi coined the term *flow* to describe these moments of full involvement. At these times self-consciousness drops away and we're free from our judging mind—we are fully engaged. We are alert, awake, and attentive.

You can identify flow experiences with a simple checklist:

FLOW CHECKLIST

- You lose awareness of time.
- You aren't thinking about yourself.
- You aren't distracted by extraneous thoughts.
- You're focused on the process rather than only on the end goal.
- You're active.
- Your activity feels effortless even if it's challenging.
- You would like to repeat the experience.

These moments of flow involve being mindful *while accomplishing something*. We tend to experience flow when our talents are optimally engaged. Whatever they might be—athletic, interpersonal, artistic, or intellectual—when our abilities are challenged fully but not overwhelmed, we experience flow. It is not surprising that mindfulness practice increases our ability to have flow experiences. By practicing being aware of present experience with acceptance, we engage more fully in everything we do.

Research suggests that these moments of flow are themselves fully satisfying. They don't lead us to want more and more or bigger and better experiences. While engaged in flow, we aren't thinking how much nicer it is elsewhere. Like other moments of mindfulness, moments of flow involve reduced self-preoccupation—they connect us to the world outside ourselves.

A Journey without Goal

There is a cosmic joke built into the pursuit of happiness. It is echoed in a cartoon I have on my desk. Two Zen monks, one old and one young, are meditating side by side. The younger monk gives the older one a quizzical look, to which the older monk replies, "Nothing happens next. This is it!"

The same way that trying to get rid of anxiety traps us in more anxiety and trying to get rid of pain traps us in more pain, *pursuing* happiness traps us in more unhappiness. This is where mindfulness practice can get particularly confusing, since it involves a paradox. Being more mindful indeed makes people happier—for reasons we've just been discussing. However, practicing mindfulness *in order to feel happy* isn't actually practicing mindfulness—since it's not necessarily accepting what's happening at the moment. And yet, if we don't practice, we're less likely to savor experience, accept what is, notice our interconnectedness, and experience flow—and therefore are less likely to be happy.

In almost all other activities that involve putting forth effort over time, we strive to reach a goal—to improve something. The idea is to wind up somewhere other than where we are right now. Mindfulness practice shows us that this striving is itself at the root of a lot of our suffering. So we experience a paradox: happiness is actually more likely to arise when we are *not* pursuing it.

This is not a call, however, to become passive, nihilistic, or disengaged—it is not about automatically resigning ourselves to circumstances. Rather it means throwing ourselves fully into life, putting all of our energies into doing whatever we're doing at the moment, but all the while letting go of our attachment to things turning out a particular way. When we run the race, we give it our all—not with an eye on the finish line so much as on the experi-

Nothing happens next. This is it.

ence of putting one foot in front of the next with all the effort we can muster.

Or, closer to the moment, as I write this book I try to craft these words well—with an eye not on how they will be judged but on how clearly they will communicate. It means putting full energy into doing what we're doing, being focused on the process rather than on the fantasy of arriving somewhere.

A Path to Well-Being

Besides being extremely useful for dealing with everyday difficulties, mindfulness practice is part of a path toward a particular sort of happiness. This happiness isn't dependent on pleasurable sensations (though we enjoy these more when they occur), and it certainly isn't based on "success" in the conventional sense. It is the more fulfilling happiness that comes from waking up.

Modern scientific research is lining up nicely with ancient wisdom to point the way to a rich and meaningful life. It is reinforcing what mindfulness practice has long revealed: savoring our experience, appreciating and embracing our place in the amazing ever-changing world, sensing our interconnection with other people, animals, and the rest of nature, and engaging our talents fully for the good of all fosters a kind of happiness that isn't dependent on fickle fortunes.

This happiness isn't the opposite of sadness, nor does it involve being free from pain. It includes feeling the full range of our human emotions while empathizing with everyone else's. It involves experiencing everything vividly, with an ease that comes from letting go of expectations, preconceptions, and worries about our particular welfare. This happiness comes from knowing that everything will change and therefore not being so shocked when it does. And it comes from really embracing *this moment*, rather than from pursuing something different in the next.

Combined with our efforts to act wisely, mindfulness practice can transform our experience of ourselves and our view of the world. It can allow us to awaken to our full potential, be more useful to others, and more completely enjoy the moments that we have together here on this planet.

It takes effort. But after all, what else is more worthwhile?

When you need more help

How to find a therapist

If worry, anxiety, depression, stress-related medical problems, unhealthy habits, or relationship troubles are making you unhappy or interfering with your ability to function, and mindfulness practices alone don't seem to be enough, consulting with a mental health professional may be a good idea. This is especially wise if the consequence of your emotional distress is likely to bring on even more emotional distress—failing at work or school because of anxiety, withdrawing from friends because of depression, losing relationships because of frequent conflicts, or damaging your health because of destructive habits.

Seeking professional help doesn't necessarily mean signing up for a long, intensive round of psychotherapy or committing to taking medications. Rather, it can be an opportunity to take a fresh look at your experience and learn about different options for working with it.

The biggest challenge is often figuring out whom to see. Usually it makes sense to choose a licensed mental health professional, since he or she should have broad knowledge about the causes of psychological distress and its treatment. Unlike seeking help for strep throat or a broken bone, however, emotional difficulties rarely have one root and therefore rarely have just one remedy. So the background and orientation of the professional you consult will likely color his or her understanding of your problem and approach to working with you.

The most important factor in getting a positive outcome is being able to trust a therapist. If possible, get a referral from a trusted friend or family member, medical doctor, or a psychotherapist you know personally. Otherwise, you can contact the referral service of your state's psychiatric, psychological, or social work association or the outpatient mental health services at your local hospital, medical center, or community mental health clinic (several referral services are listed in the Resources on page 337). If you have questions or doubts during a first meeting, try to raise them—the way the conversation unfolds will tell you a lot about how comfortable you will be working with a particular therapist.

At the present time, only some mental health professionals have a good understanding of mindfulness practice. You should feel free to ask directly if a therapist has experience in this area. While not essential, it will help the therapist guide you in using mindfulness practice along with other approaches to working with your difficulties.

There are various forms of psychotherapy, several of which were discussed earlier, which incorporate mindfulness practice. You may come across mindfulness-oriented therapists who are familiar with them. All of these approach problems in ways that are consistent with those we've been exploring:

- *Acceptance and commitment therapy* (ACT) was developed by Steven Hayes and his colleagues at the University of Nevada. It usually takes the form of individual therapy and has been shown to be helpful for a very wide range of difficulties. For more information, see *www.contextualpsychology.org/act*.

- *Dialectical behavior therapy* (DBT) was developed by Marsha Linehan and her colleagues at the University of Washington. It usually takes the form of weekly group and individual therapy and has been shown to be particularly effective for people who are readily overwhelmed by their emotions. For more information, see *www.behavioraltech.org*.

- *Mindfulness-based cognitive therapy* (MBCT) (Chapter 6) was developed in Canada by Zindel Segal and in Great Britain by Mark Williams and John Teasdale to work with recurrent depression, though it has been used successfully with anxiety and other problems as well. It usually takes the form of eight weekly group therapy sessions with daily homework. For more information, see *www.mbct.com*.

- *Mindfulness-based eating awareness training* (MB-EAT) (Chapter 9) was developed by Jeanne Kristeller and colleagues at Indiana State University to work with binge eating and other eating disorders. It usually takes the form of a 10-week course with accompanying homework. For more information, see *www.tcme.org*.

- *Mindfulness-based relapse prevention* (MBRP) (Chapter 9) was developed by Alan Marlatt and his colleagues at the University of Washington to help prevent relapses of substance abuse. It usually takes the form of eight weekly group therapy sessions with daily homework. For more information, see *www.depts.washington.edu/abrc/mbrp*.

- *Mindfulness-based stress reduction* (MBSR) (Chapter 3) was started by Jon Kabat-Zinn at the University of Massachusetts Medical Center. While not a form of psychotherapy, some psychotherapists lead MBSR groups for stress reduction. It is usually presented as an eight-week course with daily mindfulness practice assignments. For more information, see *www.umassmed.edu/cfm*.

Selecting a mental health professional can be particularly confusing because practitioners come from a variety of academic disciplines, each with its own strengths. Psychiatrists are medical doctors (MDs or DOs) specializing in psychiatric disorders who generally prescribe medications and may also provide psychotherapy, while psychiatric clinical nurse specialists (CNSs) provide similar services and often work closely with psychiatrists. Psychologists have doctoral degrees in psychology (PhD, PsyD, or EdD), and generally provide psychotherapy. They may also do psychological testing or, in a few jurisdictions, prescribe medication. Psychologists have led the development and study of mindfulness-based treatments. Clinical social workers have master's degrees in social work (MSW) and also provide psychotherapy. Their training typically includes a focus on the role of the family or wider community in emotional difficulties. Many states also license a variety of other master's-level counselors (MA or MEd) with various areas of specialization.

A well-trained mental health professional from any discipline should be able to help you understand what is causing your distress and suggest ways to resolve it. In addition to inquiring about a professional's experience with mindfulness practice or familiarity with the treatment approaches mentioned above, you might want to ask about his or her overall training and experience, areas of specialization, and general approach to treatment, as well as fees, coverage by your health insurance, office hours, and availability.

Resources

MINDFULNESS PRACTICE CENTERS

While it is certainly possible to practice mindfulness on your own, the support of a community can be a great help. Meditating with other people, receiving guidance from a teacher, and having opportunities to participate in silent retreats can all deepen your practice.

While mindfulness practices have developed in many different cultures, they've been most refined in Buddhist traditions. Most centers that teach mindfulness meditation in the West are associated with one of three broad schools of Buddhist practice:

- *Vipassana*, or insight meditation centers teach a form of meditation very similar to what is described in this book. Instructions are usually laid out in a step-by-step fashion. Most of these centers have a Western cultural atmosphere. This is a form of practice most often seen in Southeast Asia.
- *Zen* centers also teach mindfulness practice. Some provide step-by-step instructions similar to those in this book, while others suggest forms of meditation practice such as *just sitting*, which doesn't focus on a particular object of attention, or *koan* practice, which asks students to solve a riddle that has no logical answer (this helps interrupt discursive thinking). Their atmosphere may reflect their origins in Japanese, Korean, Chinese, or Vietnamese culture.
- *Tibetan Buddhist* centers teach mindfulness practice along with other forms of meditation that may involve visualization of images, recitation of mantras, tonglen practice, or prostrations (bowing). Their atmosphere often reflects their origin in Tibetan culture.

The listings below include well-known centers from these three traditions as well as several non-Buddhist organizations.

United States

Mindfulness-Based Stress Reduction

Center for Mindfulness in Medicine, Health Care, and Society
55 Lake Avenue North
Worcester, MA 01655
www.umassmed.edu/cfm

Vipassana (Insight Meditation) Tradition

Barre Center for Buddhist Studies
149 Lockwood Road
Barre, MA 01005
www.dharma.org/bcbs

Bhavana Society
Route 1, Box 218-3
High View, WV 26808
www.bhavanasociety.org

Cambridge Insight Meditation
  Center
331 Broadway
Cambridge, MA 02139
www.cimc.info

InsightLA
2633 Lincoln Boulevard, #206
Santa Monica, CA 90405-2005
www.insightla.org

Insight Meditation Community of
  Washington
PO Box 212
Garrett Park, MD 20896
www.imcw.org

Insight Meditation Society
1230 Pleasant Street
Barre, MA 01005
www.dharma.org

Metta Forest Monastery
PO Box 1419
Valley Center, CA 92082
www.watmetta.org

Mid America Dharma
455 East 80th Terrace
Kansas City, MO 64131
www.midamericadharma.org

New York Insight Meditation Center
28 West 27th Street, 10th floor
New York, NY 10001
www.nyimc.org

Spirit Rock Meditation Center
PO Box 909
Woodacre, CA 94973
www.spiritrock.org

Zen Tradition

Blue Cliff Monastery
3 Mindfulness Road
Pine Bush, NY 12566
www.bluecliffmonastery.org

Boundless Way Zen
297 Lowell Avenue
Newton, MA 02460-1826
www.boundlesswayzen.org

Deer Park Monastery
2499 Melru Lane
Escondido, CA 92026
www.deerparkmonastery.org

Upaya Zen Center
1404 Cerro Gordo Road
Santa Fe, NM 87501
www.upaya.org

Village Zendo
588 Broadway, Suite 1108
New York, NY 10012-5238
www.villagezendo.org

San Francisco Zen Center
300 Page Street
San Francisco, CA 94102
www.sfzc.org

Zen Center of San Diego
2047 Feldspar Street
San Diego, CA 92109-3551
www.zencentersandiego.org

Zen Mountain Monastery
PO Box 197
Mt. Tremper, NY 12457
www.mro.org/zmm

Tibetan Buddhist Tradition

Dzogchen Foundation
www.dzogchen.org

Naropa University
2130 Arapahoe Avenue
Boulder, CO 80302
www.naropa.edu

Shambhala Mountain Center
4921 Country Road 68C
Red Feather Lakes, CO 80545
www.shambhalamountain.org

Tenzin Gyatso Institute
PO Box 239
Berne, NY 12023
www.tenzingyatsoinstitute.org

Listing of additional Buddhist meditation centers and communities:
www.dharma.org/ims/mr_links.html

Jewish Traditions

(These vary somewhat in their degree of emphasis on mindfulness practice.)

Institute for Jewish Spirituality
330 Seventh Avenue, Suite 1902
New York, NY 10001
www.ijs-online.org

Awakened Heart Project for
   Contemplative Judaism
www.awakenedheartproject.org

Isabella Freedman Jewish Retreat
   Center
116 Johnson Road
Falls Village, CT 06031
www.isabellafreedman.org

Nishmat Hayyim
Jewish Meditation Collaborative of
   New England
1566 Beacon Street
Brookline, MA 02446
www.nishmathayyim.org

Christian Traditions (Contemplative or Centering Prayer)

Listing of programs throughout the United States and the world:

Contemplative Outreach
10 Park Place, 2nd Floor, Suite B
Butler, NJ 07405
www.contemplativeoutreach.org

Canada

Gampo Abbey
Pleasant Bay, Cape Breton
Nova Scotia, BOE 2PO
Canada
www.gampoabbey.org

Listing of other Canadian meditation centers: *www.gosit.org/Canada.htm*

Europe

Mindfulfness-Based Stress Reduction and Mindfulness-Based Cognitive Therapy

Centre for Mindfulness Research and Practice
Institute for Medical and Social Care Research
University of Wales
Bangor, LL57 1UT
UK
www.bangor.ac.uk/mindfulness

Vipassana (Insight Meditation) Tradition

Meditationszentrum Beatenberg
Waldegg
CH-3803 Beatenberg
Switzerland
www.karuna.ch

Gaia House
West Ogwell, Newton Abbot
Devon, TQ12 6EN
UK
www.gaiahouse.co.uk

Kalyana Centre
Glenahoe Castlegregory
Co Kerry
Ireland
www.kalyanacentre.com

Seminarhaus Engl
Engl 1
84339 Unterdietfurt
Bavaria
Germany
www.seminarhaus-engl.de

Listing of other European Vipassana centers: *www.mahasi.eu/mahasi/index.jsp*

Zen Tradition

Plum Village Practice Center
13 Martineau
33580 Dieulivol
France
www.plumvillage.org

Tibetan Buddhist Tradition

Shambhala Europe
Kartäuserwall 20
50678 Köln
Germany
www.shambhala-europe.org

For Shambhala centers worldwide: *www.shambhala.org/centers*

Sanctuary of Enlightened Action
Lerab Ling
34650 Roquerdonde
France
www.lerabling.org (See *www.rigpa.org* for related centers)

Australia and New Zealand

Vipassana (Insight Meditation) Tradition

Santi Forest Monastery	Bodhinyanarama Monastery
Lot 6 Coalmines Road	17 Rakau Grove, Stokes Valley
Bundanoon, NSW, 2578	Lower Hutt 5019
Australia	New Zealand
santifm1.0.googlepages.com	*www.bodhinyanarama.net.nz*

Listings of other Australian insight meditation centers:
www.bswa.org and *www.dharma.org.au*

Listing of other New Zealand insight meditation centers:
www.insightmeditation.org.nz

Zen Tradition

Listing of Zen centers in Australia:
iriz.hanazono.ac.jp/zen_centers/centers_data/australi.htm

Listing of Zen centers in New Zealand:
iriz.hanazono.ac.jp/zen_centers/centers_data/newzeal.htm

Tibetan Buddhist Tradition

Shambhala Meditation Centre Auckland
35 Scarborough Terrace
Auckland, New Zealand
www.auckland.shambhala.info

Worldwide

Listing of Buddhist meditation centers worldwide: *www.buddhanet.info/wbd*

RECORDINGS OF MINDFULNESS PRACTICE
INSTRUCTIONS AND RELATED TEACHINGS

Recordings of practices in this book and updates of resources:
www.mindfulness-solution.com

Free downloads of talks from insight meditation retreats: *www.dharmaseed.org*

Recordings from mindfulness meditation teachers: *www.soundstrue.com*

Recordings and Teaching Schedules of Selected Meditation Teachers

Mindfulness-Based Stress Reduction

Jon Kabat-Zinn: *www.umassmed.edu/cfm*, *www.mindfulnesscds.com*

Vipassansa (Insight Meditation) Tradition

Tara Brach: *www.imcw.org/tara-brach*
Jack Kornfield: *www.jackkornfield.com*
Sharon Salzberg: *www.sharonsalzberg.com*

Zen Tradition

Thich Nhat Hanh: *www.iamhome.org*, *www.plumvillage.org*

Tibetan Buddhist Tradition

Pema Chödrön: *www.shambhala.org/teachers/pema/*
Dalai Lama: *www.dalailama.com*
Lama Surya Das: *www.dzogchen.org*

Christian Tradition (Contemplative or Centering Prayer)

Father William Menninger: *www.contemplativeprayer.net*

FURTHER READING

General Mindfulness Practice

Mindfulness-Based Stress Reduction

Kabat-Zinn, J. (1994). *Wherever you go there you are: Mindfulness meditation in everyday life*. New York: Hyperion.
Kabat-Zinn, J. (2005). *Coming to our senses: Healing ourselves and the world through mindfulness*. New York: Hyperion.

Vipassansa (Insight Meditation) Tradition

Goldstein, J. (1993). *Insight meditation: The practice of freedom*. Boston: Shambhala.

Goldstein, J., & Kornfield, J. (1987). *Seeking the heart of wisdom: The path of insight meditation*. Boston: Shambhala.

Gunaratana, B. (2002). *Mindfulness in plain English*. Somerville, MA: Wisdom.

Kornfield, J. (1993). *A path with heart: A guide through the perils and promises of spiritual life*. New York: Bantam.

Kornfield, J. (2008). *The wise heart: A guide to the universal teachings of Buddhist psychology*. New York: Bantam Dell.

Rosenberg, L. (1998). *Breath by breath: The liberating practice of insight meditation*. Boston: Shambhala.

Zen Tradition

Beck, C, (1989). *Everyday zen: Love and work*. San Francisco: HarperSanFrancisco.

Hanh, T. N. (1976). *The miracle of mindfulness*. Boston: Beacon Press.

Magid, B. (2008). *Ending the pursuit of happiness: A Zen guide*. Somerville, MA: Wisdom.

Weiss, A. (2004). *Beginning mindfulness: Learning the way of awareness*. Novato, CA: New World Library.

Tibetan Buddhist Tradition

Lama Surya Das. (1997). *Awakening the Buddha within: Tibetan wisdom for the Western world*. New York: Broadway.

Trungpa, C. (2004). *Meditation in action (Shambhala Library)*. Boston: Shambhala.

Christian Tradition (Contemplative or Centering Prayer)

Keating, T. (2006). *Open mind, open heart: The contemplative dimension of the Gospel*. New York: Continuum International Group.

Pennington, M. B. (1982). *Centering prayer: Renewing an ancient Christian prayer form*. Garden City, NY: Image Books.

Jewish Tradition

Lew, A. (2005) *Be still and get going: A Jewish meditation practice for real life*. Boston: Little, Brown.

Islamic (Sufi) Tradition

Helminski, K. E. (1992). *Living presence: A Sufi way to mindfulness and the essential self*. New York: Jeremy P. Tarcher/Perigee Books.

Loving-Kindness Practice

Chodron, P. (2001). *The wisdom of no escape and the path of loving-kindness.* Boston: Shambhala.

Dalai Lama. (2001). *An open heart: Practicing compassion in everyday life.* Boston: Little Brown.

Salzberg, S. (1995). *Lovingkindness: The revolutionary art of happiness.* Boston: Shambhala.

Self-Compassion Practice

Brach, T. (2003). *Radical acceptance: Embracing your life with the heart of a Buddha.* New York: Bantam Dell.

Germer, C. K. (2009). *The mindful path to self-compassion: Freeing yourself from destructive thoughts and emotions.* New York: Guilford Press.

Mindfulness for Family and Other Relationships

Kabat-Zinn, M., & Kabat-Zinn, J. (1998). *Everyday blessings: The inner work of mindful parenting.* New York: Hyperion.

Kramer, G. (2007). *Insight dialogue: The interpersonal path to freedom.* Boston: Shambhala.

Napthali, S. (2003), *Buddhism for mothers: A calm approach to caring for yourself and your children.* Crows Nest, Australia: Allen & Unwin.

Walser, R., & Westrup, D. (2008). *The mindful couple: How acceptance and mindfulness can lead you to the love you want.* Oakland, CA: New Harbinger Press.

Mindfulness Practices for Specific Difficulties

Anger

Bankart, C. P. (2006). *Freeing the angry mind: How men can use mindfulness and reason to save their lives and relationships.* Oakland, CA: New Harbinger Press.

Eifert, G., Mckay, M., & Forsyth, J. (2006). *ACT on life not on anger: The new acceptance and commitment therapy guide to problem anger.* Oakland, CA: New Harbinger Press.

Anxiety

Brantley, J. (2003). *Calming your anxious mind.* Oakland, CA: New Harbinger Press.

Forsyth, J., & Eifert, G. (2007). *The mindfulness and acceptance workbook for anxiety.* Oakland, CA: New Harbinger Press.

Lejeune, C. (2007). *The worry trap.* Oakland, CA: New Harbinger Press.

Depression

Martin, J. (1999). *The Zen path through depression.* New York: HarperCollins.

McQuaid, J., & Carmona, P. (2004). *Peaceful mind: Using mindfulness and cognitive behavioral psychology to overcome depression.* Oakland, CA: New Harbinger Press.

Williams, M., Teasdale, J., Segal, Z., & Kabat-Zinn, J. (2007). *The mindful way through depression.* New York: Guilford Press.

Chronic Pain and Stress-Related Medical Conditions

Dahl, J., Wilson, K., Luciano, C., & Hayes, S. (2005). *Acceptance and commitment therapy for chronic pain.* Oakland, CA: New Harbinger Press.

Kabat-Zinn, J. (1990). *Full catastrophe living: Using the wisdom of your body and mind to face stress, pain, and illness.* New York: Dell.

Siegel, R. D., Urdang, M., & Johnson, D. (2001). *Back sense: A revolutionary approach to halting the cycle of back pain.* New York: Broadway. (For an introduction and worksheets, visit *www.backsense.org*)

Eating Problems

Albers, S. (2009). *Eat, drink and be mindful: How to end your struggle with mindless eating and start savoring food with intention and joy.* Oakland, CA: New Harbinger Press.

Bays, J. C. (2009). *Mindful eating: A guide to rediscovering a healthy and joyful relationship with food.* Boston: Shambhala.

Heffner, M., & Eifert, G. (2008). *The anorexia workbook: How to reclaim yourself, heal your suffering and reclaim your life.* Oakland, CA: New Harbinger Press.

Somov, P. G. (2008). *Eating the moment: 141 mindful practices to overcome overeating one meal at a time.* Oakland, CA: New Harbinger Press.

Substance Abuse Problems

Alexander, W. (1997). *Cool water: Alcoholism, mindfulness and ordinary recovery.* Boston: Shambhala.

Bien, T., & Bien, B. (2002). *Mindful recovery: A spiritual path to healing from addiction.* New York: Wiley.

Death and Dying

Halifax, J. (2008). *Being with dying: Cultivating compassion and fearlessness in the presence of death.* Boston: Shambhala.

Kumar, S. (2005). *Grieving mindfully: A compassionate and spiritual guide to coping with loss.* Oakland, CA: New Harbinger Press.

Rosenberg, L. (2000). *Living in the light of death: On the art of being truly alive.* Boston: Shambhala.

Understanding Concentration, Mindfulness, and Other Meditative Practices

Goleman, D. D., & Ram Dass. (1989). *The meditative mind: The varieties of meditative experience.* New York: HarperCollins.

Effects of Mindfulness Practice on the Brain

Begley, S. (2007). *Train your mind, change your brain.* New York: Ballantine.
Siegel, D. (2007). *The mindful brain: Reflection and attunement in the cultivation of well-being.* New York: Norton.

PSYCHOLOGICAL DISORDERS, TREATMENT OPTIONS, AND THERAPIST LISTINGS

The National Institute of Mental Health maintains a comprehensive website with descriptions of psychological disorders, treatment options, and hospital and clinic treatment resources: *www.nimh.nih.gov/health/topics/index.shtml*

If you are unable to find a mental health professional through personal contacts, your own medical doctor, or another source, website listings are also available:

Psychiatrists (choose "Psychiatry" from list):
webapps.ama-assn.org/doctorfinder/home.jsp
Psychologists: *www.findapsychologist.org* or *locator.apa.org*
Clinical social workers: *www.helppro.com/nasw*

Many commercial sites listing therapists can be found by entering "find a therapist" into a search engine. Please be aware these listings typically include individuals who are not licensed as mental health professionals.

FINDING LOCAL TWELVE-STEP PROGRAMS FOR ADDICTIONS

Alcoholics Anonymous: *www.aa.org*
Narcotics Anonymous: *www.na.org*
Gamblers Anonymous: *www.gamblersanonymous.org*

YOGA AS MINDFULNESS PRACTICE

Yoga can be an excellent form of mindfulness practice, particularly for times when the mind is restless or agitated. It is easiest to use yoga as a mindfulness practice if the poses are done slowly and meditatively. Simply bring your attention to the body sensations that arise during a pose and try to remain aware as you move from pose to pose. When the mind wanders, gently bring it back to the sensations in the body.

While it's easiest to study yoga in a class, it is possible to learn the basics using instructions from a book, DVD, or website. You might start with these resources:

Introductory Yoga Books

Ansari, M. (1999). *Yoga for beginners.* New York: Harper Perennial.

Boccio, F. (2004). *Mindfulness yoga: The awakened union of breath, body and mind.* Somerville, MA: Wisdom.

Farhi, D. (2000). *Yoga mind, body and spirit: A return to wholeness.* New York: Holt.

Kirk, M. (2006). *Hatha yoga illustrated.* Champaign, IL: Human Kinetics.

Schiffmann, E. (1996). *Yoga: The spirit and practice of moving into stillness.* New York: Pocket.

Websites Illustrating Yoga Postures

Free streaming videos of yoga practice: *www.yogatoday.com*
Clear, animated drawings of yoga postures:
   www.abc-of-yoga.com/yogapractice/postures.asp
Photographs and descriptions of yoga postures:
   www.yogabasics.com/yoga-postures.html

Introductory Yoga DVDs

Benagh, B. (2006). *Yoga for beginners.* Bethesda, MD: Bodywisdom Media.

Gormley, J. J. (2002). *Yoga for every body (with over 35 routines).* Bethesda, MD: Bodywisdom Media.

Rice, J., & Wohl, M. (2002). *Yoga for inflexible people.* Bethesda, MD: Bodywisdom Media.

Yee, R., & Saidman, C. (2009). *Yoga for beginners.* Boulder, CO: Gaiam.

RESOURCES FOR PSYCHOTHERAPISTS

Selected Readings on Mindfulness and Psychotherapy

Integrative

Didonna, F. (2008). *Clinical handbook of mindfulness.* London: Springer.

Germer, C., Siegel, R., & Fulton, P. (Eds.). (2005). *Mindfulness and psychotherapy.* New York: Guilford Press.

Hick, S., & Bien, T. (2008). *Mindfulness and the therapeutic relationship.* New York: Guilford Press.

Cognitive-Behavioral

Baer, R. (Ed.). (2006). *Mindfulness-based treatment approaches: Clinician's guide to evidence base and applications.* Burlington, MA: Academic Press.

Hayes, S., Follette, V., & Linehan, M. (Eds.). (2004). *Mindfulness and acceptance: Expanding the cognitive-behavioral tradition.* New York: Guilford Press.

Hayes, S., & Strosahl, K. (2005). *A practical guide to acceptance and commitment therapy.* New York: Springer.

Linehan, M. M. (1993). *Skills training manual for treating borderline personality disorder.* New York: Guilford Press.

Roemer, L., & Orsillo, S. (2008). *Mindfulness- and acceptance-based behavioral therapies in practice.* New York: Guilford Press.

Segal, Z., Williams, J., & Teasdale, J. (2002). *Mindfulness-based cognitive therapy for depression: A new approach to preventing relapse.* New York: Guilford Press.

Psychodynamic

Epstein, M. (1995). *Thoughts without a thinker.* New York: Basic Books.

Magid, B. (2002). *Ordinary mind: Exploring the common ground of Zen and psychotherapy.* Somerville, MA: Wisdom.

Rubin, J. (1996). *Psychotherapy and Buddhism.* New York: Plenum Press.

Safran, J. (Ed.). (2003). *Psychoanalysis and Buddhism.* Boston: Wisdom.

Young-Eisendrath, P., & Muramoto, S. (2002). *Awakening and insight: Zen Buddhism and psychotherapy.* New York: Taylor & Francis.

Selected Internet Resources on Mindfulness and Psychotherapy

The Institute for Meditation and Psychotherapy:
   www.meditationandpsychotherapy.org
Acceptance and Commitment Therapy: *www.contextualpsychology.org/act*
Dialectical Behavior Therapy: *www.behavioraltech.org*
Mindfulness-Based Cognitive Therapy: *www.mbct.com*
Mindfulness-Based Relapse Prevention: *www.depts.washington.edu/abrc/mbrp*
Mindfulness-Based Eating Awareness Training: *www.tcme.org*
The Back Sense program for treating chronic pain: *www.backsense.org*
Archives of the mindfulness and acceptance listserv of the Association for the Advancement of Behavior Therapy:
   www.listserv.kent.edu/archives/mindfulness.html

Notes

CHAPTER 1. LIFE IS DIFFICULT, *FOR EVERYONE*

Page 7   Judith Viorst's book *Necessary Losses* points out that *most* of what makes us unhappy involves difficulty dealing with the inevitability of change:

Viorst, J. (1998). *Necessary losses: The loves, illusions, dependencies, and impossible expectations that all of us have to give up in order to grow.* New York: Free Press.

Page 22   According to Dr. Nancy Etcoff, we seem to have evolved to notice and remember negative experiences more vividly than positive ones:

Lambert, C. (2007, January–February). The science of happiness: Psychology explores humans at their best. *Harvard Magazine, 109*(3), 26.

CHAPTER 2. MINDFULNESS: A SOLUTION

Page 34   Dr. Richard Davidson found that a Tibetan monk with many years of experience in mindfulness (and other) meditation practices showed more dramatic shifts toward left prefrontal activation than other subjects:

Goleman, D. (2003, February 4). Finding happiness: Cajole your brain to lean to the left. *The New York Times,* p. F5.

Page 35   After taking an eight-week mindfulness meditation course, meditating biotechnology workers had more left-sided activation, reported more improved moods, and felt more engaged in their activities than nonmeditators:

Davidson, R. J., Kabat-Zinn, J., Schumacher, J., Rosenkranz, M., Muller, D., Santorelli, S., et al. (2003). Alterations in brain and immune function produced by mindfulness meditation. *Psychosomatic Medicine, 65*(4), 564–570.

Page 36   Dr. Sara Lazar found that meditators with an average of nine years of meditation experience averaging six hours of practice per week had thicker cerebral cortexes in three areas compared to nonmeditators: the anterior insula, sensory cortex, and prefrontal cortex:

Lazar, S. W., Kerr, C., Wasserman, R. J., Gray, J. R., Greve, D., Treadway, M. T., et al. (2005). Meditation experience is associated with increased cortical thickness. *NeuroReport, 16*(17), 1893–1897.

Page 36   **Studies have shown less loss of gray matter with age among meditators, which corresponded to less loss in their ability to sustain attention—an important component of many mental tasks—compared with nonmeditating controls:**

Pagoni, G., & Cekic, M. (2007). Age effects on gray matter volume and attentional performance in Zen meditation. *Neurobiology of Aging, 28* (10), 1623–1627.

Page 36   **Dr. Lazar also found measurable changes in a part of the brain stem involved in the production of serotonin, a mood-regulating transmitter:**

Lazar, S. (2009, June 11). Personal communication.

Page 38   **Most of our psychological suffering stems from our attempts to avoid psychological suffering:**

Hayes, S. C., Wilson, K. G., Gifford, E. V., Follette, V. M., & Strosahl, K. (1996). *Journal of Consulting and Clinical Psychology, 64*(6), 1152–1168.

Page 39   **The U.S. Bureau of Labor Statistics collects data not only on what we do at work but also on what we do in our leisure time:**

U.S. Bureau of Labor Statistics. (2009). *Time spent in primary activities and percent of the civilian population engaging in each activity, averages per day by sex, 2007 annual averages.* Retrieved June 11, 2009, from United States Department of Labor, Bureau of Labor Statistics: *www.bls.gov/news.release/atus.t01.htm.*

CHAPTER 4. BUILDING A MINDFUL LIFE

Page 99   **As the writer Anne Lamott famously quipped, "My mind is a bad neighborhood I try not to go into alone":**

Lamott, A. (1997, March 13). Word by word: My mind is a bad neighborhood I try not to go into alone. Retrieved June 11, 2009, from *Salon: www.salon.com/march97/columnists/lamott970313.html.*

CHAPTER 5. BEFRIENDING FEAR: WORKING WITH WORRY AND ANXIETY

Page 118   **Why do I dwell always expecting fear and dread?**

Nanamoli, B. (Trans.), & Bodhi, B. (Ed.). (1995). Bhayabherava Sutta: Fear and dread. *The middle length discourses of the Buddha* (p. 104). Boston: Wisdom.

Page 129   **Mountain meditation:**

For an alternate version, see: Kabat-Zinn, J. (1994). *Wherever you go there you are: Mindfulness meditation in everyday life.* New York: Hyperion.

CHAPTER 6. ENTERING THE DARK PLACES: SEEING SADNESS AND DEPRESSION IN A NEW LIGHT

Page 150   **Divers who were shown lists of words both under water and on the beach were best able to recall words in the environment in which they were first learned:**

Baddeley, A. D. (1980). When does context influence recognition memory? *British Journal of Psychology, 71,* 99–104.

Page 152   **For people who had had three or more depressive episodes in the past, the chances of relapsing over the course of a year were cut in half by participating in at least four sessions of mindfulness-based cognitive therapy (MBCT):**

Ma, S., & Teasdale, J. (2004). Mindfulness-based cognitive therapy for depression: Replication and exploration of differential relapse prevention effects. *Journal of Consulting and Clinical Psychology, 72*(1), 31–40.

Teasdale, J., Segal, Z., Williams, J., Ridgeway, V., Soulsby, J., & Lau, M. A. (2000). Prevention of relapse/recurrence in major depression by mindfulness-based cognitive therapy. *Journal of Consulting and Clinical Psychology, 68*(4), 615–623.

Page 152   **MBCT was shown to be as effective as antidepressants in preventing relapses of depression and allowed many subjects to discontinue their medication:**

Kuyken, W., Byford, S., Taylor, R. S., Watkins, E., Holden, E., White, K., et al. (2008). Mindfulness-based cognitive therapy to prevent relapse in recurrent depression. *Journal of Consulting and Clinical Psychology, 76*(6), 966–978.

Page 152   **Our life is like a silent film on which we each write our own commentary.**

Williams, M., Teasdale, J., Segal, Z., & Kabat-Zinn, J. (2007). *The mindful way through depression: Freeing yourself from chronic unhappiness* (p. 21). New York: Guilford Press.

Page 156   **Some cognitive scientists have long speculated that what we call "thinking" is actually a relatively new human acquisition:**

Jaynes, J. (1976). *The origin of consciousness in the breakdown of the bicameral mind.* Boston: Houghton Mifflin.

Page 157   **The Mindful Path to Self-Compassion:**

Germer, C. K. (2009). *The mindful path to self-compassion: Freeing yourself from destructive thoughts and emotions.* New York: Guilford Press.

Page 175   **Meditators taking antidepressant medication felt that it supported their meditation practice, making it easier not to get completely caught in self-critical thought streams:**

Bitner, R., Hillman, L., Victor, B., & Walsh, R. (2003). Subjective effects of antidepressants: A pilot study of the varieties of antidepressant-induced experiences in meditators. *Journal of Nervous and Mental Disease, 191*(10), 660–667.

Page 175   **The Mindful Way through Depression:**

Williams, M., Teasdale, J., Segal, Z., & Kabat-Zinn, J. (2007). *The mindful way through depression: Freeing yourself from chronic unhappiness.* New York: Guilford Press.

CHAPTER 7. BEYOND MANAGING SYMPTOMS: TRANSFORMING PAIN AND STRESS-RELATED MEDICAL PROBLEMS

Page 177   **Some 60–90% of all physician visits are for stress-related disorders:**

Sweet, J. J., Rozensky, R. H., & Tovian, S. M. (1991). *Handbook of clinical psychology in medical settings* (p. 114). New York: Springer.

Page 181   Approximately two-thirds of people who have never suffered serious back
            pain have the same sorts of "abnormal" back structures, like herniated
            disks, that are often blamed for chronic back pain:

            Jensen, M., BrantZawadzki, M., Obucowski, N., Modic, M., Malkasian, D.,
            & Ross, J. (1994). Magnetic resonance imaging of the lumbar spine in people
            without back pain. *New England Journal of Medicine, 331*(2), 69–73.

Page 181   Millions of people who suffer chronic back pain show no "abnormalities" in
            their backs whatsoever, even after extensive testing:

            Frymore, J. W. (2008). Back pain and sciatica. *New England Journal of Medi-
            cine, 318*(5), 291–300.

Page 181   There is little relation between the mechanical success of repairs and
            whether the patient is still in pain:

            Tullberg, T., Grane, P., & Isacson, J. (1994). Gadolinium enhanced magnetic
            resonance imaging of 36 patients one year after lumbar disc resection. *Spine,
            19*(2), 176–182.

            Fraser, R., Sandhu, A., & Gogan, W. (1995). Magnetic resonance imaging
            findings 10 years after treatment for lumbar disc herniation. *Spine, 20*(6),
            710–714.

Page 181   The worldwide epidemic of chronic back pain is limited mostly to industri-
            alized nations:

            Volinn, E. (1997). The epidemiology of low back pain in the rest of the world. A
            review of surveys in low middle-income countries. *Spine, 22*(15), 1747–1754.

Page 181   Psychological stress, and particularly job dissatisfaction, predicts who will
            develop disabling back pain more reliably than do physical measures or the
            physical demands of one's job:

            Bigos S., Battie, M., Spengler., Fisher, L., Fordyce, W., Hansson, T., Nach-
            emson, & Wortley, M. (1991). A prospective study of work perceptions and
            psychosocial factors affecting the report of back injury. *Spine, 16*(1), 1–6.

Page 181   Rapidly returning to full, vigorous, physical activity is usually both safe and
            the most effective way to resolve back pain episodes:

            Hanney, W. J., Kolber, M. J., Beekhuizen, K. S. (2009). Implications for physi-
            cal activity in the population with low back pain. *American Journal of Life-
            style Medicine, 3*, 63–70.

            Rainville, J., Hartigan, C., Martinez, E., Limke, J., Jouve, C., & Finno, M.
            (2004). Exercise as a treatment for chronic low back pain. *Spine, 4*(1), 106–
            115.

Page 182   Self-treatment guide *Back Sense*:

            Siegel, R. D., Urdang, M. H,. & Johnson, D. R. (2001). *Back sense: A revolu-
            tionary approach to halting the cycle of chronic back pain.* New York: Broad-
            way Books.

Page 182   Rare medical disorders, which include tumors, infections, injuries, and
            unusual structural abnormalities, are the cause of only about one in 200
            cases of chronic back pain:

            Bigos, S., Bowyer, O., Braen, G., et al. (1994) *Acute low back problems in
            adults: Clinical Practice Guideline No. 14* (AHCPR Publication No. 95-0642).

Rockville, MD: Agency for Health Care Policy and Research, Public Health Service, U.S. Department of Health and Human Services.

Deyo, R., Rainville, J., & Kent, D. (1992). What can the history and physical examination tell us about low back pain? *Journal of the American Medical Association, 268*(6), 760–765.

Page 184   ***The Two Arrows:***

Bhikku, T. (Trans.). (2004b). *Salllatha Sutta* [The Arrow]. In *Samyutta Nikaya XXXVI6*. Retrieved June 11, 2009 from *www.accesstoinsight.org/canon/sutta/samyutta/sn36-006.html#shot.*

Page 189   **"When a man sits with a pretty girl for an hour, it seems like a minute. But let him sit on a hot stove for a minute and it's longer than any hour. That's relativity."**

Mirsky, S (2002, September). Einstein's hot time. *Scientific American, 287*(3), 81.

Page 199   **To understand the role of stress and anxiety in digestive disorders:**

Salt, W. B., & Neimark, N. F. (2002). *Irritable bowel syndrome and the mind-bodyspirit connection: 7 steps for living a healthy life with a functional bowel disorder, Crohn's disease, or colitis.* Columbus, OH: Parkview.

Page 200   **William Masters and Virginia E. Johnson developed** *sensate focus***:**

Masters, W. H., & Johnson, V. E. (1970). *Human sexual inadequacy.* New York: Bantam Books.

Page 205   **Perhaps some of the restorative function of sleep is met by mindfulness meditation:**

Kaul, P., Passafiume, J., Sargent, C., & O'Hara, B. Meditation, sleep and performance (unpublished manuscript). Cited in Nagourney, E. (2006, October 24). Perfomance: Researchers test meditation's impact on alertness. *The New York Times*, F6.

CHAPTER 8. LIVING THE FULL CATASTROPHE: MINDFULNESS FOR ROMANCE, PARENTING, AND OTHER INTIMATE RELATIONSHIPS

Page 216   ***Tao Te Ching:***

Beck, S. (2009). *Wisdom Bible.* Retrieved May 27, 2009, from Literary Works of Sanderson Beck: *www.san.beck.org/Laotzu.html#1.*

Page 217   **Eating a tangerine:**

Hanh, T. N. (1991). *Old path, white clouds: Walking in the footsteps of the Buddha* (pp. 128–129). Berkeley, CA: Parallax Press.

Page 231   **When we feel close to friends and loved ones, we experience greater energy and vitality, a greater capacity to act, increased clarity, an enhanced sense of value or dignity, and both the desire and capacity for more connection:**

Stiver, I. P., & Miller, J. B. (1997). *The healing connection.* Boston: Beacon Press.

Page 236   **"In the beginner's mind there are many possibilities, but in the expert's there are few."**
Suzuki, S. (1973). *Zen mind, beginner's mind.* New York: John Weatherhill.

CHAPTER 9. BREAKING BAD HABITS: LEARNING TO MAKE GOOD CHOICES

Page 261   **Nearly two-thirds of Americans are overweight, and one-third fit the criteria for obesity:**
Center for Disease Control. (2009). *Prevalance of overweight and obesity among adults: United States, 2003–2004.* Retrieved May 27, 2009, from National Center for Health Statistics: *www.cdc.gov/nchs/products/pubs/pubd/hestats/overweight/overwght_adult_03.htm.*

Page 261   **One to four percent of young women suffer with anorexia, bulimia, or binge eating:**
Hudson, J. I., Hiripi, E., Pope, H. G., & Kessler, R. C. (2007). The prevalence and correlates of eating disorders in the national comorbidity survey replication. *Biological Psychiatry, 61,* 346–358.

Page 265   **Thought Parade:**
Based on:
Heffner, M., Sperry, J., Eifert, G. H., & Detweiler, M. (2002). Acceptance and commitment therapy in the treatment of an adolescent female with anorexia nervosa: A case example. *Cognitive and Behavioral Practice, 9,* 232–236.

Page 268   **Mindfulness-Based Eating Awareness Training (MB-EAT) developed by Jeanne Kristeller and colleagues:**
Kristeller, J., Baer, R., & Quillian-Wolever, R. (2006). Mindfulness-based approaches to eating disorders. In R. A. Baer (Ed.), *Mindfulness-based treatment approaches.* San Diego, CA: Elsevier.
See also *The Center for Mindful Eating, www.tcme.org*

Page 268   **Approximately 8% of Americans over age 12 reported using illegal drugs in the month before they were asked and 25% smoked cigarettes. Fifty percent of us drank during the past year, while 22% have had over five drinks in a single evening. Intoxicants clearly play a big role in many of our lives:**
Substance Abuse and Mental Health Services Administration. (2004). *Results from the 2003 National Survey on Drug Use and Health: National Findings* (Office of Applied Studies, NSDUH Series H–25, DHHS Publication No. SMA 04–3964). Rockville, MD: Author.

Page 268   **While the mechanism isn't clear, it appears that regularly drinking moderate amounts of alcohol (two drinks per day for men under age 65, one drink per day for men over 65 and all women) may help to prevent cardiovascular disease and other problems:**
Mayo Clinic Staff. (2009). *Alcohol use: Why moderation is key.* Retrieved May 22, 2009, from MayoClinic.com: *www.mayoclinic.com/health/alcohol/SC00024.*

Page 273   **Mindfulness-based relapse prevention (MBRP), developed by Alan Marlatt and his colleagues at the University of Washington, has been shown to help prevent relapses of substance abuse:**

Bowen, S. W., Chawla, N., Collins, S. E., Witkiewitz, K., Hsu, S., Grow, J. C., Clifasefi, S. L., Garner, M. D., Douglas, A., Larimer, M. E., & Marlatt, G. A. (in press). Mindfulness-based relapse prevention for substance use disorders: A pilot efficacy trial. *Substance Abuse*.

See also the Addictive Behaviors Research Center of the University of Washington, *www.depts.washington.edu/abrc/index.htm.*

Page 273   *Urge Surfing for Cravings*:

Based on:

Marlatt, G. A. (1985). Cognitive assessment and intervention procedures for relapse prevention. In G. A. Marlatt & J. R. Gordon (Eds.), *Relapse prevention: Maintenance strategies in the treatment of addictive behaviors* (p. 241). New York: Guilford Press.

CHAPTER 10. GROWING UP ISN'T EASY: CHANGING YOUR RELATIONSHIP WITH AGING, ILLNESS, AND DEATH

Page 283   **"One purpose of mindfulness practice is to enjoy our old age."**

Suzuki, S. (1973). *Zen mind, beginner's mind.* New York: John Weatherhill.

Page 286   **We have *happiness set points*:**

Lykken, D., & Tellegen, A. (1996). Happiness is a stochastic phenomenon. *Psychological Science, 7*(3), 186–189.

Page 287   **In one study, scientists found that on average people ages 20–24 were sad 3.4 days a month, while those ages 65–74 were sad only 2.3 days a month:**

Wallis, C. (2005, January 7). The new science of happiness. *Time, 165*(3), A2.

Page 288   *Five Subjects for Frequent Reflection:*

Bhikku, T. (2009). *Upajjhatthana Sutta: Subjects for contemplation* (Anguttara Nikaya 5.57). Retrieved May 27, 2009, from Access to Insight: *www.accesstoinsight.org/tipitaka/an/an05/an05.057.than.html.*

Page 289   **"It is wiser to contemplate the law of impermanence than to try to repeal it."**

Rosenberg, L. (2000). *Living in the light of death: On the art of being truly alive.* Boston: Shambhala.

Page 299   **"If you don't want to die, don't be born."**

Rosenberg, L. (2000). *Living in the light of death: On the art of being truly alive.* Boston: Shambhala.

Page 300   **In mid-1800s America, it was thought to be essential to think about death every day—not to be morbid, but to take *today* seriously:**

Faust, D. G. (2008). *This republic of suffering: Death and the American Civil War.* New York: Knopf.

Page 303 *Unpleasant Parts of the Body Contemplation* and *Cemetery Contemplation:*

Bhikku, T. (2009). *Kayagata-sati Sutta: Mindfulness immersed in the body.* Retrieved May 27, 2009, from Access to Insight: *www.accesstoinsight.org/tipitaka/mn/mn.119.than.html.*

Page 305 **We sink into what psychologist and meditation teacher Tara Brach calls a *trance of unworthiness*:**

Brach, T. (2003). *Radical acceptance: Embracing your life with the heart of a Buddha.* New York: Bantam.

CHAPTER 11. WHAT'S NEXT?
THE PROMISE OF MINDFULNESS

Page 315 **Many of us climb the ladder of success only to find that it has been leaning up against the wrong wall:**

Boa, F. (1994). *The way of the myth: Talking with Joseph Campbell.* Boston: Shambhala.

Page 318 **In surveys of people who tried the *Three Good Things* exercise, most found that it significantly decreased depressive symptoms and increased positive moods for the next six months:**

Seligman, M. E., Steen, T. A., Park, N., & Peterson, C. (2005). Positive psychology progress: Empirical validation of interventions. *American Psychologist, 60*(5), 410–421.

Page 318 ***Expressing Gratitude:***

Based on:

Seligman, M. (2002). *Authentic happiness: Using the new positive psychology to realize your potential for lasting fulfillment.* New York: Free Press.

Page 319 **Albert Einstein described our challenge beautifully:**

Sullivan, W. (1972, March 29). The Einstein papers: A man of many parts. *The New York Times,* p. 1.

Page 320 **Students who spent money on others reported feeling significantly happier than those who spent money on themselves:**

Dunn, E. W., Aknin, L. B., & Norton, M. L. (2008). Spending money on others promotes happiness. *Science, 319*(21), 1687–1688.

Page 321 **The Hungarian psychologist Mihály Csíkszentmihályi coined the term *flow* to describe these moments of full involvement:**

Csíkszentmihályi, M. (1991). *Flow: The psychology of optimal experience.* New York: Harper Collins.

Index

*Available in audio at *www.mindfulness-solution.com*.

About the author

Ronald D. Siegel, PsyD, is Assistant Clinical Professor of Psychology at Harvard Medical School, where he has taught for over 25 years. He is a long-time student of mindfulness meditation and serves on the Board of Directors and faculty of the Institute for Meditation and Psychotherapy. Dr. Siegel teaches internationally about mindfulness and psychotherapy and mind–body treatment, has worked for many years in community mental health with inner-city children and families, and maintains a private clinical practice in Lincoln, Massachusetts. He is the coauthor of the self-treatment guide *Back Sense*, which integrates Western and Eastern approaches for treating chronic back pain, and coeditor of an acclaimed book for professionals, *Mindfulness and Psychotherapy*. Dr. Siegel lives in Lincoln with his wife and daughters. He regularly uses the practices in this book to work with his own busy, unruly mind.